The People's Guide to Deadly Drug Interactions

Also by Joe Graedon and Teresa Graedon

The Aspirin Handbook (with Tom Ferguson, M.D.)

Graedons' Best Medicine:
From Herbal Remedies to High-Tech Rx Breakthroughs

50+:
The Graedons' People's Pharmacy for Older Adults

The People's Pharmacy:
Totally New and Revised

Joe Graedon's The New People's Pharmacy #3:
Drug Breakthroughs of the '80s

The People's Pharmacy-2

Also by Joe Graedon

No Deadly Drug (with Tom Ferguson, M.D.)

The People's Pharmacy

The People's Guide to Deadly Drug Interactions

How to Protect Yourself from Life-Threatening
Drug/Drug, Drug/Food, Drug/Vitamin Combinations

Joe Graedon and Teresa Graedon, Ph.D.

St. Martin's Press
New York

Text design by Cassell Design Group.

Library of Congress Cataloging-in-Publication Data
Graedon, Joe
    The People's Guide to deadly drug interactions: how to protect yourself from life-threatening drug/drug, drug/food, drug/vitamin combinations /Joe Graedon and Teresa Graedon.
        p. cm.
     ISBN 0-312-13243-3 (hbk.)
     1. Drug interactions—Popular works. I. Graedon, Teresa
      II. Title
RM302.G72 1995   95-34800
615'.7045—dc20   CIP

First Edition: November 1995
10 9 8 7 6 5 4 3 2 1

ATTENTION: IMPORTANT NOTE TO READERS

This book is not intended as a substitute for the medical advice of physicians. The reader should regularly consult a physician in matters relating to his or her health and particularly in respect to any symptoms that may require diagnosis or medical attention. Certain drugs with potentially lethal interactions can be successfully used together if appropriate monitoring and other precautions are undertaken. Drug interactions can be highly controversial, and different experts may vary in their interpretations of the degree of danger.

Anyone who discovers an interaction in this book that is of concern must consult a physician before making any changes in drug therapy. **Stopping a medication can be very dangerous. Every reader must consult with his or her physician before starting or stopping any medication.** Any side effects should be reported promptly to a physician.

It is impossible to list all potentially dangerous drug interactions. Information about drug interactions remains incomplete, and new dangers are discovered all the time. In addition, the effects drugs can have vary from person to person. **The reader should not assume that because an interaction is not mentioned in this book, it is therefore safe and cannot be dangerous.**

The authors and the publisher disclaim responsibility for any adverse effects resulting directly or indirectly from the information contained in this book.

THIS BOOK IS DEDICATED TO:

DAVID AND ALENA
Wonderful children who once again had to put up with
deadlines, take-out dinners, and impatient parents

SID AND HELEN GRAEDON
Who had faith in us from the first day

HUGH TILSON
Who has dedicated his life to finding scientific answers for
elusive pharmacoepidemiological questions

HEALTH-CONSCIOUS PEOPLE
Who are trying to protect themselves from drug misadventures

Contents

Acknowledgments

Barbara Anderson, our editor, whose insight and patience made this book possible. Thanks for going to bat for us.

John Barth, who helped us better appreciate the power of words.

Angela Bowen, a fast and efficient PageMaker whiz with nimble fingers, who saved us countless hours.

Cliff Butler, an extraordinary pharmacist who always comes to our aid.

Rob and Rose Capon, wonderful colleagues who had faith in our abilities, and put forth an incredible effort to syndicate our radio show.

Maria Carmicino, a fabulous editor who keeps our syndicated newspaper column on track and out of trouble.

Keith Cassell, a wonderfully creative and imaginative designer who made this book far more readable and usable.

Pedro Cuatrecasas, simply the finest pharmaceutical researcher we know.

Ruth Day, a psychologist with a clear vision of how people learn and understand. Her insight and Duke experiments improved the accessibility of this book immeasurably. Thanks also to Teresa Allen, who assisted Dr. Day.

Mary Dorsey, a kind and caring pharmacist who responds to her beeper.

Brenden Kootsey, a computer guru who kept us humming and happy with our kangaroo and our Apple. Thanks for being so calm in the face of chaos and confusion.

Peter Lamy, the man who put the issues of geriatric pharmacology on the map.

David S. McWaters, a pharmacist and lawyer who helped more than anyone else to make this book a reality.

Karen Moseley, a great helper and a wonderful person. Thanks for keeping us on track.

Charlotte Sheedy, a fabulous agent with boundless energy and enthusiasm who helped move this book through the maze.

Stephanie Shipper, a wonderfully wise woman who opened our eyes, helped us hear, and nurtured our feelings. A whole new world awaits.

John Walker, a kind and caring man who has helped us in so many ways.

Beth Wallace, a dedicated helper with a wonderful smile and great organizational skills. Thanks for 20/20 vision.

Camille Warren, a warm and loving physician with great insight and skill. Thanks for holding our hands at a crucial moment.

Peter Welling, a superb researcher who helped us understand the importance of food and drug interactions.

Chapter One

Introduction

Would you want to play Russian roulette? Taking more than one medicine at a time could be very much like loading a gun and spinning the chamber. You may not know if a particular combination will have a lethal outcome.

When the Food and Drug Administration (FDA) set up its standards for approving medications, it did not foresee the possibility that a person might take many different pills together. The FDA, which regulates both prescription and over-the-counter drugs in the United States, does not have its own facilities and funding for drug testing; rather, it issues guidelines and examines the data produced by the companies that make the medicines. It has not required pharmaceutical manufacturers to test new compounds for interaction potential. Consequently, when a new medication is introduced, doctors may not know in advance which other drugs will be incompatible with it.

Each drug is tested under controlled conditions that don't necessarily reflect the real world in which patients take medicine. In fact, for many years most medications were given only on an empty stomach. This may have been convenient for the researchers but it has created trouble for patients. For one thing, some drugs are far better absorbed or less irritating when taken with food. And we are now learning that certain foods and beverages may create hazards when combined with other medications. Although the FDA is now beginning to ask drug companies to look at the effects of food on new drugs, most of the pharmaceuticals on drugstore shelves have few guidelines for how they should be swallowed.

It is common for people to require several different medicines to treat a number of health problems—arthritis, allergies, high blood pressure, depression, and infections, to mention just a few. Because the FDA hasn't known how to deal with the complexity of drug interactions, there is a lack of scientific information about how one drug may affect another.

There are surprisingly few systematic studies of drug interactions in the medical literature. Most of what is published evolves from case reports. An individual physician discovers an unexpected problem in one or a few patients and writes it up. Until someone decides to look further, there is no way to tell if this is truly an interaction hazard or just a coincidence.

Reporting side effects or interactions is not required by any law. Doctors are busy and many are afraid that if they raise a ruckus it may come back to haunt them in the form of a malpractice suit. FDA commissioner David Kessler has noted that "only about 1% of serious events are reported to the FDA, according to one study."[1,2] If a physician chooses not to notify the FDA or the drug companies, there's no way other doctors can learn about the situation.

Since the FDA does not have a system for gathering interaction data and drug companies have no incentive to pursue such research, it can take months or years to discover dangerous drug interactions. Hospitalizations and even deaths have occurred before the FDA realized a warning was needed. Undoubtedly, interactions have gone undetected to this day.

Even when the agency finally acknowledges that a particular drug combination poses a risk, there is no good way to bring this information to physicians' attention. It may ultimately show up in the package insert or *Physicians' Desk Reference (PDR)*, but there is no guarantee that the information will be read or appreciated. As a result, doctors must play a dangerous guessing game when they have to prescribe more than one medication.

Types of Drug Interactions

Imagine you are trying to bake a cake with two or three other people and no recipe. Only one of you can be in the kitchen at a time and so none of you knows what the others have put in the batter. Under these circumstances your cake might end up with way too much baking powder or perhaps none at all. If everyone threw in a pinch of salt the cake would taste terrible even if it looked okay. A patient with several doctors may suffer a similar fate.

A person may see three or four different specialists, all prescribing medications for various aliments. The cardiologist could have you on **Lanoxin** (digoxin) and **Vasotec** (enalapril) for your heart, the endocrinologist might have prescribed **Synthroid** (levothyroxine) for thyroid, the rheumatologist may have you on **Indocin** (indomethacin), and on your own you could be taking a multiple vitamin plus aspirin to prevent a heart attack. All these different drugs can interact with one another in a variety of ways to produce toxicity or reduce effectiveness. In the following sections we will describe the three different types of drug interactions that can cause trouble.

Additive Interactions

The drug interaction that most people are familiar with is an *additive* interaction, which occurs when one drug adds to the effect of another medication. The person who takes **Fiorinal** (aspirin, butalbital, caffeine) for a tension headache and then has a drink to relax could end up spaced out because of the combined effect of the barbiturate (butalbital) and the booze.

A century ago sailors became familiar with additive interactions when they woke up unexpectedly on a ship far from the harbor. They had been slipped a "Mickey Finn." The popular belief is that certain bartenders (in cahoots with sea captains who needed extra hands) put chloral hydrate (a sedative) in with the grog. The combination enhanced the effects of the alcohol, knocked the sailor out, and kept him asleep long enough for the ship to slip anchor.

Antagonistic Interactions

A different kind of interaction occurs when one drug cancels out the benefits of another—the $1+1=0$ effect. For example, birth control pills don't work as well when a woman takes them in conjunction with tuberculosis medicine or antiseizure drugs. She could end up unexpectedly pregnant through no fault of her own because these other drugs change the metabolism of the Pill to reduce its effectiveness. (See pages 126-131 for more details.) A similar interaction involves the popular drug **Prozac**. If it is taken in conjunction with the allergy medicine **Periactin**, **Prozac** may lose its effectiveness as an antidepressant (see page 245). Likewise, the thyroid hormone **Synthroid** may not be absorbed adequately and its effectiveness may be impaired if it is swallowed within two hours of an iron supplement (see page 93).

If a woman becomes pregnant while using birth control pills, doctors often shrug in amazement. Rather than consider a drug interaction as the culprit, they may assume that the woman was at fault for missing a dose. When an antidepressant doesn't seem to relieve depression the assumption is made that the drug isn't working for mysterious and inexplicable reasons. Doctors often chalk up such discouraging results to "biological variability." In other words, some people respond and others don't and no one knows why. Who would ever think to question breakfast as the culprit behind antidepressant failure?

A Canadian researcher has discovered that high-fiber foods can also interfere with the absorption of tricyclic antidepressants such as doxepin (**Adapin**, **Sinequan**) and desipramine (**Norpramin**).[4] Dr. Donna Stewart found that patients who had previously improved with these medications did not respond to them after switching to health-conscious diets. High levels of fiber in such foods as wheat bran, rolled oats, sunflower seeds, bran muffins, and wheat germ lowered blood levels of antidepressants. When the diets were modified, the drug levels returned to normal and the depression disappeared. (For more details see page 20.)

If a medication does not produce the anticipated benefit, phy-

Heart Drug Fails Due to Fiber

Absorption of the heart drug Lanoxin (digoxin) can be reduced when the drug is taken with high-fiber foods.[3] One physician doubled the dose of this drug for a patient who had repeated attacks of atrial fibrillation (a serious heart rhythm disturbance). The doctor should have asked about the patient's diet before changing the dose of Lanoxin. This gentleman was eating a very large bowl of oatmeal with bran every morning at the same time he took his heart pill.

sicians usually adjust the dose or change drugs. If an antidepressant fails to work, they often write a new prescription. When a blood pressure pill does not adequately control hypertension, out comes another medication, frequently at a higher cost. But sometimes the doctor may not be aware of a therapeutic failure or there may not be enough time to undo the damage of a dangerous drug interaction.

Unpredictable Interactions

Perhaps the scariest type of interaction is what we refer to as the 1+1= 3 reaction. It can take a long time to be discovered. When **Seldane** (terfenadine) was introduced in May 1985 as the first nonsedating antihistamine, it was heralded as "a major advance in the treatment of seasonal allergic rhinitis."[5] Here was a prescription allergy medicine that wouldn't make you drowsy. You could drive, work, think, or make love without feeling like a space cadet. The company bragged that side effects were no more serious with **Seldane** than with an inactive placebo, and no mention was made of any interaction with other drugs.

As a consequence, **Seldane** quickly became the world's number one allergy medicine. In the early 1990s, American doctors wrote more than 16 million prescriptions a year for this drug.[6] But something odd had begun to happen. Reports of dizziness attacks and heart palpitations began trickling in to the Food and Drug Administration (FDA). By June of 1990, enough serious cases of heart rhythm disturbances and cardiac arrest had accumulated for the FDA to call an urgent meeting. Face to face with these data, the experts finally realized that elevated levels of **Seldane,** triggered by overdose, liver disease, or *interactions with certain other drugs*, could lead to a rare but potentially lethal heart condition.

At the FDA's urging, the manufacturer of **Seldane** sent out a letter later that summer warning doctors to be wary of prescribing the antifungal drug **Nizoral** (ketoconazole) together with **Seldane**. The first report in the medical literature appeared in *The Journal of the American Medical Association* on December 5, 1990.[7] Dr. Brian Monahan and his colleagues described a healthy

"39-year-old woman who developed lightheadedness and fainting" after only ten days on **Seldane**. She was also taking **Nizoral** for a vaginal yeast infection. When they checked her electrocardiogram (ECG) they discovered a dangerous irregularity called *torsade de pointes* (a French term that describes the way the ECG points seem to twist together).

By April 1, 1992, the FDA had received 25 reports of torsades de pointes. Two of those afflicted had died and the others had to be hospitalized.[8] Of course, no one knows how many cases went unreported. When people drop dead of an apparent heart attack, it may be hard for the doctor to determine whether a medication or combination of medications could have contributed, especially if the drug is as seemingly benign as **Seldane**. Even if a doctor suspects that a patient's symptoms might be related to a combination of medicines, there is no simple way to alert others to this possibility. Getting a written report into the medical literature where other physicians can read it can take years.

Even after an interaction has been reported it might be ignored. Almost three years after the original **Seldane** alert, doctors were still prescribing this antihistamine in combination with **Nizoral** or the antibiotic erythromycin (**E.E.S.**, **E-Mycin**, **ERYC**, **EryPed**, **Ery-Tab**, **Ilosone**, **PCE**, etc.). Clinical pharmacologists at Georgetown University expressed concern that "in spite of warning letters to physicians and changes in labeling, deaths and cases of torsades de pointes continue to be reported in association with a drug that is often prescribed for what are simply uncomfortable and temporary allergic conditions."[9]

The **Seldane** story is merely one example of what can go wrong with mixing and matching medicines. It took five years for the FDA and the drug's manufacturer to realize there was a problem. After eight years, even though prescribing information

Preventable Tragedy?

"Despite regulatory action, the combination of terfenadine and ketoconazole has continued to be prescribed. The seriousness of the continued occurrence of this drug-drug interaction is illustrated in a recent report to the FDA of a 29-year-old woman who had been taking terfenadine long term for nasal congestion. She was then prescribed ketoconazole for onychomycosis [fingernail and toenail fungus]. One week later, she presented to an emergency department after 'fainting.' Both medications were continued and she suffered a fatal cardiac arrest 3 days later."

Honig, Peter K., et al. "Terfenadine-Ketoconazole Interaction: Pharmacokinetic and Electrocardiographic Consequences." *JAMA* 1993; 269:1513-1518.

was changed and "Dear Doctor" letters were sent out warning about interaction hazards, physicians kept on prescribing **Seldane** in combination with erythromycin or ketoconazole, and people continued to die.[10]

Other drugs may also interact dangerously with **Seldane**. Questions have been raised about disopyramide (**Norpace**), haloperidol (**Haldol**), pentamidine (**NebuPent**, **Pentam**), probucol (**Lorelco**), procainamide (**Pronestyl**, **Procan SR**), quinidine (**Cardioquin**, **Quinora**, **Quinidex**, **Quinaglute**), sotalol (**Betapace**), and thioridazine (**Mellaril**).[11] It might take decades before all the dangerous **Seldane** interactions are discovered. Even something as seemingly innocuous as grapefruit juice may turn out to trigger lethal heart rhythms.[12] (See pages 42 and 251 for more information.)

Protecting Yourself from Drug Interactions

- Take charge! It's your body and ultimately you are responsible for swallowing those pills. Make sure *all* your physicians know every drug you take and that they check for interaction potential. There are excellent reference books and computer programs available. Insist that they consult one of these resources.

- Ask your pharmacist for help. This person is a highly trained professional who specializes in drug information and interaction issues. Most pharmacies have computer access to interaction information. Some pharmacists may not want to scare their patients with extra precautions, so be sure to tell them everything you are taking and that you are interested in knowing about potential incompatibility.

- Check this book and report any unusual symptoms immediately. Never start or stop any medication without your doctor's knowledge and supervision. Stopping certain medications suddenly could trigger serious irregular heart rhythms, not to mention convulsions or heart attacks. In addition, discontinuing one drug may have a domino effect, in that it could increase or decrease the effects of other medicines you may be taking.

- Once a drug has been approved for general use, the Food and Drug Administration has no organized system for monitoring drug interactions, and no good way of disseminating interaction information to doctors. The *Physicians' Desk Reference (PDR)* reports some, but not all, dangerous combinations. It may take years for a deadly interaction to make its way into the standard reference books.

- Do not assume that lack of information indicates no interaction. Life-threatening interactions may go undiscovered for months or even years. If you are experiencing a strange or dangerous symptom that cannot easily be explained, ask your physician to contact the drug's manufacturer and to file a report with the FDA.

- We have found the following resources helpful in tracking down drug interactions. We have listed them in the order of their usefulness for us. If you or your physician has a question about anything you find in our book, please check these references. You will discover that there are substantial differences of opinion about the importance of certain interactions:

  Drug Interaction Facts. Tatro, David S., ed. St. Louis: Facts & Comparisons (A Wolters Kluwer Company), 1995.

  Drug Interactions & Updates Quarterly. Hansten, Philip D., John R. Horn, Mary Anne Koda-Kimble, Lloyd Y. Young, eds. Vancouver, Wash.: Applied Therapeutics, 1995.

  The Medical Letter Handbook of Adverse Drug Interactions. Rizack, Martin A., with Carol Hillman, D.M., eds. New Rochelle, N.Y.: The Medical Letter, 1994.

  Drug Facts and Comparisons. Olin, Bernie R., editor-in-chief. St. Louis: Facts & Comparisons (A Wolters Kluwer Company), 1995.

  Evaluations of Drug Interactions. Zucchero, Frederic J., Mark J. Hogan, Amy C. DeWein, eds. St. Louis: Professional Drug Systems, 1994.

  Consumer's Guide to Drug Interactions. Schein, Jeffrey R., and Philip Hansten. New York: Collier Books, 1993.

  Physicians GenR$_x$: The Complete Drug Reference. Denniston, Philip L., Jr., editor-in-chief. Smithtown, N.Y.: Physicians GenR$_x$, 1995.

Physicians' Desk Reference. Montvale, N.J.: Medical Economics Data Production Company, 1995.

Professional's Guide to Patient Drug Facts. Olin, Bernie R., editor-in-chief. St. Louis: Facts & Comparisons (A Wolters Kluwer Company), 1995.

PDR Guide to Drug Interactions, Side Effects, Indications. Mehta, Mukesh, ed. Montvale, N.J.: Medical Economics Data Production Company, 1995.

The Food and Drug Interaction Guide. Morgan, Brian L.G. New York: Simon & Schuster, 1986.

Drug Interactions Guide Book. Harkness, Richard. Englewood Cliffs, N.J.: Prentice-Hall, 1991.

References

1. Scott, H.D., et al. "Rhode Island Physicians' Recognition and Reporting of Adverse Drug Reactions." *R.I. Med. J.* 1987; 70:311–316.

2. Kessler, David A. "Introducing MEDWatch: A New Approach to Reporting Medication and Device Adverse Effects and Product Problems." *JAMA* 1993; 269:2765–2768.

3. Brown, D.D., et al. "Decreased Bioavailability of Digoxin Due to Hypercholesterolemic Interventions." *Circulation* 1978; 58:164–172.

4. Stewart, Donna E. "High-Fiber Diet and Serum Tricyclic Antidepressant Levels." *J. Clin. Psychopharmacol.* 1992; 12:438–440.

5. "Terfenadine: Separating Sedation from Relief—New Hope for Seasonal Allergic Rhinitis Sufferers." Merrell-Dow, 1985.

6. IMS America Ltd. *1992 National Prescription Audit.* Plymouth Meeting, Pa.: IMS America, 1992.

7. Monahan, Brian P., et al. "Torsades de Pointes Occurring in Association with Terfenadine Use." *JAMA* 1990; 264:2788–2791.

8. Woosley, Raymond L., et al. "Mechanism of the Cardiotoxic Actions of Terfenadine." *JAMA* 1993; 269:1532–1536.

9. Ibid., p. 1535.

10. Honig, Peter K., et al. "Terfenadine-Ketoconazole Interaction: Pharmacokinetic and Electrocardiographic Consequences." *JAMA* 1993; 269:1513–1518.

11. Woosley, op. cit., p. 1536.

12. Ibid.

Chapter Two

How to Use This Book

On the following pages you will discover scary stories and horrifying examples of dangerous, potentially lethal drug interactions. But this does not necessarily mean that the combination will be disastrous. Not everyone will experience problems because he or she swallows two theoretically incompatible medications. In many cases, interacting drugs can be used together successfully if the doctor is aware of the potential danger and takes proper precautions. You can help by knowing what to look for; that is why we wrote this book.

One way to avoid interaction problems is to ask your physician if there could be an incompatibility, and, whenever possible, to substitute a drug that is less likely to create difficulties. Remember, however, that each case is special and only your physician has the clinical experience to know if your condition requires these particular drugs. At the risk of being redundant, we emphasize that no one should ever start or stop taking any medicine without first checking with the prescribing doctor. Stopping a pill suddenly can sometimes be far more dangerous than continuing to take a medication.

Don't overreact if you read that you are taking two or three drugs that might interact in a strange, dangerous, or potentially life-threatening way. First check with both your pharmacist and physician to see what you should do. This book will alert you to the possible consequences of combining mismatched medicines. Your doctor's responsibility is to evaluate the situation in light of your special medical history.

How to Read the Guides to Dangerous Drug Interactions

The second part of this book contains detailed descriptions of a number of the most important drug interactions. We used our judgment to select the ones we thought were most common and most serious. If you asked other experts you might get a different selection. It is impossible to list every reported interaction in a book this size.

These descriptions are grouped into categories, such as antidepressants, anticoagulants, and antihistamines (the nonsedating ones, **Hismanal** and **Seldane**). Each category begins with an overview chart like the one shown on page 13. At the top of each chart, in the box, is the name of the category and some of the brand names of drugs within the category. The example shows the category of serotonin-based antidepressants with brand names of **Paxil, Prozac,** and **Zoloft**. You will notice that three columns branch out from the box labeled "Antidepressants." They are entitled "Life Threatening," "Dangerous," and "Troublesome," to indicate at a glance the level of concern about the potential interaction. The red line connects the interactions that are potentially lethal to the box at the top of the page. Serious, but not necessarily deadly, interactions are labeled "Dangerous" and are connected with a pink line. The gray line leads to those interactions that could cause discomfort or trouble. (You will find a key titled "Levels of Hazard" on each of these charts.)

In the pages following each overview chart, we detail the interactions between the medications. For example, on page 15 you will see a guide to the possible interactions between serotonin-based antidepressants such as **Paxil, Prozac**, and **Zoloft**, and MAO inhibitor antidepressants such as **Nardil** and **Parnate**. Under each drug category you will find a brief description of how it is used and instructions on how it is best taken

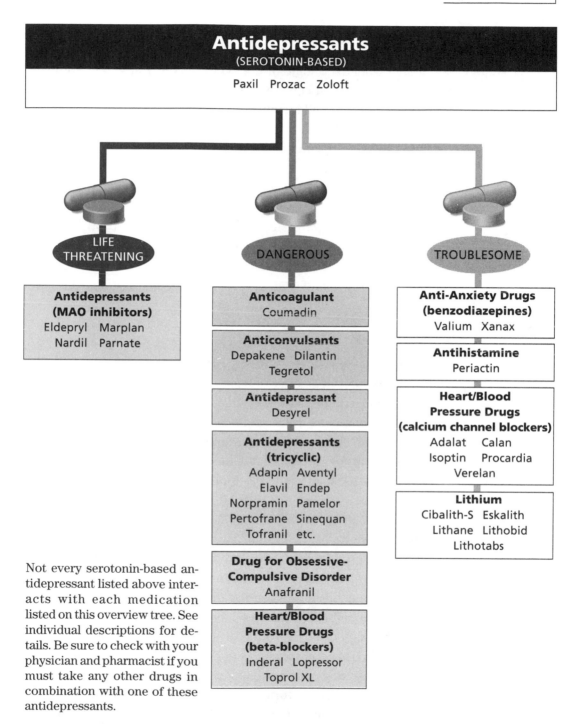

Antidepressants
(SEROTONIN-BASED)

Paxil   Prozac   Zoloft

LIFE THREATENING

Antidepressants (MAO inhibitors)
Eldepryl   Marplan
Nardil   Parnate

DANGEROUS

Anticoagulant
Coumadin

Anticonvulsants
Depakene   Dilantin
Tegretol

Antidepressant
Desyrel

Antidepressants (tricyclic)
Adapin   Aventyl
Elavil   Endep
Norpramin   Pamelor
Pertofrane   Sinequan
Tofranil   etc.

Drug for Obsessive-Compulsive Disorder
Anafranil

Heart/Blood Pressure Drugs (beta-blockers)
Inderal   Lopressor
Toprol XL

TROUBLESOME

Anti-Anxiety Drugs (benzodiazepines)
Valium   Xanax

Antihistamine
Periactin

Heart/Blood Pressure Drugs (calcium channel blockers)
Adalat   Calan
Isoptin   Procardia
Verelan

Lithium
Cibalith-S   Eskalith
Lithane   Lithobid
Lithotabs

Not every serotonin-based antidepressant listed above interacts with each medication listed on this overview tree. See individual descriptions for details. Be sure to check with your physician and pharmacist if you must take any other drugs in combination with one of these antidepressants.

LEVELS OF HAZARD: LIFE THREATENING   DANGEROUS   TROUBLESOME

(with food or on an empty stomach). The box labeled *interaction* in the center of the page describes the nature of the interaction and summarizes some of the symptoms to watch for. Not every interaction has specific side effects, but we try to indicate what precautions should be taken.

Please note that **Prozac** and **Paxil** are sometimes prescribed in combination with other types of antidepressants, even though there are indications that such combinations are occasionally dangerous. For some patients, however, this may represent the best treatment. The potential hazards are worth noting, so that you and your doctor can be alert for any sign of difficulty. Remember, if you become concerned about anything you read here, be sure to *discuss it with your doctor*, so you can understand your treatment and what to do if you detect symptoms of a problem.

How Not to Use This Book

This book contains a summary of many important drug interactions, but it is *not* a bible in which you will find every hazard. You must understand that there is no organized, scientific system for establishing dangerous chemical incompatibilities. Sometimes serious adverse drug reactions are missed or go unreported. Even when an article appears in the medical literature its findings may be ignored or take years to get into reference books or computer data banks.

Once an interaction makes it into the medical manuals there is still uncertainty about the clinical significance of the situation. Physicians and researchers and drug manufacturers often argue for years about the relevance of a particular report. For example, when the cholesterol-lowering drugs **Mevacor** (lovastatin) and **Lopid** (gemfibrozil) are prescribed together, they have on occasion been reported to produce a potentially life-threatening disorder called rhabdomyolysis. In this condition muscle tissue breaks down, resulting in pain, weakness, and possibly even kidney failure. Despite horror stories in the medical literature, admonitions against the combination by experts at the Food and Drug Administration, and strong warnings in the *Physicians' Desk Reference (PDR)*, many cardiologists believe they can combine these drugs

Antidepressants

(SEROTONIN-BASED)

Antidepressants

(MAO INHIBITORS)

BRAND NAME	GENERIC NAME
Paxil	paroxetine
Prozac	fluoxetine
Zoloft	sertraline

DESCRIPTION

These antidepressants block the reuptake into brain cells of serotonin, a chemical messenger. Because they work differently from older antidepressants, they have different side effects and indications. Prozac is also prescribed for obsessive-compulsive disorder and for bulimia. Older people and those with kidney or liver problems may need reduced doses. Prozac is metabolized slowly and may linger weeks after discontinuation.

INSTRUCTIONS

Prozac, Paxil, and Zoloft are usually taken once a day, often in the morning. Prozac may be taken without regard to meals. Taking it with food may reduce stomach upset. A few patients experience serious weight loss on these medications. If this occurs, the doctor should be notified.

BRAND NAME	GENERIC NAME
Eldepryl	selegiline
Marplan	isocarboxazid
Nardil	phenelzine
Parnate	tranylcypromine

DESCRIPTION

These medications were among the earliest antidepressants to be developed, and still work very well for some patients. Eldepryl, a drug used to treat Parkinson's disease, also has some monoamine oxidase (MAO) inhibitor activity and may interact with serotonin-based antidepressants. These drugs are slow to start acting, and may last in the body for a few weeks after medication is stopped.

INSTRUCTIONS

MAO inhibitors can interact in dangerous ways with tyramine-containing foods and beverages. See page 47. Consult your doctor before taking other prescription or over-the-counter drugs. Notify him or her if you notice a skin rash, severe headache, yellow eyes or skin, or dark urine. Do not stop this medicine unless your doctor so advises.

· INTERACTION

When a patient does not get adequate relief of depression from one medication, the doctor may add a different antidepressant. The literature accompanying serotonin-based antidepressants warns against this combination. *Fatalities have resulted from this interaction.* Some people who have received this combination experience "serotonin syndrome," a very serious, potentially lethal reaction. Because these drugs last in the body for quite some time, at least two weeks should pass after discontinuing an MAO inhibitor before starting on Prozac, Zoloft, or Paxil. The manufacturer of Prozac recommends waiting five weeks after stopping Prozac before beginning an MAO inhibitor antidepressant. For Zoloft and Paxil, at least two weeks should elapse after stopping the serotonin-based antidepressant before beginning Marplan, Nardil, or Parnate. Eldepryl may also interact with the serotonin-based antidepressants.

Symptoms of Serotonin Syndrome

Severe shivering, agitation, confusion, restlessness, muscle twitches or rigidity, diarrhea, elevated temperature, sweating, changes in blood pressure, and coma. Notify your doctor at once if you experience any of these symptoms.

Never take or stop medication without your doctor's advice.

INTERACTION

LIFE THREATENING

safely with careful medical supervision. Who's right? Maybe there is no one right answer. All we can say is that we don't want you to be an unsuspecting guinea pig.

The point is that there are no clear rules when it comes to drug interactions. And there is no good place to turn for guidance. The FDA and the drug companies have left us dangling. Reference books disagree on the facts and their importance.

That makes it virtually impossible for anyone to reassure you that a particular combination is 100 percent safe . . . or warn you that it is definitely hazardous in every case. For example, most interaction guides caution that combining aspirin with the prescription anticoagulant **Coumadin** (warfarin) can be quite dangerous (though some texts are more adamant than others). Information for patients in the *PDR* says unequivocally to avoid salicylates (e.g., aspirin). The fear has been that severe bleeding episodes could occur, leading to fatal hemorrhaging.

The risk is real, but there is a growing realization that cautious physicians can prescribe these two drugs in low doses to prevent heart attack and stroke and that both together might turn out to be better than either alone. A huge study called CARS (Coumadin Aspirin Reinfarction Study) is underway to determine if 3 mg of **Coumadin** combined with a baby aspirin (80 mg) can safely protect the heart and brain from blood clots without causing dangerous bleeding problems. Careful monitoring is critical with such a regimen, though, so anyone taking aspirin and **Coumadin** will need expert supervision and frequent blood tests to determine prothrombin time (a measure of bleeding vulnerability).

We hope you understand that we could not include every troublesome, dangerous, or even life-threatening interaction in this book. Our primary references list thousands of potentially problematic drug combinations. One example of a drug interaction we did not discuss, although it is extremely serious and has been associated with deaths, is the combination of **Coumadin** and **Atromid-S** (clofibrate). The reason is that **Atromid-S**, a cholesterol-lowering compound, is prescribed infrequently compared to other such medications. For the same reason, we also left out the interactions of **Coumadin** with **Rythmol** (propafenone), a heart medicine, and with **Antabuse** (disulfiram), a drug that is sometimes given to alcoholics to prevent them from consuming alcohol.

We have generally not covered injectable drugs, which would be administered in the doctor's office or in a hospital. For example, flu vaccine has been reported to interact with **Coumadin** in some patients, and monitoring of prothrombin time is advised. In such a situation, make sure the prescribing physician knows all other medications you are taking.

As you can now tell, evaluating complex combinations is like focusing on a moving target. You never know where it will be next. What was "true" last year may no longer be true this year. Goodness knows what the experts will declare next year. We estimate that more than 20,000 interactions are mentioned in the medical literature. There is no way to include all of them in this work and many are of interest primarily to academic researchers who spend little time with real patients. There are others that have not yet been discovered.

This book is a starting point to alert you to potential dangers, but we don't know your individual situation. No one should ever start or stop any medication without first checking with a physician. Also consult your pharmacist. Chances are good that he or she can look up your medications on a computer to see if there are any flagged interactions. Don't forget to mention any over-the-counter remedies or nutritional supplements you may be taking.

Safety Checklist

Dear Doctor/Pharmacist,

To assist me in taking my medicines properly, and to reduce the risk of dangerous drug interactions, please help me answer these questions:

1) What is the name of my medicine?

brand: _____

generic: _____

2) What is the dose? _____

3) What time(s) should I take this medicine?

_____am   _____ am
_____ pm   _____ pm   _____ pm

4) Should I take this medicine:

☐ with food?
☐ at least one hour before or two hours after eating?

5) Are there any special foods I should avoid?

6) Are there any vitamins or supplements I should avoid?

7) Are there any precautions or warnings I should know about?

8) Are there any contraindications that would make this drug inappropriate?

9) Which other medicines should I avoid?

10) Are there any OTC remedies I should avoid?

11) What side effects are common with my medicine?

12) Are there any symptoms that are so serious you would want to know about them immediately?

Photocopy this page and take it to your health care provider.

Chapter Three

Lethal Drug/Drug Combinations

What makes a drug interaction dangerous? Lots of combinations create unpleasant consequences. For example, the broad-spectrum antimicrobial drug **Flagyl** (metronidazole) is prescribed for certain digestive tract and vaginal infections and also as part of an exciting new treatment against infectious ulcers. If someone taking **Flagyl** were to drink alcohol, the result might be nausea, flushing, rapid heart beat, and vomiting. This is uncomfortable, but probably not life threatening.

We're more concerned about incompatibilities that have already resulted in one or more reported deaths. We are equally worried about situations that could be so serious someone might die. Since these are often indirect, they may be overlooked and unreported.

The older person who is taking **Valium** (diazepam) or **Xanax** (alprazolam) for nervousness may be a little less steady than his younger counterpart. If he were to receive a prescription for **Tagamet** (cimetidine) for bad heartburn or ulcer pain, the stomach drug could delay elimination of the anti-anxiety agent from the body. That in turn could lead to increased sedation and dizziness as blood levels climbed. If this resulted in a fall and a broken hip, it could be a death sentence for the older person.

Drug interactions can kill in two ways. First, two or more incompatible chemicals can produce an unexpected, disastrous reaction in the body. If you gave a child a chemistry set and turned her loose without an instruction booklet, she might have a great time mixing one chemical with another and watching colors change—until she happened on an explosive combination. Your body won't blow up when you combine chemicals in it, but there have been situations in which blood pressure climbed so high that an artery blew out, resulting in hemorrhage and death.

People also die if one drug blocks another that is crucial to survival. Someone taking an epilepsy drug could have a fatal accident if a competing medicine alters the anticonvulsant's effectiveness. An infection that progresses because an antibiotic is inactivated could be lethal. An anticoagulant prescribed to prevent blood clots may not thin the blood adequately as a result of an interaction. The resulting stroke might be a killer.

Therapeutic failures are hard to track. For example, people who are depressed sometimes commit suicide. If someone takes his life while on an antidepressant, the automatic assumption is made that the medicine wasn't strong enough to overcome feelings of hopelessness. Family and friends are left wondering what went wrong and what more they might have done. Few would think to look for an interaction as a contributing factor in such a suicide.

The Case of the Bran Muffins

We were intrigued to read about the 42-year-old woman who, like her father, had suffered from severe depression. Over nine years she had four bad bouts of the blues that required antidepressant therapy. Her psychiatrist had prescribed 75 mg of desipramine (Norpramin) with excellent results.

The physician was puzzled when her patient didn't improve on this drug a fifth time. The dose was the same but after three weeks the patient wasn't getting any better. Blood tests revealed that less than half the usual amount of desipramine was circulating in her body; this was too little to be effective.

Upon questioning, the patient said her family doctor had recommended bran to overcome constipation. She was eating only a bran muffin at breakfast and another at lunch. The fiber dramatically interfered with the absorption of her medicine. Thanks to an alert psychiatrist, the patient gave up the muffins, her blood levels returned to normal, and the depression soon lifted.

Stewart, Donna E. "High-Fiber Diet and Serum Tricyclic Antidepressant Levels." *J. Clin. Psychopharmacol.* 1992; 12:438–440.

Antidepressant (MAO Inhibitor) Hazards

When a depressed patient doesn't seem to be getting better on a particular antidepressant, the physician may add another type of drug to the program. There are several different kinds of medicines to choose from. They work through distinct pathways in the brain and affect separate neurochemicals, such as serotonin, dopamine, and norepinephrine. Combining the wrong classes of antidepressants can lead to disaster.

In one case a physically healthy 34-year-old engineer was being treated with **Parnate** (tranylcypromine) for serious depression. Although this drug had worked in the past, this time the engineer was still feeling extremely depressed, even suicidal. His doctor added **Anafranil** (clomipramine), hoping that the two drugs together would be helpful. Instead, the engineer felt awful. After two doses he felt nauseated and began sweating profusely. When he called his doctor to complain about these symptoms, he was reassured and told to keep taking both medications.

The combination of **Anafranil** and **Parnate** led to further problems. The engineer became confused and anxious; other symptoms included rapid heart beat, shivering, fever, and breathing difficulty. Two days later he was admitted to the hospital and put in intensive care where he lost consciousness. His condition deteriorated rapidly and he died 30 hours later.[1] Apparently these two drugs triggered hemorrhaging throughout his body.

This isn't the first time an antidepressant has killed someone because of a bad interaction. The class of medications called MAO (monoamine oxidase) inhibitors includes **Nardil** (phenelzine), **Marplan** (isocarboxazid), and **Parnate** (tranylcypromine). These drugs are prescribed for a range of problems including depression, agoraphobia (fear of crowds), panic, and bulimia (an eating disorder that involves bingeing).

Deaths have been reported when other types of antidepressants are prescribed with MAO inhibitors. For example, tricyclic antidepressants such as those in the box can be extremely dangerous in combination with MAO inhibitors.

Tricylic Antidepressants

Asendin	(amoxapine)
Aventyl	(nortriptyline)
Elavil	(amitriptyline)
Norpramin	(desipramine)
Pamelor	(nortriptyline)
Sinequan	(doxeprin)
Surmontil	(trimipramine)
Tofranil	(imipramine)
Vivactil	(protriptyline)

Symptoms of the interaction include confusion, fever, rapid heart rate, fast breathing, sweating, agitation, seizures, flushing, headache, and coma. It is safest to allow at least two weeks after stopping an MAO inhibitor before starting one of these other antidepressants.

Even some of the newer medications for depression such as **Prozac** (fluoxetine) and **Zoloft** (sertraline) may provoke a severe interaction when taken with MAO inhibitors.[2, 3, 4] People may develop restlessness, nausea, shivering, double vision, confusion, and uncontrollable muscle contractions. Deaths have been reported.[5] Because **Prozac** lasts a long time in the body, its manufacturer recommends allowing at least five weeks to pass between stopping **Prozac** and starting any MAO inhibitor.

Prozac Interactions

Other drugs that may interact with Prozac include other antidepressants like **Desyrel** (trazodone), **Tofranil** (imipramine), **Norpramin** (desipramine), and **Pamelor** (nortriptyline); pain relievers like **Talwin** (pentazocine); anti-anxiety agents like **Valium** (diazepam) and **Xanax** (alprazolam); major tranquilizers such as **Haldol** (haloperidol); and the antiseizure drug **Tegretol** (carbamazepine).[6] (See page 236 for specifics.)

A number of other prescription drugs can interact in a dangerous or life-threatening way with MAO inhibitors. Perhaps the most famous case is that of Libby Zion. This 18-year-old woman was admitted to New York Hospital on the evening of March 4, 1984, with a fever and an earache. Although she told physicians that she had been taking **Nardil** for depression, they administered a pain reliever called **Demerol** (meperidine) to calm her down. Instead, it made her more agitated. Because she was thrashing around, hospital personnel tried to control her with a restraining jacket and tied her hands and feet to the bed. Her condition continued to deteriorate and by 6:30 A.M. her temperature had reached 108°F. Libby Zion died around 7:45 A.M.

The physician on duty did not realize that **Nardil** and **Demerol** do not mix. This combination can cause agitation, seizures, and fever, and lead to coma or death. The cause of Libby Zion's tragic death remains controversial, but it is clear that she never should have been given **Demerol**. On February 6, 1995, a jury technically awarded Libby Zion's parents $750,000 for their daughter's pain and suffering.

People find it hard to believe that certain foods can be lethal in combination with medicine. Yet someone taking **Nardil** or

Parnate could die if they ate cheddar cheese, pepperoni, pickled herring, guacamole, or even soy sauce. Such foods contain a substance called tyramine that, in combination with these drugs, can raise blood pressure so high it could cause a stroke. For a more complete discussion of this interaction, turn to Chapter 4.

Over-the-counter remedies can also be hazardous in combination with MAO inhibitors. Nonprescription diet pills and cold remedies contain the decongestant phenylpropanolamine (PPA). It is found in everything from **Acutrim**, **Dexatrim**, and **Stay Trim** to **Alka-Seltzer Plus Night-Time Cold Medicine**, **Contac 12 Hour Capsules**, **Dimetapp Cold and Flu Caplets**, and **Tylenol Cold Effervescent Tablets**. One patient on **Nardil** developed a severe heart rhythm disturbance and another died when they added cold remedies containing PPA.[7] Pseudoephedrine (an ingredient in **Actifed**, **Advil Cold and Sinus**, **Dristan Sinus Caplets**, **NyQuil**, **Sudafed**, etc.) has been implicated in stroke and death when taken with an MAO inhibitor such as **Nardil**.

Cough medicine could also be dangerous in conjunction with MAO inhibitors. One 26-year-old woman on **Nardil** died after swallowing two ounces of cough syrup containing dextromethorphan.[8] Another person experienced an adverse reaction after taking two teaspoons of a cough medicine together with **Marplan**.[9] The culprit appears to be dextromethorphan, an ingredient found in most over-the-counter cough remedies. Nausea, dizziness, muscle spasms, and loss of consciousness are symptoms of this interaction.

Digitalis Dangers

Lanoxin (digoxin) is one of the most commonly prescribed, herb-based medicines in the world. It is derived from digitalis, the foxglove plant, which has a long history of medicinal use. Digitalis was used by the ancient Egyptian and Roman physicians as a heart tonic. Today digoxin is employed primarily to treat congestive heart failure and certain heart rhythm disturbances such as atrial fibrillation and flutter. Although digoxin started to fall into disfavor in the 1980s, new research suggests that this time-honored agent still plays a significant role in heart treatment.

Getting the dose of digoxin correct is tricky, however, and can be a little like walking a tightrope. Too much digoxin can be extremely hazardous. Symptoms can include loss of appetite, nausea, vomiting, diarrhea, headache, confusion, depression, weakness, drowsiness, disturbed vision, and disorientation. Hallucinations, seizures, and ultimately life-threatening disruptions of heart rhythm can be consequences of digoxin toxicity. Death can be the ultimate result of overdose.

Because digoxin levels can be altered by other drugs, a physician might not realize that an older person is getting too much of this medicine. Symptoms may be attributed to aging or to the underlying heart problem. Let's face it, confusion, weakness, and disorientation might be mistaken for the onset of Alzheimer's disease. If someone dies suddenly of an apparent heart attack, most people would assume this unfortunate event occurred despite his many medicines, rather than because of them.

Because people taking **Lanoxin** often have other heart problems, they may also be using other heart medications. Quinidine (**Cardioquin, Quinalan, Quinaglute, Quinidex, Quinora**) is frequently prescribed for a variety of arrhythmias. But quinidine and digoxin is a dangerous mix unless the cardiologist is extremely careful. Quinidine can increase blood levels of digoxin into the danger zone.[10] It took more than 60 years for physicians to discover this dangerous interaction. Doctors who believe they can anticipate trouble just by doing blood tests may be kidding themselves and putting their patients at risk. New research suggests that even when serum digoxin levels are in the so-called normal therapeutic range, electrocardiograms may show evidence of toxicity.[11]

Another heart drug that may cause life-threatening problems in conjunction with **Lanoxin** is **Cordarone** (amiodarone). **Cordarone** may cause digoxin levels to soar into the toxic range. In addition, when some patients took this combination their hearts stopped beating (asystole).[13] Their lives were saved, but the sight of an electrocardiogram strip showing only a flat line can be very scary.

Diuretic Dangers

Physicians consider water pills (diuretics) so safe and effective that they are among the most widely used drugs in the world. Such medications are frequently the first step in treating high blood

Drugs That May Increase Digoxin Levels[12]

(Never stop Lanoxin [digoxin] or any other medicine without careful
medical supervision. Have your doctor and pharmacist evaluate the interaction
potential of digoxin with the following medications.)

Achromycin V (tetracycline)	**Ery-Tab** (erythromycin)	**Rythmol** (propafenone)
Adalat (nifedipine)*	**Erythrocin** (erythromycin)	**Sandimmune** (cyclosporine)
Calan (verapamil)	**Ilosone** (erythromycin)	**Sporanox** (itraconazole)
Cardizem (diltiazem)*	**Isoptin** (verapamil)	**Tambocor** (flecainide)
Cordarone (amiodarone)	**Minocin** (minocycline)	**Terramycin** (oxytetracycline)
Declomycin (demeclocycline)	**Orinase** (tolbutamide)	**Valium** (diazepam)
E.E.S. (erythromycin)	**PCE** (erythromycin))	**Vascor** (bepridil)*
E-Mycin (erythromycin)	**Plaquenil** (hydroxychloroquine)	**Verelan** (verapamil)
ERYC (erythromycin)	**Procardia** (nifedipine)*	**Vibramycin** (doxycycline)
EryPed (erythromycin)	**Quinamm** (quinine)	**Xanax** (alprazolam)*

*These interactions are controversial and confusing. Please ask your doctor to monitor your progress
carefully for any signs of toxicity.

pressure and may be used to combat fluid buildup due to many different causes, including congestive heart failure.

It is quite common for people with serious heart trouble to be taking both **Lanoxin** and a diuretic such as **Lasix** (furosemide). The trouble is that many water pills deplete the body of minerals, including sodium, potassium, and magnesium. We can probably do without the sodium, but both potassium and magnesium are crucial for normal heart function. Cortisone (**Cortone**) and similar drugs such as betamethasone (**Celestone**), dexamethasone (**Decadron**), hydrocortisone (**Cortef**, **Hydrocortone**), prednisone, prednisolone (**Delta-Cortef)**, and methylprednisolone (**Medrol**) may also deplete potassium, so close monitoring is essential if this combination is necessary.

Physicians are aware that low potassium levels can make digitalis-type drugs extremely hazardous, even lethal. The heart can suddenly stop beating. That's why doctors are usually very careful to monitor blood levels of this mineral when someone is on **Lanoxin**. If potassium drops too low they may prescribe a potassium supplement (**K-Lor, K-Lyte, K-Tab, Micro-K, Slow-K**, etc.) or switch the patient to a potassium-preserving diuretic such as **Dyazide, Moduretic,** or **Maxzide**.

Too Much Potassium
(Hyperkalemia)

• Serum potassium above 5mEq/L
• Palpitations, heart rhythm changes
• Tingling or numbness in lips, feet, or hands
• Breathing difficulty
• Weakness
• Slow pulse
• Confusion

Too Little Potassium
(Hypokalemia)

• Serum potassium below 3.5 mEq/L
• Irregular pulse
• Muscle cramps
• Breathing difficulty
• Weakness

If all this sounds complicated, hang on to your seat. It gets worse. The problem is that too *much* potassium may be just as hazardous as too little and can also cause cardiac arrest. Think about Goldilocks and the porridge. Getting it just right is not easy. Combining diuretics such as **Aldactone, Aldactazide, Dyazide, Maxzide,** or **Moduretic** (which keep potassium levels up) with heart and blood pressure pills such as **Accupril** (quinapril), **Altace** (ramipril), **Capoten** (captopril), **Lotensin** (benazepril), **Monopril** (fosinopril), **Prinivil** (lisinopril), **Vasotec** (enalapril), and **Zestril** (lisinopril) can be very tricky. It is not uncommon for people taking digoxin to be taking such medications as well, but this combination can lead to a buildup of excess potassium that may trigger life-threatening changes in heart rhythms. People who use potassium-containing salt substitutes could also end up in trouble.

When people are on diuretics, magnesium levels may also drop. This mineral is often overlooked, but it can be as important as potassium for people on **Lanoxin**. Make sure your physician is checking your blood magnesium as well as potassium if you are on digoxin and a diuretic. That way he or she may be able to spot a problem before it becomes life-threatening. For additional information see the diuretic section in the Guides to Dangerous Drug Interactions at the end of this book (pages 296 and 304).

Arthritis Drug Interactions

Millions of people rely on their daily dose of pain medicine to make it through the day. These drugs are used for everything from tennis elbow and bursitis to headaches and arthritis. They are called nonsteroidal anti-inflammatory drugs, or NSAIDs for short. While they can relieve discomfort, they can also do nasty things to the stomach, kidneys, and liver.

It is estimated that every year at least 70,000 people are hospitalized because of digestive diseases brought on by NSAIDs. Experts report that these medications are responsible for anywhere between 7,600 and 20,000 deaths annually.[14, 15]

Anticoagulants

Blood thinners such as **Coumadin** (warfarin) save lives. They prevent blood clots that can lead to strokes and heart attacks. But thinning the blood too much can lead to life-threatening hemorrhage. Up to a third of those on long-term anticoagulant therapy experience bouts of serious bleeding. [16]

That's cause for concern by itself, but add an arthritis drug to the mix and you are playing with fire. Anti-inflammatory drugs often cause stomach irritation and ulceration. When someone taking one of these pain relievers also takes an anticoagulant such as **Coumadin,** the risk of a bleeding ulcer becomes much greater. This could be a deadly complication, especially in older people.

Methotrexate

NSAIDs create extra problems when they are mixed with certain other medications. Some of these interactions may be fatal. One in particular concerns us. It is the combination of anti-inflammatory drugs and methotrexate (**Abitrexate**, **Folex**, **Rheumatrex**), a powerful chemotherapeutic agent for cancer treatment. In recent years it has gained much wider use against psoriasis and rheumatoid arthritis. The problem is that cases of serious toxicity are cropping up. There have even been deaths reported.

A few people who took both methotrexate and a drug such as **Ansaid, Butazolidin, Indocin, Naprosyn, Orudis,**

NSAIDs	
NAME	GENERIC
Advil	ibuprofen
Aleve	naproxen
Anaprox	naproxen
Ansaid	flurbiprofen
Butazolidin	phenylbutazone
Clinoril	sulindac
Dolobid	diflunisal
Feldene	piroxicam
Indocin	indomethacin
Indocin SR	
Lodine	etodolac
Meclomen	meclofenamate
Motrin	ibuprofen
Motrin IB	
Nalfon	fenoprofen
Naprosyn	naproxen
Nuprin	ibuprofen
Orudis	ketoprofen
Relafen	nabumetone
Rufen	ibuprofen
Tolectin	tolmetin
Voltaren	diclofenac

Anticoagulants and NSAIDs

"Our data show that compared with nonusers of either drug, concurrent users of NSAIDs and oral anticoagulants had nearly a 13-fold increase in the risk of developing hemorrhagic peptic ulcer disease and that approximately 10% of the hospitalizations for hemorrhagic ulcer disease in users of anticoagulants were attributable to NSAID exposure. These findings provide clear evidence that NSAIDs increase the risk of hemorrhagic complications in elderly users of anticoagulants, and they should be used with extreme caution in patients receiving anticoagulants."

Shorr, Ronald I., et al. "Concurrent Use of Nonsteroidal Anti-Inflammatory Drugs and Oral Anticoagulants Places Elderly Persons at High Risk for Hemorrhagic Peptic Ulcer Disease." *Arch. Intern. Med.* 1993; 153:1665-1670.

or even aspirin have experienced complications such as diarrhea, fever, severe ulceration of the mouth and gastrointestinal tract, nausea, vomiting, kidney failure, blood abnormalities due to bone marrow damage, and death.[17] Apparently NSAIDs can boost blood levels of methotrexate, sometimes to dangerous levels.

If you suffer from severe arthritis or psoriasis, you should be alert to the dangers of this interaction because these medications might be prescribed together for someone with your condition. No one seems to know how often this interaction proves fatal, and it may be quite rare. Nevertheless, it is serious enough to warrant careful attention. Unless a physician is monitoring methotrexate closely it could be a recipe for disaster when combined with NSAIDs.

Lithium

People who suffer from bipolar mood disorder (previously called manic-depression) are usually treated with lithium (**Cibalith-S**, **Eskalith**, **Lithobid**, **Lithonate**, **Lithotabs**). This medication is supposed to smooth out the wild mood swings typical of this problem, blunting the highs and interrupting the lows.

Under the best of conditions, lithium can be a difficult drug. Adverse reactions may include thirst, hand tremor, nausea, irregular heart rhythms, muscle twitches, dizziness, slurred speech, con-

<table>
<tr><td colspan="2" align="center">**Signs of
Lithium Poisoning**</td></tr>
<tr><td>diarrhea</td><td>vomiting</td></tr>
<tr><td>drowsiness</td><td>incoordination</td></tr>
<tr><td>weakness</td><td>confusion</td></tr>
<tr><td>slurred speech</td><td>blurred vision</td></tr>
<tr><td>blackouts</td><td>seizures</td></tr>
<tr><td>kidney failure</td><td>coma</td></tr>
<tr><td colspan="2" align="center">death</td></tr>
</table>

fusion, forgetfulness, hair loss, fatigue, and impotence. Fortunately, such complications are rare when blood levels are carefully controlled.But many arthritis medicines may interfere with normal elimination of lithium and lead to toxicity.[18, 19, 20]

Thiazide diuretics such as hydrochlorothiazide may also raise lithium levels and lead to symptoms of overdose. Careful monitoring is essential!

Be Vigilant

There are far too many possible interactions for your doctor to know them all by heart. Anytime you add another medication to what you are already taking, ask her to look it up to see if it is compatible. Then make sure you ask the pharmacist as well. Don't overlook vitamins, minerals, or nonprescription drugs. Remember, even something as seemingly innocuous as a cold or allergy remedy could be lethal in combination with an antidepressant such as **Nardil** (an MAO inhibitor). (See page 98 for more details.)

Hospitalization is another potential risk. You would think that a place with so many health professionals would be good protection against the kind of problems we are talking about in this book, but bureaucracies can create confusion. In hospitals it is quite possible for the left hand not to know what the right hand is doing. People often get more medicines in a hospital than they do at home. Some experts have estimated that the average hospital patient receives nine different drugs simultaneously. And surgery poses special risks. A "simple" antibiotic such as tetracycline could interact with the general anesthetic **Penthrane** (methoxyflurane) to cause kidney damage. Three deaths have been reported as a result of this combination.[21]

The following table lists drugs that have been reported to interact in especially hazardous ways. Some of these combinations have resulted in fatal outcomes. There is not enough space to discuss every serious interaction in this book, but we make this information available to you so that you can check with your pharmacist and physician about your particular situation. Remember, NEVER start or stop any medication without medical supervision. If you want further details on the nature of some of the most common and serious interactions, check the individual drug listings in Guides to Dangerous Drug Interactions at the back of this book.

Hazardous Drug Interactions*

*Each person may react differently, and your doctor may have an excellent reason to prescribe certain drugs together. Be sure to discuss your individual situation with your physician.

THIS DRUG	CAN INTERACT WITH
Advil (ibuprofen)	**Coumadin** (warfarin)
Advil (ibuprofen)	lithium
Advil (ibuprofen)	methotrexate
Aldactone (spironolactone)	potassium supplements/salt substitutes
Aleve (naproxen)	**Coumadin** (warfarin)
Aleve (naproxen)	lithium
Aleve (naproxen)	methotrexate
Anafranil (clomipramine)	**Hismanal** (astemizole)
Anafranil (clomipramine)	**Nardil** (phenelzine)
Anafranil (clomipramine)	**Parnate** (tranylcypromine)
Anafranil (clomipramine)	**Prozac** (fluoxetine)
Anafranil (clomipramine)	**Seldane** (terfenadine)
Anaprox (naproxen)	**Coumadin** (warfarin)
Anaprox (naproxen)	lithium
Anaprox (naproxen)	methotrexate
Ansaid (flurbiprofen)	**Coumadin** (warfarin)
Ansaid (flurbiprofen)	methotrexate
Antabuse (disulfiram)	**Coumadin** (warfarin)
Anturane (sulfinpyrazone)	**Coumadin** (warfarin)
Asendin (amoxapine)	**Nardil** (phenelzine)
Asendin (amoxapine)	**Parnate** (tranylcypromine)
aspirin	**Coumadin** (warfarin)
Bactrim (co-trimoxazole)	**Coumadin** (warfarin)
barbiturates	**Coumadin** (warfarin)
Bronkaid tablets (theophylline, etc.)	**Cipro** (ciprofloxacin)
Bronkaid tablets (theophylline, etc.)	**Noroxin** (norfloxacin)
Bronkaid tablets (theophylline, etc.)	**Tagamet** (cimetidine)
Butazolidin (phenylbutazone)	**Coumadin** (warfarin)
Butazolidin (phenylbutazone)	methotrexate
Calan (verapamil)	**Lanoxin** (digoxin)
Cardioquin (quinidine)	**Cordarone** (amiodarone)
Cardioquin (quinidine)	**Lanoxin** (digoxin)

THIS DRUG	CAN INTERACT WITH
Cardizem (diltiazem)	**Cordarone** (amiodarone)
Catapres (clonidine)	**Norpramin** (desipramine)
Catapres (clonidine)	**Pertofrane** (desipramine)
Catapres (clonidine)	**Tofranil** (imipramine)
Choloxin (dextrothyroxine)	**Coumadin** (warfarin)
Cipro (ciprofloxacin)	theophylline
Cordarone (amiodarone)	**Cardizem** (diltiazem)
Cordarone (amiodarone)	**Coumadin** (warfarin)
Cordarone (amiodarone)	**Lanoxin** (digoxin)
Cordarone (amiodarone)	quinidine
Cordarone (amiodarone)	**Sandimmune** (cyclosporine)
Coumadin (warfarin)	androgens (male hormones)
Coumadin (warfarin)	**Antabuse** (disulfiram)
Coumadin (warfarin)	**Anturane** (sulfinpyrazone)
Coumadin (warfarin)	aspirin and other NSAIDs
Coumadin (warfarin)	**Bactrim** (co-trimoxazole)
Coumadin (warfarin)	barbiturates
Coumadin (warfarin)	**Butazolidin** (phenylbutazone)
Coumadin (warfarin)	**Choloxin** (dextrothyroxine)
Coumadin (warfarin)	**Cordarone** (amiodarone)
Coumadin (warfarin)	**Danazol** (danocrine)
Coumadin (warfarin)	**Diflucan** (fluconazole)
Coumadin (warfarin)	**Flagyl** (metronidazole)
Coumadin (warfarin)	**Monistat** (miconazole)
Coumadin (warfarin)	**Nolvadex** (tamoxifen)
Coumadin (warfarin)	**Septra** (co-trimoxazole)
Coumadin (warfarin)	**Tagamet** (cimetidine)
Cytovene (ganciclovir)	**Retrovir** (zidovudine)
Danocrine (danazol)	**Coumadin** (warfarin)
Darvocet-N (propoxyphene/APAP)	**Tegretol** (carbamazepine)
Darvon (propoxyphene)	**Tegretol** (carbamazepine)
Demerol (meperidine)	**Nardil** (phenelzine)
Demerol (meperidine)	**Parnate** (tranylcypromine)
Desyrel (trazodone)	**Prozac** (fluoxetine)
dextromethorphan	**Nardil** (phenelzine)
dextromethorphan	**Parnate** (tranylcypromine)
Diflucan (fluconazole)	**Coumadin** (warfarin)

THIS DRUG	CAN INTERACT WITH
Diflucan (fluconazole)	**Hismanal** (astemizole)
Diflucan (fluconazole)	**Seldane** (terfenadine)
Dilantin (phenytoin)	isoniazid
Duraquin (quinidine)	**Cordarone** (amiodarone)
Dyazide (triamterene+HCTZ)	potassium supplements/salt substitutes
E.E.S. (erythromycin)	**Hismanal** (astemizole)
E.E.S. (erythromycin)	**Mevacor** (lovastatin)
E.E.S (erythromycin)	**Norpace** (disopyramide)
E.E.S. (erythromycin)	**Pravachol** (pravastatin)
E.E.S. (erythromycin)	**Seldane** (terfenadine)
E.E.S (erythromycin)	**Tegretol** (carbamazepine)
E.E.S (erythromycin)	**Zocor** (simvastatin)
Effexor (venlafaxine)	**Parnate** (tranylcypromine)
Elavil (amitriptyline)	**Eldepryl** (selegiline)
Elavil (amitriptyline)	**Isuprel** (isoproterenol)
Elavil (amitriptyline)	**Nardil** (phenelzine)
Elavil (amitriptyline)	**Parnate** (tranylcypromine)
Eldepryl (selegiline)	**Elavil** (amitriptyline)
Eldepryl (selegiline)	**Luvox** (fluvoxamine)
Eldepryl (selegiline)	**Paxil** (paroxetine)
Eldepryl (selegiline)	**Prozac** (fluoxetine)
Eldepryl (selegiline)	**Vivactil** (protriptyline)
Eldepryl (selegiline)	**Zoloft** (sertraline)
E-Mycin (erythromycin)	**Hismanal** (astemizole)
E-Mycin (erythromycin)	**Mevacor** (lovastatin)
E-Mycin (erythromycin)	**Norpace** (disopyramide)
E-Mycin (erythromycin)	**Pravachol** (pravastatin)
E-Mycin (erythromycin)	**Seldane** (terfenadine)
E-Mycin (erythromycin)	**Tegretol** (carbamazepine)
E-Mycin (erythromycin)	**Zocor** (simvastatin)
ERYC (erythromycin)	**Hismanal** (astemizole)
ERYC (erythromycin)	**Mevacor** (lovastatin)
ERYC (erythromycin)	**Norpace** (disopyramide)
ERYC (erythromycin)	**Pravachol** (pravastatin)
ERYC (erythromycin)	**Seldane** (terfenadine)
ERYC (erythromycin)	**Tegretol** (carbamazepine)

THIS DRUG	CAN INTERACT WITH
ERYC (erythromycin)	**Zocor** (simvastatin)
EryPed (erythromycin)	**Hismanal** (astemizole)
EryPed (erythromycin)	**Mevacor** (lovastatin)
EryPed (erythromycin)	**Norpace** (disopyramide)
EryPed (erythromycin)	**Pravachol** (pravastatin)
EryPed (erythromycin)	**Seldane** (terfenadine)
EryPed (erythromycin)	**Tegretol** (carbamazepine)
EryPed (erythromycin)	**Zocor** (simvastatin)
Ery-Tab (erythromycin)	**Hismanal** (astemizole)
Ery-Tab (erythromycin)	**Mevacor** (lovastatin)
Ery-Tab (erythromycin)	**Norpace** (disopyramide)
Ery-Tab (erythromycin)	**Pravachol** (pravastatin)
Ery-Tab (erythromycin)	**Seldane** (terfenadine)
Ery-Tab (erythromycin)	**Tegretol** (carbamazepine)
Ery-Tab (erythromycin)	**Zocor** (simvastatin)
Eskalith (lithium)	NSAIDs
Flagyl (metronidazole)	**Coumadin** (warfarin)
Folex (methotrexate)	NSAIDs
Haldol (haloperidol)	**Prozac** (fluoxetine)
Hismanal (astemizole)	**Diflucan** (fluconazole)
Hismanal (astemizole)	erythromycin
Hismanal (astemizole)	**Luvox** (fluvoxamine)
Hismanal (astemizole)	**Nizoral** (ketoconazole)
Hismanal (astemizole)	**Prozac** (fluoxetine)
Hismanal (astemizole)	**Sporanox** (itraconazole)
Imuran (azathioprine)	**Zyloprim** (allopurinol)
Indocin (indomethacin)	**Coumadin** (warfarin)
Indocin (indomethacin)	lithium
Indocin (indomethacin)	methotrexate
isoniazid	**Dilantin** (phenytoin)
Isoptin (verapamil)	**Lanoxin** (digoxin)
Isuprel (isoproterenol)	**Elavil** (amitriptyline)
K-Dur (potassium)	potassium-sparing diuretics
K-Tab (potassium)	potassium-sparing diuretics
Klor-Con (potassium)	potassium-sparing diuretics
Lanoxin (digoxin)	**Cardioquin** (quinidine)
Lanoxin (digoxin)	**Cordarone** (amiodarone)

THIS DRUG	CAN INTERACT WITH
Lanoxin (digoxin)	**Quinaglute** (quinidine)
Lanoxin (digoxin)	**Quinalan** (quinidine)
Lanoxin (digoxin)	**Quinidex** (quinidine)
Lanoxin (digoxin)	quinidine
Lanoxin (digoxin)	**Quinora** (quinidine)
Lanoxin (digoxin)	**Rythmol** (propafenone)
Lanoxin (digoxin)	**Sandimmune** (cyclosporine)
Lanoxin (digoxin)	**Vascor** (bepridil)
Lanoxin (digoxin)	**Verelan** (verapamil)
Larodopa (levodopa)	**Nardil** (phenelzine)
Larodopa (levodopa)	**Parnate** (tranylcypromine)
lithium	**Indocin** and other NSAIDs
Lithobid (lithium)	NSAIDs
Lithonate (lithium)	NSAIDs
Lithotabs (lithium)	NSAIDs
Lopid (gemfibrozil)	**Mevacor** (lovastatin)
Luvox (fluvoxamine)	**Eldepryl** (selegiline)
Luvox (fluvoxamine)	**Hismanal** (astemizole)
Luvox (fluvoxamine)	**Nardil** (phenelzine)
Luvox (fluvoxamine)	**Parnate** (tranylcypromine)
Luvox (fluvoxamine)	**Seldane** (terfenadine)
Maxzide (triamterene + HCTZ)	potassium supplements/salt substitutes
methotrexate	**Indocin** and other NSAIDs
Mevacor (lovastatin)	**Biaxin** (clarithromycin)
Mevacor (lovastatin)	erythromycin
Mevacor (lovastatin)	**Lopid** (gemfibrozil)
Mevacor (lovastatin)	niacin
Mevacor (lovastatin)	**Sandimmune** (cyclosporine)
Micro-K (potassium)	potassium-sparing diuretics
Midamor (amiloride)	potassium supplements/salt substitutes
Moduretic (amiloride + HCTZ)	potassium supplements/salt substitutes
Monistat (miconazole)	**Coumadin** (warfarin)
Motrin (ibuprofen)	**Coumadin** (warfarin)
Motrin (ibuprofen)	lithium
Motrin (ibuprofen)	methotrexate

THIS DRUG	CAN INTERACT WITH
Naprosyn (naproxen)	**Coumadin** (warfarin)
Naprosyn (naproxen)	lithium
Naprosyn (naproxen)	methotrexate
Nardil (phenelzine)	**Anafranil** (clomipramine)
Nardil (phenelzine)	**Asendin** (amoxapine)
Nardil (phenelzine)	**Demerol** (meperidine)
Nardil (phenelzine)	dextromethorphan
Nardil (phenelzine)	diet pills/decongestants
Nardil (phenelzine)	**Elavil** (amitriptyline)
Nardil (phenelzine)	**Larodopa** (levodopa)
Nardil (phenelzine)	**Norpramin** (desipramine)
Nardil (phenelzine)	phenylpropanolamine
Nardil (phenelzine)	**Prozac** (fluoxetine)
Nardil (phenelzine)	pseudoephedrine
Nardil (phenelzine)	**Tofranil** (imipramine)
Nizoral (ketoconazole)	**Hismanal** (astemizole)
Nizoral (ketoconazole)	**Seldane** (terfenadine)
Nolvadex (tamoxifen)	**Coumadin** (warfarin)
Noroxin (norfloxacin)	theophylline
Norpace (disopyramide)	erythromycin
Norpramin (desipramine)	**Catapres** (clonidine)
Norpramin (desipramine)	**Nardil** (phenelzine)
Norpramin (desipramine)	**Parnate** (tranylcypromine)
Norpramin (desipramine)	**Prozac** (fluoxetine)
Nuprin (ibuprofen)	**Coumadin** (warfarin)
Nuprin (ibuprofen)	lithium
Nuprin (ibuprofen)	methotrexate
Orudis (ketoprofen)	**Coumadin** (warfarin)
Orudis (ketoprofen)	methotrexate
Pamelor (nortriptyline)	**Prozac** (fluoxetine)
Parnate (tranylcypromine)	**Anafranil** (clomipramine)
Parnate (tranylcypromine)	**Asendin** (amoxapine)
Parnate (tranylcypromine)	**Demerol** (meperidine)
Parnate (tranylcypromine)	dextromethorphan
Parnate (tranylcypromine)	diet pills/decongestants
Parnate (tranylcypromine)	**Effexor** (venlafaxine)

THIS DRUG	CAN INTERACT WITH
Parnate (tranylcypromine)	**Elavil** (amitriptyline)
Parnate (tranylcypromine)	**Larodopa** (levodopa)
Parnate (tranylcypromine)	**Luvox** (fluvoxamine)
Parnate (tranylcypromine)	**Norpramin** (desipramine)
Parnate (tranylcypromine)	**Paxil** (paroxetine)
Parnate (tranylcypromine)	phenylpropanolamine
Parnate (tranylcypromine)	**Prozac** (fluoxetine)
Parnate (tranylcypromine)	pseudoephedrine
Parnate (tranylcypromine)	**Tofranil** (imipramine)
Parnate (tranylcypromine)	**Zoloft** (sertraline)
Paxil (paroxetine)	**Eldepryl** (selegiline)
Paxil (paroxetine)	**Nardil** (phenelzine)
Paxil (paroxetine)	**Parnate** (tranylcypromine)
PCE (erythromycin)	**Hismanal** (astemizole)
PCE (erythromycin)	**Mevacor** (lovastatin)
PCE (erythromycin)	**Norpace** (disopyramide)
PCE (erythromycin)	**Pravachol** (pravastatin)
PCE (erythromycin)	**Seldane** (terfenadine)
PCE (erythromycin)	**Tegretol** (carbamazepine)
PCE (erythromycin)	**Zocor** (simvastatin)
Pertofrane (desipramine)	**Catapres** (clonidine)
phenylpropanolamine	**Nardil** (phenelzine)
phenylpropanolamine	**Parnate** (tranylcypromine)
potassium-sparing diuretics	**Micro-K** (potassium)
potassium-sparing diuretics	**Slow-K** (potassium)
potassium supplements/salt substitutes	**Dyazide** (triamterene + HCTZ)
potassium supplements/salt substitutes	**Maxzide** (triamterene + HCTZ)
potassium supplements/salt substitutes	**Midamor** (amiloride)
potassium supplements/salt substitutes	**Moduretic** (amiloride + HCTZ)
potassium-wasting diuretics	**Lanoxin** (digoxin)
Primatene Tablets (theophylline, etc.)	**Cipro** (ciprofloxacin)
Primatene Tablets (theophylline, etc.)	**Noroxin** (norfloxacin)
Primatene Tablets (theophylline, etc.)	**Tagamet** (cimetidine)
Prozac (fluoxetine)	**Anafranil** (clomipramin)
Prozac (fluoxetine)	**Desyrel** (trazodone)
Prozac (fluoxetine)	**Eldepryl** (selegiline)

THIS DRUG	CAN INTERACT WITH
Prozac (fluoxetine)	**Haldol** (haloperidol)
Prozac (fluoxetine)	**Nardil** (phenelzine)
Prozac (fluoxetine)	**Norpramin** (desipramine)
Prozac (fluoxetine)	**Pamelor** (nortriptyline)
Prozac (fluoxetine)	**Parnate** (tranylcypromine)
Prozac (fluoxetine)	**Tegretol** (carbamazepine)
Prozac (fluoxetine)	**Tofranil** (imipramine)
Prozac (fluoxetine)	**Valium** (diazepam)
Prozac (fluoxetine)	**Xanax** (alprazolam)
pseudoephedrine	**Nardil** (phenelzine)
pseudoephedrine	**Parnate** (tranylcypromine)
Purinethol (mercaptopurine)	**Zyloprim** (allopurinol)
Quinaglute (quinidine)	**Cordarone** (amiodarone)
Quinaglute (quinidine)	**Lanoxin** (digoxin)
Quinalan (quinidine)	**Cordarone** (amiodarone)
Quinalan (quinidine)	**Lanoxin** (digoxin)
Quinidex (quinidine)	**Cordarone** (amiodarone)
Quinidex (quinidine)	**Lanoxin** (digoxin)
quinidine	**Cordarone** (amiodarone)
quinidine	**Lanoxin** (digoxin)
Quinora (quinidine)	**Cordarone** (amiodarone)
Quinora (quinidine)	**Lanoxin** (digoxin)
Retrovir (zidovudine)	**Cytovene** (ganciclovir)
Rheumatrex (methotrexate)	NSAIDs
Sandimmune (cyclosporine)	**Cordarone** (amiodarone)
Sandimmune (cyclosporine)	**Lanoxin** (digoxin)
Seldane (terfenadine)	**Diflucan** (fluconazole)
Seldane (terfenadine)	erythromycin
Seldane (terfenadine)	**Luvox** (fluvoxamine)
Seldane (terfenadine)	**Nizoral** (ketoconazole)
Seldane (terfenadine)	**Prozac** (fluoxetine)
Seldane (terfenadine)	**Sporanox** (itraconazole)
Septra (co-trimoxazole)	**Coumadin** (warfarin)
Slo-bid (theophylline)	**Tagamet** (cimetidine)
Slow-K (potassium)	potassium-sparing diuretics
Slo-bid (theophylline)	**Cipro** (ciprofloxacin)

THIS DRUG	CAN INTERACT WITH
Slo-bid (theophylline)	**Noroxin** (norfloxacin)
Sporanox (itraconazole)	**Hismanal** (astemizole)
Sporanox (itraconazole)	**Seldane** (terfenadine)
Tagamet (cimetidine)	**BiCNU** (carmustine)
Tagamet (cimetidine)	**Coumadin** (warfarin)
Tagamet (cimetidine)	theophylline
Tedral (theophylline, etc.)	**Cipro** (ciprofloxacin)
Tedral (theophylline, etc.)	**Noroxin** (norfloxacin)
Tedral (theophylline, etc.)	**Tagamet** (cimetidine)
Tegretol (carbamazepine)	**Biaxin** (clarithromycin)
Tegretol (carbamazepine)	**Darvocet-N** (propoxyphene/APAP)
Tegretol (carbamazepine)	**Darvon** (propoxyphene)
Tegretol (carbamazepine)	erythromycin
Tegretol (carbamazepine)	**Tagamet** (cimetidine)
Theo-Dur (theophylline)	**Cipro** (ciprofloxacin)
Theo-Dur (theophylline)	**Noroxin** (norfloxacin)
Theo-Dur (theophylline)	**Tagamet** (cimetidine)
theophylline	**Tagamet** (cimetidine)
Tofranil (imipramine)	**Catapres** (clonidine)
Tofranil (imipramine)	**Marplan** (isocarboxazid)
Tofranil (imipramine)	**Nardil** (phenelzine)
Tofranil (imipramine)	**Parnate** (tranylcypromine)
Tofranil (imipramine)	**Prozac** (fluoxetine)
Tolectin (tolmetin)	**Coumadin** (warfarin)
Tolectin (tolmetin)	methotrexate
Valium (diazepam)	**Prozac** (fluoxetine)
Vivactil (protriptyline)	**Eldepryl** (selegiline)
Voltaren (diclofenac)	**Coumadin** (warfarin)
Voltaren (diclofenac)	lithium
Voltaren (diclofenac)	methotrexate
Xanax (alprazolam)	**Prozac** (fluoxetine)
Zoloft (sertraline)	**Eldepryl** (selegiline)
Zoloft (sertraline)	**Nardil** (phenelzine)
Zoloft (sertraline)	**Parnate** (tranylcypromine)
Zyloprim (allopurinol)	**Imuran** (azathioprine)
Zyloprim (allopurinol)	**Purinethol** (mercaptopurine)

References

1. Tackley, R.N., and B. Tregaskis. "Fatal Disseminated Intravascular Coagulation Following a Monoamine Oxidase Inhibitor/Tricyclic Interaction." *Anaesth.* 1987; 42:760–763.

2. Westermeyer, Joseph. "Fluoxetine-Induced Tricyclic Toxicity: Extent and Duration." *J. Clin. Pharmacol.* 1991; 31:388–392.

3. Otton, S. Victoria, et al. "Inhibition by Fluoxetine of Cytochrome P450 2D6 Activity." *Clin. Pharmacol. Ther.* 1993; 53:401–409.

4. Reidenberg, Marcus M. "Clinical Pharmacology." *JAMA* 1993; 270:192–194.

5. Hansten, Philip D., and John R. Horn. *Drug Interactions & Updates.* Malvern, Pa.: Lea & Febiger, 1993, pp. 491–492.

6. Otton, op. cit.

7. Ibid.

8. Rivers, N., et al. "Possible Lethal Reaction Between Nardil and Dextromethorphan." *Can. Med. Assoc. J.* 1970; 103:85.

9. Sovner, R., et al. "Interaction Between Dextromethorphan and Monoamine Oxidase Inhibitor Therapy with Isocarboxazid." *N. Engl. J. Med.* 1988; 319:1671.

10. Reiffel, J.A., et al. "A Previously Unrecognized Drug Interaction Between Quinidine and Digoxin." *Clin. Cardiol.* 1979; 2:40–42.

11. Mordel, Amnon, et al. "Quinidine Enhances Digitalis Toxicity at Therapeutic Serum Digoxin Levels." *Clin. Pharmacol. Ther.* 1993; 53:457–462.

12. Tatro, David S., et al. *Drug Interaction Facts.* St. Louis, Mo.: Facts and Comparisons, 1993.

13. Klein, H.O., et al. "Asystole Produced by the Combination of Amiodarone and Digoxin." *Am. Heart J.* 1987; 113: 399–400.

14. Fries, James F. "NSAID Gastropathy: Epidemiology." *J. Musculoskeletal Med.* 1991: 8(2):21–28.

15. Paulus, H.E. "FDA Arthritis Advisory Committee Meeting: Post-Marketing Surveillance of Non-Steroidal Anti-Inflammatory Drugs." *Arthritis Rheum.* 1985; 28:1168–1169.

16. Levine, M.N., et al. "Hemorrhagic Complications of Long-Term Anticoagulant Therapy." *Chest* 1989; 95:26S–36S.

17. Hansten, Philip D., et al., eds. *Drug Interactions and Updates Quarterly.* Vancouver, Wa.: Applied Therapeutics, 1993, pp. 415–418.

18. Herschberg, S.N., and F.S. Sierles. "Indomethacin-Induced Lithium Toxicity." *Am. Fam. Phys.* 1983; 28(2):155–157.

19. Reiman, N.I.W., and J.C. Frolich. "Effects of Diclofenac on Lithium Kinetics." *Clin. Pharmacol. Ther.* 1981; 30:348–352.

20. Simard, M., et al. "Lithium Carbonate Intoxication." *Arch. Int. Med.* 1989; 144:36–46.

21. Kuzucu, E.Y. "Methoxyflurane, Tetracycline, and Renal Failure." *JAMA* 1970; 211:1162.

Chapter Four

Eat, Drink, and Be Wary! Food/Drug Interactions

Who would ever guess that taking your blood pressure medicine with grapefruit juice instead of orange juice could make you sick? Or that licorice could be lethal when eaten with **Lanoxin** or **Lasix**? How could cheddar cheese, pepperoni pizza, or pickled herring combined with an antidepressant create a hypertensive crisis? Yet all of these interactions are real and could lead to disaster.

Hidden Hazards of Grapefruit Juice

Most people don't think twice about how they swallow their pills. But the beverage used to wash them down or the food that is eaten at the same time may produce unexpected, even fatal, results. Grapefruit juice contains ingredients called flavonoids (naringenin, quercetin, kaempferol). Naringenin has a profound impact on the metabolism of certain drugs. It appears to affect the action of a crucial liver enzyme.[1]

Calcium channel blockers such as felodipine (**Plendil**) and nifedipine (**Adalat, Procardia**) have become extremely popular for treating high blood pressure and angina. But grapefruit juice can dramatically increase the concentration of such medications.[2] One study examined blood levels of **Plendil** taken with Old South grapefruit juice, with water, and with Minute Maid orange juice.

While neither water nor orange juice had a measurable impact on blood levels of the drug, grapefruit juice tripled the amount of drug in the circulation.[3] Increased blood levels of the drug were associated with headaches, flushing, and light-headedness. Nifedipine bioavailability was boosted by 134 percent.

People who take drugs such as nifedipine and verapamil (**Calan**, **Isoptin**, and **Verelan**) are rarely told what beverages to avoid. Because grapefruit juice can affect the rate at which the drugs are metabolized, boosting their levels in the bloodstream, the possibility of side effects is increased. Be prudent: choose another liquid for swallowing those pills.

As far as we know, the complications associated with **Plendil** and **Procardia** are not life threatening. But concern has been raised that **Seldane** and **Seldane-D** (terfenadine) may also interact with grapefruit juice.[4] Because the flavonoids in grapefruit juice can interfere with the liver enzyme that processes the antihistamine terfenadine, some individuals might end up with unusually high levels of **Seldane** circulating in the body. In susceptible people, this could provoke a dangerous change in heart rhythm called "torsade de pointes."[5]

So far as we know, there haven't been any deaths or hospitalizations attributed to grapefruit juice in combination with **Seldane**—yet. Until recently, however, doctors didn't know that they should even ask their patients if they drank grapefruit juice, and it's certainly not something that would show up on a patient's medical record. As difficult as it may be to get information about drug/drug interactions, it is even more difficult to try to track down drug/food interactions. Researchers have just begun to investigate the grapefruit juice connection.[6, 7, 8] Dr. David Flockhart at Georgetown University Medical Center is an authority on this interaction. His research suggests that grapefruit juice can indeed have an important impact on both **Seldane** and **Hismanal**.[9] We urge you not to contribute to medical science by getting written up in a case report. Choose something else with which to swallow your **Seldane**.

Sandimmune (cyclosporine) is a powerful immune-suppressing drug that is frequently prescribed for patients who have received organ transplants. It has also been tried experimentally for a range of serious health problems including Crohn's disease, lupus, multiple sclerosis, rheumatoid arthritis, and severe psoriasis. The dose of **Sandimmune** has to be adjusted carefully and frequent tests of kidney and liver function are crucial. Adverse reactions such as kidney problems, high blood pressure, diarrhea, tremor, numbness, and convulsions may occur.

Since this medicine has to be diluted in a beverage, people are frequently advised to disguise the flavor with milk or juice. If they select grapefruit juice, however, it could have a profound impact on the blood levels of the medicine. Researchers at the University of California, San Francisco, have found that an ingredient in grapefruit juice slows the liver's ability to metabolize cyclosporine. A study with transplant patients shows that an eight-ounce glass of grapefruit juice together with the cyclosporine can boost blood levels of the drug by about one third, on average.[10] Such an increase could lead to toxicity if blood levels are not monitored very carefully. On the other hand, some scientists have suggested that this interaction could be used to the patient's advantage. Because **Sandimmune** is very expensive, a patient whose dose is lowered through coadministration with grapefruit juice might be able to achieve the desired effect with less medicine. One individual told us that over a period of several months, his doctors reduced his dose of cyclosporine gradually to about half of his initial dose. This is not a do-it-yourself project, and requires extremely careful monitoring and close coordination with the transplant follow-up team.

Although orange juice does not appear to interact with **Plendil**, **Procardia**, **Seldane**, or **Sandimmune**, it may affect aluminum absorption from some common antacids. For decades, researchers assumed that the aluminum in antacids was not absorbed into the body. Doctors became alarmed, however, when they discovered that an aluminum overload was responsible for dementia in kidney dialysis patients when they were given aluminum antacids or when the water was not purified to remove aluminum. While no research demonstrates a causal connection, this mineral is also found in higher concentrations in the brains of Alzheimer's disease victims.

Aluminum remains very controversial, but it appears prudent to minimize the amount of aluminum absorbed into the body. Taking an aluminum-containing antacid with orange juice increases aluminum absorption substantially. British scientists at the Institute of Food Research found that "there was an approximately 10-fold increase in 24 hour urinary aluminium excretion following the **Aludrox** plus orange juice." They concluded, "**Aludrox** and other aluminium-containing medicines should not be taken together with citric acid because of the increase in aluminium absorption. Patients should therefore be advised not to consume food or drinks containing citric acid (such as citrus fruits and juices) at the same time as their antacid preparation but to leave an interval of at least 2–3 hours between them."[11]

Another fruit juice interaction involves antibiotics. Penicillin and erythromycin should not be taken with citrus juice or soft drinks, because these acidic beverages could interfere with proper absorption and effectiveness of the drug.

Liabilities of Licorice

Licorice lovers of the world, beware! Your favorite candy could be a killer. The ingredient in natural licorice that gives people problems is glycyrrhizin. It has been used as a drug for centuries. Folk wisdom has it that licorice can be helpful against indigestion and ulcers.[12] Russian researchers suggest that it lowers cholesterol in rabbits.[13] Chinese scientists find that it controls coughs. Japanese investigators are looking into the immune-stimulating properties of this herbal remedy.[14]

So far, so good. Licorice sounds terrific, and, as connoisseurs ourselves, we were delighted to learn about these benefits. But too much licorice can cause serious medical complications. Regular indulgence in more than an ounce of natural black licorice daily can lead to muscle pain, fluid retention, weakness, hormonal imbalance, fatigue, hypertension, sexual complications, paralysis, and, worst of all, potassium depletion. There is a case of one woman who experienced cardiac arrest because her licorice binges produced excessive potassium loss from her system.[15]

People can really get themselves into serious trouble if they are on diuretics that deplete potassium and if they also indulge in

Where to Look for Licorice

Candy
Smokeless tobacco products
Cough drops
Chinese medicine
Sweetening additive in foods and drinks

licorice treats. This combination has been reported to produce dangerously low potassium levels, leading to such adverse reactions as weakness, muscle pain, and paralysis.[16, 17]

If a regular licorice eater were also taking **Lanoxin** (digoxin), it could easily become a prescription for disaster. Irregular heart rhythms and cardiac arrest are a distinct possibility. One reader of our syndicated newspaper column wrote to tell us that she had an extreme reaction to such a combination: "The doctors in the emergency room had no idea what was wrong, but a friend of my granddaughter's asked about licorice. Not one doctor ever heard of such a thing. Since then I have heard of several people who have had this problem."

Don't assume that licorice is found only in candy. We heard from another reader who wondered about smokeless tobacco: "My husband chews tobacco. Since he started, his blood pressure has really gone up. Is there any licorice in this product?" The answer is yes. Licorice is frequently used to flavor tobacco and it can be absorbed into the body. Licorice also appears in other unlikely places. As one woman told us, "For years I sucked on licorice 'chips' from England to relieve chronic throat irritation. They worked fine for my throat, but I ended up with hypertension and went into a coma. Beware of licorice!"

Treacherous Tyramine: The Cheese Effect

There are a few drugs that absolutely demand that you pay strict attention to what you eat because of the potential for a fatal drug/food interaction. The MAO (monoamine oxidase) inhibitors are unquestionably the most notorious, because they can interact with a substance called tyramine, which is found in certain foods. This interaction can cause extreme elevations in blood pressure and has led to fatalities.

By the time physicians realized that these medications could interact with common foods such as cheddar cheese, avocado, pepperoni, salami, and soy sauce, scores of people had experienced strokes and at least 15 had died.[18] And those were the reported cases. No one knows how many strokes and deaths went unreported.

What makes this reaction so bizarre is that the tyramine content of a food can vary dramatically. For example, liver is safe if it is very fresh. But a liver pâté that has sat around for a few days may contain a hazardous level of tyramine for someone taking an MAO inhibitor. A firm avocado may be okay, while a ripe one might be high enough in tyramine to induce a hypertensive crisis.[19]

When MAO inhibitors first became popular for treating depression, physicians had no idea of the dangers. Anecdotes started accumulating in the medical literature. In 1964 Welsh physicians reported the following case:

> On September 3, 1963, a 40-year-old man was put on Parnate (tranylcypromine) for serious depression. A month later he complained of a slight headache but ate supper with his family. He consumed beef casserole, cheese, and crackers. The cheese was cheddar, Caerphilly (a Welsh cheese similar to cheddar), and some Danish blue. During the night he felt much worse. He was dizzy, nauseated, and his headache was unbearable. By morning he felt well enough to eat breakfast with his family and consumed two or three large slices of cheese. Shortly thereafter he became distressed and incoherent. He started bleeding from his nose and was agitated, aggressive, and confused. By the time he got to the hospital he was incoherent, his temperature was 104.5°F, and his pulse and blood pressure were elevated. He died at 8:30 P.M. On autopsy his brain was found to be swollen with intense vascular congestion. The physicians concluded that it was the combination of the cheese and his medicine that killed him.
>
> Cuthill, J.M., et al. "Death Associated with Tranylcypromine and Cheese." *Lancet* 1964; i:1076–1077.

Physicians began to realize that certain foods, especially cheese, could get patients into trouble when eaten in conjunction with an MAO inhibitor. In 1965 a fascinating episode took place at a psychiatric hospital in Hartford, Connecticut. On the afternoon of October 21, a patient complained of severe headache, nausea, dizziness, and heart palpitations shortly after eating lunch. His blood pressure was also elevated. Within an hour, five other patients "experienced similar severe symptoms." Some blood pressures reached stratospheric levels with systolic numbers soaring over 200 (normal is around 120).

The similarity of the reactions led physicians to question what these patients had in common. All six had eaten chicken livers for lunch and they were all on **Parnate**. The leftover chicken livers were analyzed, and they turned out to be quite high in tyramine. This incident raised medical awareness that chicken livers (especially if not perfectly fresh) in combination with an MAO inhibitor could trigger a dangerous hypertensive crisis.[20]

Foods That May Interact with MAO Inhibitors

Avocados	Fish (pickled, salted,
Bananas (overripe)	or smoked)
Beef liver (stored)	Gruyère cheese
Blue cheese	Meat concentrate (in gravy
Bologna	or soup)
Brick cheese	Miso soup
Brie	Mozarella cheese
Brewer's yeast	Parmesan cheese
Broad beans	Pepperoni
Caffeine (large quantities)	Protein dietary supplements
Camembert	Provolone cheese
Caviar	Romano cheese
Chartreuse liqueur	Roquefort cheese
Cheddar	Salami
Chianti	Soy sauce
Chicken liver (stored)	Stilton cheese
Chocolate (large quantities)	Summer sausage
Drambuie liqueur	Vermouth
Emmenthaler cheese	Yeast extract (Marmite, etc.)
Figs (canned or overripe)	Yeast supplements

Because this reaction is so serious, there are at least four types of foods that must be strictly avoided while taking an MAO inhibitor. They include **broad bean pods** (also known as fava beans or Italian green beans—not ordinary green beans or lima beans); **yeast concentrates** such as Marmite, as well as brewer's yeast and yeast supplements; salted, smoked, or pickled fish, especially

Signs of Hypertensive Crisis

Severe headache	Chills
Stiff neck	Pale appearance
Palpitations	Chest pain
Anxiety	Sweating
High blood pressure	Collapse
	Coma

pickled herring; and **aged cheeses**, including blue types such as Stilton and Roquefort, soft varieties such as Camembert or Brie, and other popular kinds including cheddar, Swiss, brick, and Parmesan. Cottage cheese, farmer's cheese, and cream cheese, or Neufchâtel, aren't aged and therefore pose little if any threat.[21]

Other tyramine-containing foods warrant caution. The action of bacteria on protein produces tyramine, so any meat, including fish or chicken, should be avoided if you are not convinced of its freshness. This warning usually extends to liver pâtés and chopped chicken liver if they have been stored any length of time, and to aged sausages such as salami, pepperoni, and bologna. One young man on **Nardil** had a hypertensive reaction to the spicy chicken nuggets he ate in a restaurant, presumably due to the MSG in the seasoning mix.[22] Fermented soybean products, such as miso, and oriental fish or shrimp pastes may pose hazards.

Chianti wine is high in tyramine, and one person died from an MAO inhibitor/vermouth interaction, so it is smart to avoid Chianti and vermouth. Experts counsel moderation when it comes to other drinks: not more than one or two bottles of beer or eight ounces of wine. Nonalcoholic brands may contain relatively high levels of tyramine and are not a good substitute. Some imported beers are also high in tyramine and ought to be avoided. Since not all brands have been tested, it is wise to eschew them all.

As a result of these kinds of reactions, MAO inhibitors such as **Nardil** (phenelzine) and **Parnate** (tranylcypromine) lost their luster in the 1970s and 1980s. The tricyclic class of antidepressants became far more popular because they seemed safer. But in recent years there has been a resurgence of interest in the MAO inhibitors. For one thing, not everyone responds to one class of medicine. Some people may actually get better faster on a drug like **Nardil** or **Parnate** than with **Elavil** (amitriptyline) or even **Prozac** (fluoxetine). Another reason is that physicians have found that MAO inhibitors may help some patients who suffer from eating disorders such as bulimia (in which people may binge and then throw up the food they have eaten). They may also be beneficial in treating panic attacks, agoraphobia, obsessive-compulsive disorder, posttraumatic stress syndrome, and narcolepsy.

Antidepressants aren't the only medications that possess the ability to block the enzyme monoamine oxidase—and therefore require users to follow a diet low in tyramine. Another such drug is isoniazid, a tuberculosis medication being used with increasing frequency as TB makes a comeback. Brand names include **Laniazid**, **Nydrazid**, **Rifamate**, and **Rimactane/INH**. Others include the antibiotic **Furoxone** (furazolidone); **Matulane** (procarbazine), a chemotherapeutic agent used against cancer; and the blood pressure pill **Eutonyl** (pargyline). All of these drugs can interact with tyramine-containing foods to cause stimulation and raised blood pressure. Any person taking a drug that blocks the enzyme monoamine oxidase should avoid or restrict the foods in the table on page 47.

Hazards of Healthy Foods

We often seem to fall into the habit of thinking about certain foods as especially good for us. When something fits into our mental category of "health," we encourage people to clean their plate, and eat that food often. The idea that anyone could overdose on broccoli, spinach, or brussels sprouts is almost unthinkable. But in combination with particular medications, a wonderful Dr. Jekyll food could turn into a dangerous Mr. Hyde.

Salt Substitutes

One example of a "healthy" food that can potentially cause harm is the salt substitute. By now, most people are aware that too much sodium in the diet can be dangerous, especially when there's a tendency to fluid retention or high blood pressure. As a result, those worried about their blood pressure may turn to using one of the salt alternatives found in the grocery store. A good idea? Yes, but only if they are not also taking medicine that leads to potassium buildup in the body. Most of the salt substitutes rely on potassium to provide the missing "salty" flavor.

> One man was admitted to the Veterans Administration Hospital in Madison, Wisconsin, "complaining of sudden onset of shortness of breath, severe weakness, and dizziness." He had been taking Lasix (furosemide), Aldactone (spironolactone), and digoxin. On admission the physicians noted the patient "appeared lethargic, and weak, with labored respirations." His blood pressure was dangerously low and his pulse was only 12 to 15 beats per minute. The electrocardiogram revealed a person on the verge of cardiac arrest. His serum potassium level was perilously high—7.8.
>
> Intensive treatment saved his life but the physicians were puzzled as to how he could have ended up in such a state. Then, they reported "the patient's wife told us that her husband was liberally using a commercially available salt substitute for several days prior to admission."
>
> Yap, Vicente, et al. "Hyperkalemia with Cardiac Arrhythmia: Induction by Salt Substitutes, Spironolactone, and Azotemia." *JAMA* 1976; 236:2775–2776.

What happened to this Wisconsin patient was a drug/food interaction between his salt substitute and the potassium-sparing diuretic **Aldactone**. Other drugs that can also cause a dangerous elevation of potassium in combination with either a salt substitute or potassium supplement include **Accupril, Altace, Aldactone, Aldactazide, Capoten, Dyazide, Lotensin, Maxzide, Moduretic, Monopril, Prinivil, Vasotec**, and **Zestril**. If you are taking any of these drugs, make sure to check with your physician about any salt substitutes and have your blood level of potassium monitored frequently.

Overdosing on Oatmeal

After years of hearing that eating oatmeal is "the right thing to do," it is difficult to imagine that anything so wholesome could cause trouble. But one reader must have had an inkling when he wrote: "I take **Lanoxin** to control atrial fibrillation [an irregular heart rhythm that can lead to blood clots that cause strokes]. I have had nine attacks within the last four years. Three of those attacks were within just one month. Since then, my doctor increased the **Lanoxin** from 0.25 to 0.50 mg. Are there any liquids, foods, fruits, vegetables, or vitamins that may interfere with the

Lanoxin being effective in controlling the heartbeat? (I eat a very large dish of Mother's oats and bran every morning.)"

Bran, oatmeal, and other high-fiber foods may interfere with absorption of the crucial heart medicine **Lanoxin** (digoxin). Because it can be tricky to get the dose of **Lanoxin** adjusted properly, anything that affects its absorption may reduce this drug's effectiveness. According to clinical pharmacologist Brian F. Johnson, M.D., and his colleagues, ". . . concurrent administration of digoxin tablets with a meal high in fiber content has been demonstrated to decrease the extent of absorption. This may be a frequent problem in view of the current campaigns of medical organizations and manufacturers to promote greater consumption of fiber-rich foods."[23] These researchers found that **Lanoxicaps** were not as strongly affected by fiber as **Lanoxin** tablets. Don't stop your cereal suddenly, however. If you do, blood levels of digoxin could soar and lead to toxicity. Consult with your doctor to develop a plan for adjusting your diet and dosage.

Large amounts of fiber can interfere with other drugs as well, including certain antidepressants. When antidepressants are affected, mood disorders may not respond.[24] Because of the potential for suicide, this drug/food interaction must be taken seriously.

Broccoli, Brussels Sprouts, and Blood Clots

It doesn't seem fair that eating healthy food like oatmeal could get people into trouble with their medicine. How about those old standbys liver and spinach, together with today's vegetable superstars—broccoli, cabbage, and brussels sprouts? These healthy foods are all quite rich in vitamin K, and while they are indeed nutritious, they could have a dangerous impact on a person taking a blood-thinning drug such as **Coumadin** (warfarin).

Coumadin works partly by counteracting the vitamin K essential to the blood's clotting action. But when it is overwhelmed by too much vitamin K from a huge helping of kale or kohlrabi, the usual dose might be inadequate. The consequence could be a life-threatening blood clot in the brain, lung, or heart. All of the vegetables in the entire cabbage family, as well as asparagus, lettuce, and the already-mentioned liver, are high in vitamin K; these foods should be eaten only in modest quantities by anyone on

Coumadin. Periodic blood tests (prothrombin times) are also a good idea.

Although it is not usually thought of as rich in vitamin K, large quantities of avocado can also reduce the effectiveness of **Coumadin**.[25] As with vitamin-K–rich foods, overindulging could be a mistake with serious consequences. It would, at least in theory, be possible for someone taking **Coumadin** to experience a dangerous blood clot as a result of pigging out on too much guacamole.

When Milk Does a Body Harm

Health-conscious dieters know that milk and other dairy products have many nutritional benefits, especially for women trying to maintain adequate calcium intake. But dairy products can interact with certain antibiotics to render them virtually useless. Milk can reduce blood levels of tetracyclinelike drugs such as **Achromycin V**, as well as **Cipro** (ciprofloxacin) and **Noroxin** (norfloxacin) by 50 percent or more. That's enough to sabotage their impact.

A woman taking tetracycline for a *Chlamydia* infection (a very common sexually transmitted disease that can cause infertility) might not realize her medicine was ineffective when taken within an hour of her breakfast yogurt. Someone with the life-threatening tick-borne disease Rocky Mountain spotted fever could continue to get sicker or even die if he took his tetracycline in the morning and then had milk in his coffee or pancakes made with powdered milk.

Another medicine that may not do its job effectively when taken with milk or dairy products is **Didronel** (etidronate). This drug is being prescribed for osteoporosis prevention. But if calcium is consumed within two hours of taking **Didronel**, the medicine cannot be absorbed adequately.

Milk can also interfere with the planned action of laxatives containing bisacodyl, such as **Carter's Little Pills**, **Dulcolax,** or **Fleet**. Normally, these pills are coated to keep them from dissolving in the acid environment of the stomach, so that they go to work in the lower intestine. Drinking milk at the same time as you take the drug may lower stomach acidity enough that the coating dissolves there. This could result in stomach irritation and a big bellyache.

Coffee Complaints

Most of us have learned how much coffee we can handle before getting into trouble with jitters, insomnia, or heart palpitations. But some drugs may interact with caffeine to give you more of a java jolt than expected. **Cipro** (ciprofloxacin), **Penetrex** (enoxacin), and **Noroxin** (norfloxacin) may all slow elimination of caffeine from the body and produce unexpected stimulation. Even oral contraceptives and the popular stomach medicine **Tagamet** (cimetidine) could give someone more clout from their cup. That may be okay during a morning coffee break but could be an unwelcome effect at bedtime.

Anyone taking the asthma drug theophylline (**Bronkaid** tablets, **Bronkodyl**, **Primatene** tablets, **Slo-bid**, **Theo-Dur**) should limit caffeine from all sources. Since theophylline and caffeine are chemical cousins and produce similar effects in the body (caffeine can even help open airways), taking them together would be like getting an overdose.

Caffeine can crop up in some of the most unexpected places. You might not even realize that you are taking a hefty dose of caffeine when you swallow two **Bayer Select Headache Pain Relief** pills. But at 130 mg of caffeine per dose, you would be getting the equivalent of a strong cup of coffee. Be suspicious of herbal products that claim to boost energy. They may contain naturally occurring caffeinelike ingredients that could interact with other medications.

Coffee and tea can get some people into trouble in an entirely different way. Both beverages (but especially tea) may interact with supplements taken to combat iron deficiency anemia. The tannins in the tea grab on to the iron in the supplement and keep it from being absorbed. Whether the iron is in a pill all by itself,

---

Sources of Caffeine

Anacin (32mg/pill)
Bayer Select Headache (65mg/pill)
BC Powder (32mg/powder)
Coffee 8 oz (100 to 150 mg/cup)
Cola beverages 12 oz (38-46 mg)
Excedrin (65mg/pill)
Midol Max-Strength (60mg/pill)
NoDoz (100mg/tab)
Tea 6 oz brewed 3 minutes (36 mg)
Vanquish (33mg/pill)
Vivarin (200mg/pill)

such as **Feosol** or **Femiron**, or combined with other nutrients as a vitamin supplement with iron, it will be wasted if it is taken at breakfast with coffee or tea.

Iced tea lovers will also have to be wary. Someone who has a healthy spinach salad or an egg salad sandwich will not absorb the iron if they drink iced tea with their lunch. In fact, tea is so effective at blocking iron absorption it is sometimes prescribed for people with excess iron buildup in the blood.

Food and Asthma Medications

One of the strangest drug/food interactions we have ever heard of is the alteration of asthma medicine by meat cooked over coals. Theophylline (**Bronkaid** tablets, **Bronkodyl**, **Primatene** tablets, **Slo-bid**, **Theobid**, **Theo-Dur**, **Theolair**, **Theo-24**, **Uniphyl,** etc.) is eliminated from the body up to 42 percent more rapidly when a person has been eating a diet high in char-broiled foods.[26] Apparently the compounds formed when food is "blackened" by grilling make the liver work harder and faster. This means that some medicines, particularly theophylline, may not work as well as they should. That could lead to worsening of symptoms or an asthma attack.

Another potential interaction that is undeniably peculiar involves red peppers. Experiments with rabbits indicate that a hot pepper suspension (perhaps along the lines of **Tabasco** sauce?) increases the blood levels of theophylline for quite some time after the two substances are taken together.[27] We have no idea whether this could spell trouble for jalapeño junkies, but be forewarned.

Food can also make certain asthma preparations far more hazardous. Drug companies have developed slow-release theophylline for the sake of convenience. Products such as **Theo-24**, **Theochron**, **Theo-X**, and **Uniphyl** are designed to linger in the body so that only one or two doses will be needed in a day. In some cases, food can change the rate of release and raise the risk of side effects. When **Theo-24**, for example, is taken with a high-fat breakfast (or within an hour of such a meal) absorption and blood levels of the drug are boosted substantially. Symptoms such as nausea, vomiting, loss of appetite, anxiety, irritability, headache, palpitations, and muscle contractions could occur after a meal containing fried eggs, bacon, buttered toast, or whole milk. Taking a different theophylline product, however, may have the opposite effect. If someone swallows **Theolair** with a high-fat breakfast, it may reduce the amount of theophylline available to fight asthma symptoms.

There is some evidence that **Uniphyl** absorption increases when the drug is swallowed at mealtime, but the effect is not nearly so impressive as that seen with **Theo-24.** Maintaining consistency (same time of day, same type of food) seems logical. The situation is so complicated that you should check and double-check with both your physician and your pharmacist as to exactly how your brand of theophylline should be taken. Then follow the instructions consistently. Always taking this medicine the same way, whether it is with food or without, will help the doctor establish the proper dose, and should lower the likelihood of unpleasant surprises.

Pudding and Dilantin

Patients who don't swallow pills well may sometimes be given their medicine crushed and mixed with food to mask the taste. A research team in San Antonio discovered that it made a big difference whether that food was applesauce or vanilla pudding. Some ingredient in the pudding interfered with the absorption of **Dilantin Infatabs** (phenytoin) so that the appropriate dose did not get into the bloodstream. The resulting blood levels were only half as high as those achieved when the **Dilantin Infatabs** were mixed in applesauce.[28]

The researchers found that a similar interaction occurred when phenytoin was administered with a special solution used for tube feeding. The common ingredients include caseinates, corn oil starch, coconut oil, and carrageenan. Many foods may contain one or more of these ingredients, but we do not know if they would also interact with **Dilantin Infatabs**.

Which Medicines to Take with Food—or Without Food

The next time you get a prescription from your physician that says "take three times a day," it's time to arrange a conference with your doctor and pharmacist. Such instructions are woefully inadequate. Find out if you should be taking your medicine with meals or on an empty stomach, and if there are any specific foods or beverages that might interfere with its proper action. You have learned that such simple pleasures as licorice, grapefruit juice, chicken nuggets, and vanilla pudding can have unexpected and undesirable consequences when taken with certain drugs.

You would think that physicians have ready access to basic dosing instructions. After all, how you take your pills can have a profound effect on how well they get into your bloodstream and work in your body. Despite the importance of this essential information, it's not readily available. Only a few entries in the *Physicians' Desk Reference* specify how a pill should be swallowed in relation to meals.

The problem goes back to when the Food and Drug Administration set up its guidelines for drug testing. To keep things simple, the scientists wanted the drugs given at the same time and in the same way to everyone in a laboratory setting. That usually meant on an empty stomach. While this might have made sense once, it has nothing to do with real life. Who has time to get up early so you can take your pill an hour before breakfast? Fitting it in two hours after a meal in the midst of a hectic afternoon is just as improbable.

Because the FDA was slow to recognize the importance of the food/drug connection, and even slower to require research on the issue, the available data is sketchy at best. There is no one place doctors can check, and if they search the literature as we did, they will discover confusion and contradiction. This is also a constantly changing arena. Acetaminophen, for example, is one of the most common drugs in the world. It is not only available as **Anacin-3**, **Tylenol**, and **Panadol**, but also can be found in hundreds of OTC combination products. Although acetaminophen has been used for decades, it wasn't until 1994 that researchers discovered that fasting greatly enhanced its potential to cause liver damage.[29] This may not be an esoteric concern. When people are sick with the flu or are suffering from chronic pain, they may not feel like eating for days. The acetaminophen/food question demonstrates how important this whole issue is and how badly it has been neglected.

We contacted most major pharmaceutical manufacturers to ask them how their most popular drugs should be taken. In a shocking number of cases we learned there were inadequate or no data available. Frequently the companies had no recommendations as to how and with what their medicines should be swallowed.

We have gathered the information we were able to find into the following table. If your doctor gives you other instructions, check with her and your pharmacist to find out if they know something we don't. There may be special circumstances that apply in your case. Make sure you ask them to fill out the form on page 18, which specifies instructions on taking your medication.

Medicines that are to be taken without food should be swallowed at least one hour before eating or two hours afterward ("on an empty stomach"). If a medication upsets your stomach, you may experience less discomfort if you take it with food. Consult your physician and pharmacist as to whether that is appropriate. Other medications may be absorbed best with food, and the kind of food you take it with (high fat versus low fat) might make a difference.

In the table that begins on page 59, drugs that are absorbed better with food are marked with a single asterisk. This is somewhat unusual, because food often delays or interferes with drug absorption. Better absorption generally increases the levels of a medication in the bloodstream and enhances the effectiveness of the drug. It may also increase the risk of side effects. Drugs that are marked with a double asterisk are absorbed better without food, but may cause stomach upset. If you experience stomach distress, please check with your doctor to see if you should take your medicine with food to reduce this side effect. Drug companies that make certain diabetes medications often advise that these be taken 15 to 30 minutes before a meal. Such drugs are marked with a triple asterisk in the table.

Food and Drug Compatibility

DRUG	TAKE WITH FOOD	TAKE WITHOUT FOOD	TAKE WITHOUT REGARD TO FOOD
Accutane	■		
acetaminophen			■
acetaminophen + codeine	■		
acetazolamide	■		
Achromycin V		■	
Actifed	■		
Adalat		■	
Adapin	■		
Advil	■		
Agoral		■	
Alazine	■*		
Aldactazide	■*		
Aldactone	■*		
Aldoclor	■*		
Aldoril	■		
Allerest	■		
allopurinol	■		
Alupent	■		
Amcill		■	
aminophylline	■		
amitriptyline	■		
amoxicillin		■	
Amoxil			■
ampicillin		■	
Anacin-3			■
Anafranil	■		
Anaprox	■		
Antivert	■		
Anturane	■		
APAP			■
Apresazide	■*		
Apresoline	■*		
Aralen	■		

* Absorbed better with food.
** Absorbed better without food; may be taken with food to reduce stomach upset.
*** To be taken 15 to 30 minutes before a meal.

DRUG	TAKE WITH FOOD	TAKE WITHOUT FOOD	TAKE WITHOUT REGARD TO FOOD
Aristocort	■		
Artane	■		
A.S.A. Enseals			■
Ascriptin w/Codeine	■		
Asendin	■		
aspirin	■		
aspirin (coated)		■	
Atabrine	■		
atenolol			■
Ativan	■		
Atromid-S	■		
Augmentin			■
Aventyl	■		
Azo Gantanol		■	
Azo Gantrisin		■	
Azolid	■		
Azulfidine	■		
Bactocill		■	
Bactrim		■**	
Beepen-VK		■**	
Benadryl	■		
Benemid	■		
Bentyl	■		
Benylin	■		
benztropine	■		
betamethasone	■		
Betapen-VK		■**	
bethanechol		■	
Bicillin		■	
Bonine	■		
Brethine	■		
Bricanyl	■		
brompheniramine	■		
Bronkodyl	■		

* Absorbed better with food.
** Absorbed better without food; may be taken with food to reduce stomach upset.
*** To be taken 15 to 30 minutes before a meal.

DRUG	TAKE WITH FOOD	TAKE WITHOUT FOOD	TAKE WITHOUT REGARD TO FOOD
Butazolidin	■		
Calan SR	■		
calcium carbonate	■		
Capoten		■	
Carafate		■	
Cardioquin	■		
Cardizem		■	
Cardizem SR			■
Ceclor		■**	
Ceftin	■*		
Celestone	■		
cephalexin			■**
chlorothiazide	■*		
chlorpheniramine	■		
chlorpromazine	■		
Chlor-Trimeton	■		
chlorzoxazone	■		
Cipro		■**	
Claritin		■	
Cleocin			■
Clinoril	■		
clofibrate	■		
cloxacillin		■	
Cloxapen		■	
codeine	■		
Cogentin	■		
Cognex		■**	
Colace	■		
ColBenemid	■		
Colestid			■
Compazine	■		
Corgard			■
Cortef	■		
cortisone	■		

* Absorbed better with food.
** Absorbed better without food; may be taken with food to reduce stomach upset.
*** To be taken 15 to 30 minutes before a meal.

DRUG	TAKE WITH FOOD	TAKE WITHOUT FOOD	TAKE WITHOUT REGARD TO FOOD
Corzide	■*		
Coumadin			■
Cuprimine		■	
Darvocet-N 100	■*		
Darvon	■*		
Darvon Compound	■*		
Decadron	■		
Declomycin		■	
Delta-Cortef	■		
Deltapen-VK		■**	
Deltasone	■		
Demulen			■
Depakene	■		
Depen		■	
desipramine	■		
Desyrel	■		
dexamethasone	■		
DiaBeta	■***		
Diabinese	■		
Dialose	■		
Diamox	■		
dicloxacillin	■		
dicumarol	■*		
dicyclomine	■		
Didrex		■	
Didronel		■	
diethylpropion		■	
digoxin	■		
Dilantin	■*		
dimenhydrinate	■		
Dimetane	■		
Dimetapp	■		
diphenhydramine	■		
dipyridamole		■	

* Absorbed better with food.
** Absorbed better without food; may be taken with food to reduce stomach upset.
*** To be taken 15 to 30 minutes before a meal.

DRUG	TAKE WITH FOOD	TAKE WITHOUT FOOD	TAKE WITHOUT REGARD TO FOOD
Diupres	■*		
Diuril	■*		
docusate	■		
Dolene	■*		
Dolobid	■		
Dopar		■**	
doxepin	■		
doxycycline	■		
Dramamine	■		
Drixoral	■		
Dulcolax		■	
Duricef			■
Duvoid		■	
Dyazide	■*		
Dycill		■	
Dymelor	■		
Dynapen		■	
Dyrenium	■*		
Ecotrin		■	
Edecrin	■		
E.E.S.	■		
Elavil	■		
Elixophyllin	■		
Empirin w/Codeine	■		
E-Mycin			■
Endep	■		
Entex LA	■		
Equanil	■		
Eramycin		■	
ERYC		■	
Erypar		■	
EryPed	■*		
Erythrocin		■	
erythromycin		■	

* Absorbed better with food.
** Absorbed better without food; may be taken with food to reduce stomach upset.
*** To be taken 15 to 30 minutes before a meal.

DRUG	TAKE WITH FOOD	TAKE WITHOUT FOOD	TAKE WITHOUT REGARD TO FOOD
erythromycin estolate	■		
erythromycin ethylsuccinate	■		
erythromycin stearate		■	
Esimil	■		
Eskalith	■*		
Evac-Q-Kwik		■	
Fastin		■	
Feldene	■		
Femiron	■		
Feosol	■		
Fergon	■		
Fer-in-Sol	■		
Fiorinal w/Codeine	■		
Flagyl	■		
Flexeril	■		
Fulvicin	■*		
Furadantin	■*		
Furalan	■*		
furosemide		■**	
Gantanol		■	
Gantrisin		■	
Gastrocrom	1/2 hour before meals and at bedtime		
Geocillin		■	
Glucotrol	■***		
Grifulvin	■*		
Grisactin	■*		
Gris-PEG	■*		
griseofulvin	■*		
Halcion			■
Haldol	■		
haloperidol	■		
Hexadrol	■		
Hismanal		■	

* Absorbed better with food.
** Absorbed better without food; may be taken with food to reduce stomach upset.
*** To be taken 15 to 30 minutes before a meal.

DRUG	TAKE WITH FOOD	TAKE WITHOUT FOOD	TAKE WITHOUT REGARD TO FOOD
hydralazine	■*		
hydrochlorothiazide	■		
hydrocodone	■		
hydrocortisone	■		
Hygroton	■		
Ibuprin	■		
ibuprofen	■		
Ilosone	■*		
imipramine	■		
Imuran	■		
Inderal	■*		
Inderide	■*		
Indocin	■		
indomethacin	■		
INH		■	
iron	■		
Ismelin	■		
isoniazid		■	
Isoptin		■	
Isordil		■	
Kaochlor	■		
Kaon	■		
Kato	■		
Kay Ciel	■		
Keflex			■**
Kenacort	■		
K-Lor	■		
Klorvess	■		
Klotrix	■		
K-Lyte	■		
labetalol	■*		
Laniazid		■	
Lanoxicaps			■
Lanoxin	■		

* Absorbed better with food.
** Absorbed better without food; may be taken with food to reduce stomach upset.
*** To be taken 15 to 30 minutes before a meal.

DRUG	TAKE WITH FOOD	TAKE WITHOUT FOOD	TAKE WITHOUT REGARD TO FOOD
Larodopa		■**	
Larotid		■	
Lasix		■**	
Ledercillin VK		■**	
levodopa		■**	
Levothroid		■	
Levsin		■	
Levsinex		■	
Libritabs	■		
Librium	■		
Lincocin		■	
lithium	■*		
Lithobid	■*		
Lithonate	■*		
Lithotabs	■*		
Lodine	■		
Lo/Ovral	■		
Lopid	■***		
Lopressor	■*		
Lorabid		■	
Lorelco	■*		
Lozol	■		
Ludiomil	■		
Macrodantin	■*		
Mandelamine	■		
maprotiline	■		
Marax	■		
Maxzide			■
meclizine	■		
Meclomen	■		
Medrol	■		
Mellaril	■		
meprobamate	■		
methenamine	■		

* Absorbed better with food.
** Absorbed better without food; may be taken with food to reduce stomach upset.
*** To be taken 15 to 30 minutes before a meal.

DRUG	TAKE WITH FOOD	TAKE WITHOUT FOOD	TAKE WITHOUT REGARD TO FOOD
methylprednisolone	■		
Meticorten	■		
metoprolol	■		
metronidazole	■		
Mevacor	■*		
Mexitil	■		
Micro-K	■		
Micronase	■***		
Midamor	■*		
milk of magnesia		■	
Miltown	■		
Moduretic	■*		
Motrin	■		
Motrin IB	■		
Mysoline	■		
Nafcil		■	
nafcillin		■	
Nalfon	■		
Naprosyn	■		
Nardil	■		
Naturetin			■
Navane	■		
NegGram		■	
niacin	■		
Nicobid	■		
Nicolar	■		
nitrofurantoin	■*		
Nitrostat		■	
Nizoral	■*		
Noctec	■		
Normodyne	■*		
Norpramin	■		
nortriptyline	■		
Nuprin	■		

* Absorbed better with food.
** Absorbed better without food; may be taken with food to reduce stomach upset.
*** To be taken 15 to 30 minutes before a meal.

DRUG	TAKE WITH FOOD	TAKE WITHOUT FOOD	TAKE WITHOUT REGARD TO FOOD
Nydrazid		■	
Omnipen		■	
Orinase		■**	
Ornade	■		
Ortho-Novum			■
oxacillin		■	
Oxalid	■		
Oxsoralen	■*		
Oxycodan	■		
oxycodone	■		
oxyphenbutazone	■		
oxytetracycline		■	
Pamelor	■		
Panmycin		■	
papaverine	■		
Paraflex	■		
paraminosalicylic acid	■		
Parnate	■		
P.A.S.	■		
Pavabid	■		
Paxipam	■		
PBZ	■		
PCE		■	
Pediazole	■*		
penicillamine		■	
penicillin G		■	
penicillin V		■	
penicillin V K		■**	
pentaerythritol tetranitrate		■	
Pentids		■	
Pen-V		■**	
Pen-Vee K		■**	
Pepcid			■

* Absorbed better with food.
** Absorbed better without food; may be taken with food to reduce stomach upset.
*** To be taken 15 to 30 minutes before a meal.

DRUG	TAKE WITH FOOD	TAKE WITHOUT FOOD	TAKE WITHOUT REGARD TO FOOD
Percocet	■		
Percodan	■		
Periactin	■		
Peritrate		■	
Permitil	■		
Persantine		■	
Pertofrane	■		
phentermine		■	
phenylbutazone	■		
phenytoin	■*		
Placidyl	■		
Plaquenil	■		
Polycillin		■	
Polymox		■	
Pondimin		■	
Ponstel	■		
potassium	■		
prednisolone	■		
prednisone	■		
Preludin		■	
Premarin	■		
primidone	■		
Principen		■	
Prinivil			■
Priscoline	■		
Pro-Banthine		■	
probenecid	■		
procainamide		■**	
Procan SR		■**	
Procardia		■	
Prolixin	■		
Proloprim			■
Pronestyl		■**	

* Absorbed better with food.
** Absorbed better without food; may be taken with food to reduce stomach upset.
*** To be taken 15 to 30 minutes before a meal.

DRUG	TAKE WITH FOOD	TAKE WITHOUT FOOD	TAKE WITHOUT REGARD TO FOOD
propantheline		■	
propoxyphene w/acetaminophen	■		
propranolol	■*		
Propulsid	■***		
Prostaphlin		■	
Protostat	■		
Provera	■		
Prozac			■**
Quadrinal	■		
Quibron-T	■		
Quinaglute	■		
Quinidex	■		
quinidine	■		
quinine	■		
Quinora	■		
Reglan	30 min before meals		
reserpine	■		
Rifadin		■	
Rifamate		■	
rifampin		■	
Rimactane		■	
Ritalin	Children: At mealtime Adults: 30 to 45 min before meals		
Rondomycin		■	
Rufen	■		
Rythmol	■		
Salutensin	■		
Sandimmune	■		
Seldane			■
Seldane-D	■		
Septra		■**	
Ser-Ap-Es	■*		
Serax	■		

* Absorbed better with food.
** Absorbed better without food; may be taken with food to reduce stomach upset.
*** To be taken 15 to 30 minutes before a meal.

DRUG	TAKE WITH FOOD	TAKE WITHOUT FOOD	TAKE WITHOUT REGARD TO FOOD
Serpasil	■		
Sinequan	■		
Slo-bid			■
Slow-K	■		
Somophyllin	■		
Sorbitrate		■	
Spectrobid		■	
spironolactone	■*		
Sporanox	■*		
Stelazine	■		
sulfamethoxazole		■	
sulfasalazine	■		
sulfinpyrazone	■		
sulfisoxazole		■	
Sumycin		■	
Surmontil	■		
Synalgos	■		
Synthroid		■	
Tagamet	■		
Talwin Compound	■		
TAO		■	
Tavist-D	■		
Tedral	■		
Tegison	■		
Tegopen		■	
Tegretol	■*		
Tenoretic			■
Tenormin			■
Tenuate		■	
Tepanil		■	
Terramycin		■	
tetracycline		■	
Tetralan		■	

* Absorbed better with food.
** Absorbed better without food; may be taken with food to reduce stomach upset.
*** To be taken 15 to 30 minutes before a meal.

DRUG	TAKE WITH FOOD	TAKE WITHOUT FOOD	TAKE WITHOUT REGARD TO FOOD
Theo-24		■	
Theo-Dur	■		
Theo-Dur Sprinkle		■	
Theobid	■		
Theolair	■		
theophylline	■		
thioridazine	■		
Thorazine	■		
Thyrolar		■	
Ticlid	■*		
Tofranil	■		
Tolectin		■**	
Tolinase	■		
Trandate	■*		
Tranxene	■		
Trental	■		
triamcinolone	■		
triamterene	■		
Triavil	■		
trifluoperazine	■		
trihexyphenidyl	■		
Trilafon	■		
Trimox			■
Tuss-Ornade	■		
Tylenol			■
Tylenol w/codeine	■		
Tylox	■		
Unipen		■	
Uniphyl	■*		
Unipres	■*		
Urecholine		■	
Uri-Tet		■	
Urobiotic-250		■	
Valium	■		

* Absorbed better with food.
** Absorbed better without food; may be taken with food to reduce stomach upset.
*** To be taken 15 to 30 minutes before a meal.

DRUG	TAKE WITH FOOD	TAKE WITHOUT FOOD	TAKE WITHOUT REGARD TO FOOD
valproic acid	■		
Vasotec			■
V-Cillin K		■**	
Veetids		■**	
Velosef			■
Vibramycin	■		
Vicodin	■		
Videx		■	
Visken			■
Vivactil	■		
Voltaren	■		
Wyamycin S		■	
Wygesic	■		
Xanax	■		
Zantac	■		
Zestril			■
Zoloft	■*		
Zovirax			■
Zyloprim	■		

* Absorbed better with food.
** Absorbed better without food; may be taken with food to reduce stomach upset.
*** To be taken 15 to 30 minutes before a meal.

References

1. Guengerich, F.P., and D.H. Kim. "In Vitro Inhibition of Dihydropyridine Oxidation and Aflatoxin B1 Activation in Human Liver Microsomes by Naringenin and Other Flavonoids." *Carcinogen* 1992; 11:2275–2279.

2. Edgar, B., et al. "Acute Effects of Drinking Grapefruit Juice on the Pharmacokinetics and Dynamics of Felodipine—and its Potential Clinical Relevance." *Eur. J. Clin. Pharmacol.* 1992; 42:313–317.

3. Bailey, David G., et al. "Interaction of Citrus Juices with Felodipine and Nifedipine." *Lancet.* 1991; 337:268–270.

4. Woosley, Raymond L., et al. "Mechanism of the Cardiotoxic Actions of Terfenadine." *JAMA* 1993; 269:1532–1536.

5. Ibid., pp. 1535–1536.

6. Soons, P.A., et al. "Grapefruit Juice and Cimetidine Inhibit Stereoselective Metabolism of Nitrendipine in Humans." *Clin. Pharmacol. Ther.* 1991; 50:394–403.

7. Miniscalco, A., et al. "Inhibition of Dihydropyridine Metabolism in Rat and Human Liver Microsomes by Flavonoids Found in Grapefruit Juice." *J. Pharmacol. Exp. Ther.* 1992; 261:1195–1199.

8. Fuhr, Uwe, et al. "Inhibitory Effect of Grapefruit Juice and Its Bitter Principal, Naringenin, on CYP1A2 Dependent Metabolism of Caffeine in Man." *Br. J. Clin. Pharmacol.* 1993; 35:431–436.

9. Flockhart, David. Personal communication, November 16, 1993.

10. Ducharme, M.P., et al. "Trough Concentrations of Cyclosporine in Blood Following Administration with Grapefruit Juice." *Br. J. Clin. Pharmacol.* 1993; 36:457–459.

11. Fairweather-Tait, S., et al. "Orange Juice Enhances Aluminium Absorption from Antacid Preparation." *European J. Clin. Nutr.* 1994; 46:71–73.

12. Tarnawski, Andrzej, et al. "Cytoprotective Drugs: Focus on Essential Fatty Acids and Sucralfate." *Scand. J. Gastroenterol.* 1987; 22(Suppl. 127):39–43.

13. Mezenova, T.D. "Hypolipidemic Activity of Licorice Root Extract." *Pharm. Chem. J._(USSR)* 1984; 17:275–277.

14. Shinada, Masahiro, et al. "Enhancement of Interferon-√ Production in Glycyrrhizin-Treated Human Peripheral Lymphocytes in Response to Concanavalin A and to Surface Antigen of Hepatitis B Virus (42241)." *Proc. Soc. Exp. Biol. Med.* 1986; 181:205–210.

15. Bannister, B., et al. "Cardiac Arrest Due to Licorice Induced Hypokalemia." *Br. Med. J.* 1977; 2:738–739.

16. Shintani, Shuzo, et al. "Glycyrrhizin (Licorice)-Induced Hypokalemic Myopathy." *Eur. Neurol.* 1992; 32:44–51.

17. Farese, Robert V., et al. "Licorice-Induced Hypermineralocorticoidism." *N. Engl. J. Med.* 1991; 325:1223–1227.

18. Baldessarini, Ross J. "Drugs and the Treatment of Psychiatric Disorders," in *Goodman and Gilman's The Pharmacological Basis of Therapeutics*, 8th ed. Gilman, Alfred, et al., eds. New York: Pergamon, 1990, pp. 417.

19. Generali, J.A., et al. "Hypertensive Crisis Resulting from Avocados and a MAO Inhibitor." *Drug Intell. Clin. Pharm.* 1981; 15:904–906.

20. Hedberg, David L., et al. "Six Cases of Hypertensive Crisis in Patients on Tranylcypromine after Eating Chicken Livers." *Am. J. Psychiatry.* 1966; 122:933–937.

21. Brown, Candace, et al. "The Monoamine Oxidase Inhibitor-Tyramine Interaction." *J. Clin. Pharmacol.* 1989; 29:529–532.

22. Pohl, R., et al. "Reaction to Chicken Nuggets in a Patient Taking an MAOI." *Am. J. Psychiatry* 1988; 145:651.

23. Johnson, Brian F., et al. "The Effect of Dietary Fiber on the Bioavailability of Digoxin in Capsules." *J. Clin. Pharmacol.* 1987; 27:487–490.

24. Stewart, Donna E. "High-Fiber Diet and Serum Tricyclic Antidepressant Levels." *J. Clin. Psychopharmacol.* 1992; 12:438–440.

25. Wells, Philip S., et al. "Interactions of Warfarin with Drugs and Food." *Ann. Int. Med.* 1994; 121:676–683.

26. Kappus, A., et al. "Effect of Charcoal-Broiled Beef on Antipyrine and Theophylline Metabolism." *Clin. Pharmacol. Ther.* 1978; 23:445–449.

27. Bouraoui, A., et al. "Effects of Capsicum Fruit on Theophylline Absorption and Bioavailability in Rabbits." *Drug-Nutrient Interactions* 1988; 5:345–350.

28. Jann, M. W., et al. "Interaction of Dietary Pudding with Phenytoin." *Pediatrics* 1986; 78:952–953.

29. Whitcomb, David C., et al. "Association of Acetaminophen Hepatoxicity with Fasting and Ethanol Use." *JAMA* 1994; 272:1845–1850.

Chapter Five

Drug/Vitamin and Drug/Mineral Interactions

People often take their vitamins for granted. They don't think of them as medicines and may not mention them when the doctor asks what else they are taking. In fact, some people are afraid to discuss vitamin supplements with their physician because they worry that he or she will be scornful or dismissive. Sometimes this concern is justified. Many medical schools do not give nutrition an important place in the curriculum; some do not teach it at all. As a consequence, the doctor may not know much more than the patient about vitamins, minerals, and their potential impact on health.

Treating nutritional supplements casually or keeping them a secret from the physician could be a mistake, however. Some medications are known to interact with minerals or vitamins in a negative manner, but the doctor or pharmacist probably won't think to give you advice on avoiding these dangers unless he or she knows you take vitamins. The popularity of vitamin and mineral supplements has increased dramatically over the past decade or so, as women try to prevent osteoporosis with extra calcium and vitamin D, as middle-aged baby boomers learn that beta carotene pills may reduce the risk of heart attack or cancer, and as other people take high doses of vitamin C to prevent and treat the common cold. With more and more people popping vitamin pills, the potential for interactions with popular drugs also increases.

How Drugs Affect Nutrition

Unfortunately, researchers have not devoted enormous amounts of time and energy to the study of how nutrients interact with drugs, partly because the practical benefits are not immediately apparent. The Food and Drug Administration has not required drug companies to spend the time or resources required to uncover such interactions. Federal bureaucrats generally have been skeptical about the need for supplements or the existence of nutritional problems. Unless people start developing classic deficiency diseases such as scurvy, pellagra, or beriberi, no one is likely to worry.

Such clear-cut and dramatic cases of deficiency disease are almost unknown in the United States today. We have heard that there were cases of pellagra on hospital wards in the American South until the early 1960s, but none has been seen for decades. In some impoverished pockets of the country there still may be children suffering from the weak bones of rickets, or people with gums and old scars bleeding from scurvy. But there may be millions more people with deficiencies far more subtle.

One careful study showed that the potent ulcer and heartburn medicine **Prilosec** (omeprazole) can reduce absorption of vitamin B_{12} dramatically.[1] **Zantac** (ranitidine) and **Tagamet** (cimetidine) may also affect vitamin B_{12} absorption. Over a long period of time, it is certainly possible that the chronic depletion of vitamin B_{12} could have a negative effect on a person's health, even resulting in pernicious anemia. Neurological problems may also result. Symptoms to be alert for include burning tongue or feet, numbness or tingling, depression, and irritability.

Some deficiencies may be so common that they are hardly noticed. Several studies over the past few years have demonstrated a strong link between high blood levels of homocysteine and low levels of the B vitamins folic acid, B_6 and B_{12}.[2, 3]

You may be wondering what homocysteine is and why anyone would get excited about it. This toxic amino acid has gotten relatively little public attention, but it may be almost as important as cholesterol in determining who is at risk of heart attack, stroke, or other vascular diseases:

"Why should we care about homocysteine? Early studies showed that individuals with very high levels of homocysteine (due to genetic metabolic defects) often died of severe vascular disease in their teens or twenties. More recent work has shown that even moderately elevated levels are associated with increased risk of cardiovascular disease . . . an elevated homocysteine concentration may contribute to a substantial fraction of myocardial infarctions [heart attacks] (and perhaps other cardiovascular outcomes) in the United States."

Stampfer, Meir J., and Willett, Walter C. "Homocysteine and Marginal Vitamin Deficiency: The Importance of Adequate Vitamin Intake." (Editorial) *JAMA* 1993; 270:2726–2727.

The suggestion of a connection between vitamin intake, homocysteine levels, and the risk of heart attack is not brand new. It was presented to the public over a decade ago in the fascinating book, *Beyond Cholesterol: Vitamin B₆, Arteriosclerosis, and Your Heart*, by Edward R. Gruberg and Stephen A. Raymond, but despite this, the hypothesis has not captured people's attention as cholesterol has. Not only does this recent research, part of the far-reaching Framingham study, confirm the connection between low B-vitamin levels and high levels of homocysteine, but it also indicates that inadequate B-vitamin status may be far more common than expected, at least among the elderly.

Biochemists have known for years that certain medications can alter nutritional balance, creating a relative deficiency of one vitamin or another. A number of drugs reduce the levels of vitamin B₆ and folic acid circulating in the bloodstream. Anticonvulsants, especially **Dilantin**, are the best-known culprits, but oral contraceptives; estrogen replacement drugs such as **Premarin**, **Estrace,** and **Estraderm**; aspirin; and blood pressure drugs such as **Apresoline**, **Dyazide**, and **Maxzide** may also lower the amounts of one or another of these crucial B vitamins in the body. Cholesterol medicines such as **Questran**, corticosteroids, the potent rheumatoid arthritis medicine methotrexate, and even alcohol can also have this effect.

Eminent epidemiologists Meir J. Stampfer and Walter C. Willett point out that we can't even be sure that low B-vitamin levels are responsible for high homocysteine, but "several investigators have demonstrated that elevated levels of homocysteine can often be normalized with nutritional supplements, particularly with folate; thus, the associations observed by Selhub et al. are very likely to be causal."[4]

So far as we know, researchers have not yet examined the possibility that many of these medications might be indirectly connected to high homocysteine levels and an elevated risk of heart attack. This appears theoretically possible, though. What a shame it would be if people were taking medicines such as **Dyazide** or even **Premarin** to protect their hearts, and these drugs ended up lowering folate levels, raising homocysteine, and thus increasing the risk of a heart attack. If you want to err on the side of caution, you might check whether the medication you take could affect your nutritional status. The table at the end of this chapter is a good place to start. Another precaution might be vitamin supplements. Drs. Gruberg and Raymond recommended an intake of 10 to 25 mg of vitamin B_6 supplement daily, because the average American diet rarely supplies more than 2 mg of this vitamin. Various experts suggest that supplementation of folic acid, for whatever reason, usually should be 400 to 800 micrograms (0.4 to 0.8 mg) daily.

How Supplements Affect Drugs

Doctors and pharmacists are unquestionably interested in one type of interaction between nutrients and drugs. When nutritional supplements interfere with a medication and make it less effective, they tend to sit up and take notice. You should, too, because taking a medicine with supplements that counteract it is a waste of money and potentially damaging to your health. One of the clearest examples of such an interaction is tetracycline and calcium.

Mineral Supplements and Tetracycline

Tetracycline is one of the most commonly prescribed antibiotics in the world. It is cheap and quite effective for treating all kinds of maladies from acne to sexually transmitted diseases. It is the drug of choice against a *Chlamydia* infection, which can cause scarring of the fallopian tubes and infertility. Tetracycline is also the primary treatment for Rocky Mountain spotted fever, a potentially deadly disease transmitted by wood ticks.

When tetracycline (**Achromycin V**, **Sumycin**, etc.) or one of its common relatives (**Declomycin [demeclocycline]**, **Terramycin [oxytetracycline]**, etc.) is dispensed by a pharmacist, it usually comes with a warning on the label to avoid milk and dairy products. Calcium can inactivate tetracycline and prevent its absorption into the bloodstream.

The patient may not realize that antacids, laxatives, and, most important, nutritional supplements should also be shunned. Few physicians and pharmacists realize how many women now swallow calcium pills to prevent osteoporosis. In addition, they may be taking vitamin and mineral supplements with iron, magnesium, and zinc. These minerals can all bind to tetracycline, forming an insoluble precipitate and preventing the drug's absorption if they are taken with it. How many people take their supplements and antibiotic together? Most of us find it much easier just to swallow the whole handful of pills at once and forget about it until it's time for the afternoon dose of tetracycline. But once you learn about minerals, you won't want to take them at the same time as this antibiotic.

A woman being treated for *Chlamydia* infection might not know it was not clearing up. Her doctor might not realize it, either. Weeks and months could go by before he discovered the problem, and by then serious complications that can lead to infertility might be in progress.

An even more dangerous situation could occur if a person had Rocky Mountain spotted fever. This disease can kill if it is not treated quickly and appropriately, preferably with tetracycline. Inactivating the antibiotic by taking a vitamin and mineral supplement with it could lead to tragedy, although we don't know of any actual fatalities due to this potential oversight.

Another class of antibiotics also interacts poorly with mineral supplements. The quinolones, including **Cipro**, **Floxin**, **Maxaquin**, **Noroxin**, and **Penetrex**, are not absorbed efficiently if the minerals calcium, zinc, or iron are taken at the same time. Certain vitamin and mineral formulations now feature zinc because of its reputation for speeding healing and protecting against macular degeneration (an eye disorder). A number of antacids also contain minerals and should be avoided when a person is taking one of these strong new antibiotics. See page 103 for a more complete discussion.

B Vitamin Supplements and Anticonvulsants

As we mentioned, the epilepsy medicine **Dilantin** (phenytoin) can lower folic acid and vitamin B_6 levels in the body. If it were severe enough, this interaction could lead to blood abnormalities; it is possible that it might contribute to high homocysteine levels as well. Correcting the vitamin deficit requires medical supervision, however, because high levels of either folic acid or vitamin B_6 might interfere with the efficacy of the medication and result in seizures. This is why communicating with the doctor is so crucial. Although he may be well aware that 80 mg of vitamin B_6 can halve the effectiveness of the anticonvulsant, he may not know that the patient is taking this vitamin on her own to treat premenstrual symptoms. Supplementation with folic acid or vitamin B_6 can also diminish the effectiveness of barbiturates, especially phenobarbital. Since the risk of a seizure is so serious, no one on these anticonvulsants should take supplements containing the B vitamins for any reason unless the doctor is supervising.

Vitamins E and K and Coumadin

Vitamins also interact in a dangerous manner with the anticoagulant **Coumadin** (warfarin). Vitamin E has been praised for its antioxidant properties and is getting attention for its possible role in preventing heart disease. Investigators have documented that vitamin E supplements seem to lower the risk of heart disease by about one third and boost the cardioprotective action of beta carotene.[5] Vitamin E, like aspirin, also helps blood flow freely by promoting factors that prevent clots. Vitamin E could create havoc when taken with **Coumadin**, because this vitamin apparently adds to the effect of the blood thinner. Clearly, if you take an anticoagulant, don't undertake self-treatment with vitamin E. Your doctor should be monitoring any such supplementation very closely.

Vitamin K has the opposite effect on **Coumadin**, but fortunately it is not widely available as a supplement. If you are on this anticoagulant, though, keep in mind that excessive amounts of foods rich in vitamin K (mostly vegetables, but also some other foods such as liver) can block the activity of **Coumadin** and allow clots to form. Rather than avoid these healthy foods altogether, it makes most sense to try to keep your intake fairly constant from one day and one week to the next. If you plan to alter your diet, ask your doctor to monitor your prothrombin time a little more closely. See pages 51 and 196 for summaries of these **Coumadin** interactions.

Foods Rich in Vitamin K (more than 50 mcg/100 g)

Bran	Liver
Broccoli	Mung Beans
Cabbage	Oats
Cauliflower	Seaweed
Chick-peas	Soybean Oil
Corn Oil	Soybeans
Eggs	Spinach
Lentils	Turnip Greens
Lettuce	Watercress

Source: Adapted from Pennington, Jean A. T., ed. *Bowes & Church's Food Values of Portions Commonly Used,* 15th ed. New York: Harper & Row, 1989.

Another nutritional supplement that interacts with **Coumadin** (warfarin) is something called coenzyme Q_{10} (ubiquinone). This is a natural substance found in the body. It has become a very hot item in health food stores and mail-order vitamin catalogs. Research suggests that this antioxidant may be beneficial in helping to treat congestive heart failure, cardiovascular conditions, gum disease, and a number of other disorders. How effective it is remains to be determined, but judging from sales figures, this is a very successful product taken by lots of folks.

Researchers in Sweden have observed that when patients on a stable regimen of **Coumadin** to prevent blood clots started taking coenzyme Q_{10}, their bleeding time changed significantly. Their blood became more prone to clotting, and the **Coumadin** appeared less effective.[6] This interaction could be extremely dangerous, because a person might have a life-threatening clot as a consequence. Anyone taking coenzyme Q_{10} together with **Coumadin** should consult a physician before stopping the supplement. Sudden discontinuation of coenzyme Q_{10} might trigger an unexpected alteration in clotting time.

Potentially Dangerous Nutrient/Nutrient Interactions

Potassium and Vitamin B$_{12}$

Relatively few doctors or patients are aware that prescription potassium supplements such as **K-Dur**, **K-Tab**, **Micro-K,** and **Slow-K** can interfere with the absorption of vitamin B$_{12}$. This vitamin is stored in the body and does not become depleted quickly, so a short course of potassium therapy poses little cause for concern. But long-term use—by people taking diuretic blood pressure pills who are simultaneously prescribed potassium supplements, for example—could eventually result in depletion of body stores of this crucial vitamin. Ask your doctor to evaluate your situation, as injections are usually the most effective means of supplementing vitamin B$_{12}$.

Beta Carotene, Vitamin E, and Alcohol

Little red capsules of beta carotene are probably among the hottest items on the vitamin shelf these days. Some researchers hypothesize that this precursor to vitamin A may help protect the body against a number of different cancers, and that it may help reduce the risk of heart attack. As a result, there may be millions of people taking it in the hope of warding off heart disease or cancer.

This probably makes good sense. Beta carotene is an excellent antioxidant, and the toxicity of this vitamin building block is very low. It is, for example, far safer than preformed vitamin A, which is stored in the body and can build up to dangerous levels. Beta carotene has one important and little-known interaction, however. Long-term supplementation (15 mg daily up to 60 mg) lowers blood levels of vitamin E significantly. These two antioxidants seem to work together, for beta carotene protects from heart attack most strongly when people also have high vitamin E levels.[7] Therefore, it would be prudent, if you plan to take beta carotene as a preventive measure, to take vitamin E as well. This should keep your levels of both antioxidants in the normal range or above.

Beta carotene is also reported to interact negatively with alcohol. The combination may increase liver damage well over that found with alcohol alone. The research was done in baboons who were given a substantial dose of alcohol as a proportion of their daily calories over an extended period of time.[8] As a consequence, we don't have good information on how much alcohol might trigger this response in humans. It is chilling, however, to think of someone maintaining a moderate drinking habit (between one and three drinks a day) because of research showing this may reduce the risk of heart disease, and adding a beta carotene supplement for the same reason. Liver disease is devastating, so if you drink regularly, it might be prudent not to make beta carotene a habit.

Drug/Nutrient Interactions

The table of Drug/Nutrient Interactions on the following pages summarizes information on how drugs affect nutrient status and which nutritional supplements may interfere with optimal drug benefits. This field is still evolving and we expect more information to become available over the next several years. (The table does not include discussion of most cancer drugs, however, as these are administered primarily in the hospital under close supervision. Many of them have significant effects on nutritional status, but in some cases that contributes to their effectiveness.) Please remember to keep your physician informed of your concerns and of any supplements you plan to take in conjunction with prescribed medications.

Drug/Nutrient Interactions

DRUG	INTERACTION	NUTRIENT
Acne Medicine **Accutane**	Because **Accutane** is related to vitamin A, taking these two compounds together could increase toxicity. Avoid this combination.	**Vitamin A**
Alcohol	Research in baboons indicates that beta carotene can increase the liver damage caused by chronic alcohol intake. Alcohol has numerous effects on the body. Some of these, such as changes in liver and intestinal function, may impact several nutrients. One consequence of long-term alcohol abuse is brain damage—Wernicke-Korsakoff syndrome. Lack of the B vitamin thiamine plays an important role in the development of this problem. Absorption or utilization of vitamins B_6, B_{12}, and C is affected by regular alcohol intake. In addition, drinkers may absorb too much iron and too little zinc, putting additional stress on the system. These nutritional problems occur when a person drinks alcohol too much or too often.	**Beta Carotene** **Folic Acid** **Thiamine** **Vitamin B_6** **Vitamin B_{12}** **Vitamin C** **Iron** **Zinc**
Aluminum-Based Antacids **Di-Gel** **Gelusil** **Maalox** **Mylanta** **Riopan,** and others	The aluminum and magnesium in antacids can form a complex with phosphate and deplete the body of calcium. Weakened bones may result. Anyone at risk of osteoporosis should be cautious about this interaction. Aluminum-based antacids may inactivate thiamine. Don't take them at mealtime.	**Calcium** **Phosphate** **Thiamine**
Antibiotics **Bactrim** **Mandol** **Moxam** Neomycin **Septra** and others	Broad-spectrum antibiotics can mess up the good intestinal bacteria that make vitamin K. In some people this could lead to unusual bleeding. Check with your physician and pharmacist to see whether vitamin K supplementation is a good idea.	**Vitamin K**

DRUG	INTERACTION	NUTRIENT
Quinolones **Cipro** **Floxin** **Maxaquin** **Noroxin** **Penetrex**	These high-powered antibiotics may not work as well as expected if they are taken at the same time as certain minerals. This includes antacids as well as nutritional supplements. Check with your doctor and pharmacist, because this interaction could be serious.	**Calcium** **Iron** **Zinc**
Tetracyclines **Achromycin** **Aureomycin** **Minocin** **Panmycin** **Terramycin** and others	Calcium and other minerals can combine with tetracyclines so that the antibiotics are not absorbed into the body. Make sure you don't take any mineral supplements or mineral-containing antacids within two hours of a tetracycline pill. Long-term use of tetracycline may deplete these nutrients and require supplementation. Expert Daphne Roe, M.D., suggests 5 mg of riboflavin, 100 to 200 mg vitamin C, and 800 to 1,500 mg calcium daily, to be taken at least two hours before or after the tetracycline.	**Calcium** **Iron** **Magnesium** **Riboflavin** **Vitamin C** **Zinc**
Arthritis *Medicines* Aspirin **Anacin** **Ascriptin** **Bayer** **Bufferin** **Excedrin** and others	Studies suggest aspirin may block vitamin C from getting into cells. Questions remain about the importance of this interaction. Until more is known, it seems logical to increase daily consumption of vitamin-C–containing foods or consider a supplement (50 to 100 mg) while taking aspirin regularly. It is not clear whether extra vitamin C will correct this imbalance. Folic acid levels are lower when people rely on large doses of aspirin. Regular users may need a folic acid supplement. Check with your physician for the right amount. Dr. Roe suggests 0.4 to 1.0 mg. Small amounts of blood are regularly lost from the stomach when aspirin is taken. This can add up over time and deplete the body of iron. This actually may be beneficial for people at risk of heart disease since some research suggests that excess iron increases the risk of heart attack. If anemia results, however, iron supplementation (20 to 50 mg) may be necessary. A blood test is needed for this diagnosis.	**Vitamin C** **Folic Acid** **Iron**

DRUG	INTERACTION	NUTRIENT
Indomethacin **Indocin**	Indomethacin irritates the stomach lining even more than aspirin. Over time, continued low-level blood loss could lead to iron deficiency. If anemia occurs, a supplement of 20 to 50 mg of iron daily may be needed.	**Iron**
Methotrexate **Folex** **Methotrate** **Mexate** **Rheumatrex**	Methotrexate affects the intestinal wall so that these nutrients are not absorbed efficiently. Nutritional imbalances may result. Since methotrexate is being used more aggressively against arthritis, psoriasis, and cancer, it is essential that patients discuss this issue with their physicians.	**Folic Acid** **Vitamin B_{12}** **Beta Carotene**
Penicillamine **Cuprimine** **Depen**	Penicillamine may not be as well absorbed if it is taken at the same time as iron or magnesium. Supplements often contain these minerals, so it may make sense to wait several hours before you take your multivitamin preparation. This medicine may also deplete the body of copper or zinc, causing a loss of the sense of taste. Ask about supplements, including 24- to 100-mg tablets of vitamin B_6.	**Iron** **Magnesium** **Copper** **Zinc** **Vitamin B_6**
Beta Carotene	As people learn more about the potential benefits of antioxidant vitamins, many are taking beta carotene at levels much higher than those normally found in the vegetables in their diets. Regular doses of beta carotene (from 15 to 60 mg daily) can lead, over a period of months, to lowered levels of vitamin E in the blood. Because vitamin E is itself an important antioxidant, it might be wise to add a supplement of 100 to 400 IU if you are taking beta carotene.	**Vitamin E**
Birth Control Pills **Demulen** **Norlestrin** **Ortho-Novum** **Ovcon** **Ovral** **Tri-Norinyl** and others	Women using combination oral contraceptives may need more of these vitamins. Both folic acid and B_6 levels may be low, and too little vitamin B_6 could be responsible for depression. Ask your doctor about a supplement.　　Vitamin C (1 gram or more) may increase blood levels of estrogen. Side effects may become more noticeable. This interaction is controversial and may not be significant.	**Vitamin B_6** **Folic Acid** **Vitamin E** **Vitamin C**

DRUG	INTERACTION	NUTRIENT
Blood Pressure Medicines ACE Inhibitors **Accupril** **Altace** **Capoten** **Lotensin** **Monopril** **Prinivil** **Vasotec** **Zestril**	These popular blood pressure medications tend to maximize potassium levels. This is fine unless a person is getting extra potassium through a potassium supplement or a potassium-based salt substitute. Too much of this important mineral is just as bad as not enough. If you are taking one of these medicines, you should probably avoid extra potassium unless your doctor is supervising closely. Your physician should periodically test your blood levels of potassium.	**Potassium**
Hydralazine-containing **Apresazide** **Apresoline** Hydralazine **Ser-Ap-Es** and others	This medicine can deplete the body of vitamin B_6 through its effect on an essential enzyme. Reduced vitamin B_6 may result in depression or nerve damage (leading to numbness or tingling of hands or feet). Supplementation may be advisable. Dr. Daphne Roe suggests 25 to 100 mg daily.	**Vitamin B_6**
Loop Diuretics **Bumex** **Edecrin** **Lasix**	These strong diuretics (water pills) may cause the loss of important minerals from the body. Periodic blood tests are essential to see whether supplements are needed.	**Calcium** **Magnesium** **Potassium**
Thiazide Diuretics **Aldoril** **Diuril** Hydrochlorothiazide **HydroDIURIL** **Ser-Ap-Es** and others	These diuretics promote urination. Minerals are often lost in the process. This could actually prove counterproductive, since both potassium and magnesium appear to help regulate blood pressure. Periodic blood checks to keep track of mineral levels are a good idea.	**Magnesium** **Potassium** **Zinc**
Triamterene-containing **Dyazide** **Dyrenium** **Maxzide**	Folic acid deficiency could become a problem unless a supplement (0.4 to 1.0 mg) is taken. These drugs conserve potassium. Taking a potassium supplement at the same time could result in an overload of this mineral.	**Folic Acid** **Potassium**
Blood Thinners **Coumadin** **Panwarfin** Warfarin	Very large amounts (5 grams or more) of vitamin C could interfere with the effectiveness of this medicine. This interaction is uncertain.	**Vitamin C**

DRUG	INTERACTION	NUTRIENT
Blood Thinners *(italic)* **Coumadin** **Panwarfin** Warfarin	Vitamin E itself acts as an anticoagulant, and the combination may thin the blood too much and lead to bruises or excessive bleeding. Less than 400 IU daily does not appear to be a problem. Vitamin K counteracts these medications and makes them less effective. Don't go overboard on foods high in this vitamin (see list on page 83). For any of these interactions, your doctor can check bleeding time with a test.	**Vitamin E** **Vitamin K**
Cholesterol Medicines **Cholybar** **Colestid** **Questran**	"Bile acid sequestrants" such as **Questran** can interfere with the absorption of fats and fat-soluble vitamins. Some animal studies suggest that vitamin E and even iron absorption may also be adversely affected. Because of their impact on vitamin K, these drugs could cause complications in combination with blood thinners. Blood tests are advised. Supplements of 2,000 to 5,000 IU vitamin A, 200 to 800 IU vitamin D, and 0.4 to 1.0 mg folic acid should be taken at a different time from the cholesterol medicine.	*Fat-Soluble Vitamins* **Vitamin A** **Vitamin D** **Vitamin E** **Vitamin K** *Water-Soluble Vitamins* **Vitamin B$_{12}$** **Folic Acid**
Colchicine **ColBenemid**	Absorption of these nutrients may be impaired. Check with your physician about supplementation.	**Vitamin B$_{12}$** **Beta Carotene** **Magnesium** **Potassium**
Corticosteroids **Aristocort** **Cortef** **Decadron** **Delta-Cortef** **Deltasone** **Kenacort** **Medrol** Prednisone and others	Cortisonelike drugs can deplete the body of vitamin D$_3$ and interfere with calcium absorption and metabolism. Long-term use may result in bone loss. Such medications may also lead to depletion of potassium and vitamins B$_6$, B$_{12}$, or folic acid. Check with your doctor about a supplement.	**Calcium** **Vitamin D$_3$** **Potassium** **Vitamin B$_6$** **Vitamin B$_{12}$** **Folic Acid**
Epilepsy Drugs Barbiturates Phenobarbital	Either folic acid or vitamin B$_6$ supplements can reduce blood levels of this anticonvulsant, potentially leading to seizures. If supplementation is needed, it should be carefully monitored.	**Folic Acid** **Vitamin B$_6$**

DRUG	INTERACTION	NUTRIENT
Epilepsy Drugs Barbiturates Phenobarbital	Barbiturates such as phenobarbital interfere with the normal metabolism of vitamin D, and as a consequence calcium may be lost from bones. Rickets or osteomalacia are a hazard. Check with your doctor about vitamin D supplements.	**Vitamin D** **Calcium**
Dilantin	Patients on Dilantin (phenytoin) may become deficient in folic acid or vitamin B_6. Supplementation is very tricky, however, and must be directed by a knowledgeable physician. Too much folic acid (more than 2 mg/day) or vitamin B_6 can interfere with effectiveness so that the drug would fail to prevent seizures. At doses of 80 mg daily of vitamin B_6, Dilantin is only 50 percent as effective as it is without the vitamin B_6. Periodic blood tests for anemia are needed.	**Folic Acid** **Vitamin B_6**
	Dilantin interferes with vitamin D, and thus with calcium. The consequence could be rickets in children or osteomalacia (weak bones) in adults. A supplement of 400 to 800 IU of vitamin D daily is appropriate.	**Vitamin D** **Calcium**
	Blood levels of vitamin K may be reduced. A supplement of 1 to 5 mg daily may be advisable. Ask your doctor.	**Vitamin K**
Mysoline	Levels of vitamin K may be lower. The doctor might prescribe a supplement of 1 to 5 mg daily to overcome this.	**Vitamin K**
	Like other barbiturates, Mysoline (primidone) alters the metabolism of vitamin D and can lead to the loss of calcium from bones. A vitamin D supplement (400 to 800 IU daily) may be necessary.	**Calcium** **Vitamin D**
Etidronate **Didronel**	Minerals such as calcium, magnesium, and iron react with this medicine to prevent its absorption if they are taken within 2 hours of taking the drug. However, the drug changes vitamin D metabolism, so adequate calcium and vitamin D intake must be maintained.	**Calcium** **Iron** **Magnesium** **Vitamin D**

DRUG	INTERACTION	NUTRIENT
Hormone Replacement Therapy **Estrace** **Estratab** **Menest** **Premarin** and others	Women using estrogen replacement therapy may need more of these vitamins. Both folic acid and B_6 levels may be low, and too little vitamin B_6 could be responsible for depression. Ask your doctor about a supplement such as 1.5 to 5 mg vitamin B_6 and 0.4 to 1.0 mg folic acid.	**Vitamin B_6** **Folic Acid** **Vitamin E**
Iron **Femiron** **Feosol** **Fer-in-Sol** **Mol-Iron** and others	Taking a calcium supplement at the same meal with an iron supplement or a multivitamin containing iron can reduce the amount of iron absorbed. To minimize interference, take these pills at different times.	**Calcium**
Laxatives Mineral Oil **Agoral** **Mikinol** **Neo-Cultol** and others	Regular use of a mineral oil laxative interferes with proper absorption of the fat-soluble vitamins. A lack of vitamin D can affect calcium and phosphate balance, and bone loss may occur.	***Fat-Soluble Vitamins*** **Vitamin A** **Vitamin D** **Vitamin E** **Vitamin K**
Phenolphthalein **Ex-Lax** **Feen-a-mint** **Modane** **Tablets** and others	Regular use of these laxatives may interfere with vitamin D and calcium metabolism, eventually weakening bones.	**Calcium** **Vitamin D**
Levodopa **Dopar** **Larodopa**	Vitamin B_6 can reduce the effectiveness of this anti-Parkinson's disease drug. Supplementation should be avoided.	**Vitamin B_6**
Major Tranquilizers Chlorpromazine **Thorazine** Fluphenazine **Permitil** **Prolixin** and others	The B vitamins riboflavin and B_{12} (cyanocobalamin) may become depleted. A supplement may be required to prevent deficiency. A high dose of vitamin C reduced the serum level of Prolixin in one case, however, so caution is suggested. Dr. Daphne Roe suggests 2 to 5 mg of riboflavin daily.	**Riboflavin** **Vitamin B_{12}** **Vitamin C**

DRUG	INTERACTION	NUTRIENT
Potassium **Kaon-Cl** **Klotrix** **K-Tab** **Micro-K** **Slow-K** and others	Potassium supplements can interfere with the absorption of vitamin B_{12}. Because these medications are often taken for many weeks or months, a deficiency of this crucial vitamin could develop. Research has shown that some older people show cognitive or neurological effects of inadequate vitamin B_{12} even before their blood tests show a deficiency.	**Vitamin B_{12}**
Sleeping Pills **Doriden**	Long-term use of this sleeping pill can interfere with vitamin D metabolism, which in turn affects calcium balance. The result could be osteomalacia, or weakened bones. A vitamin D supplement might be appropriate.	**Vitamin D** **Calcium**
Sulfasalazine **Azulfidine**	This medicine for inflammatory bowel disease interferes with the proper absorption of folic acid. Talk to your doctor about a supplement in the range of 0.4 to 1 mg daily.	**Folic Acid**
Thyroid Hormone Levothyroxine **Levo-T** **Levothroid** **Levoxine** **Synthroid**	Iron supplements taken at the same time as thyroid replacement hormone can reduce the hormone's effectiveness, as judged by blood tests and clinical symptoms. Take these pills at different times.	**Iron**
Tuberculosis Drugs Isoniazid **INH** **Laniazid** **Nydrazid** **Rifamate**	Deficiencies of niacin and vitamin B_6 are possible, and may require supplementation. Do *not* take supplements without supervision, as too much vitamin B_6 might diminish the effectiveness of the drug. (Recommended daily doses range from 6 to 50 mg of B_6, and from 15 to 25 mg of niacin.) Drug-induced changes in vitamin D metabolism may also affect calcium and phosphate balance. Check with your doctor about a vitamin D supplement of 400 or 800 IU daily.	**Niacin** **Vitamin B_6** **Vitamin D** **Calcium** **Phosphate**
Para-aminosalicylate **P.A.S.**	A vitamin B_{12} deficiency is possible. Folic acid may also become depleted. Ask your doctor if supplements are advisable.	**Vitamin B_{12}** **Folic Acid**

DRUG	INTERACTION	NUTRIENT
Ulcer Medicines **Prilosec** **Tagamet** **Zantac**	These acid-suppressing drugs, and possibly others including Axid and Pepcid, can reduce the absorption of vitamin B_{12} that is chemically bound to protein. The effect may depend upon dose and seems to disappear after the drug is discontinued. Ask your doctor about supplementation.	**Vitamin B_{12}**
Tagamet **Zantac**	A controversial theory suggests that reducing acid as effectively as these medications do could allow bacteria to survive in the stomach. These "bugs" may produce carcinogenic chemicals called nitrosamines, which might increase the risk of stomach cancer. We suggest vitamin insurance: the antioxidants vitamin C (500 mg 3 or 4 times daily) and vitamin E (400 IU daily) may help protect the stomach.	**Vitamin C** **Vitamin E**
Urinary *Anti-Infectives* **Furadantin** **Furalan** **Macrodantin** and others	Nitrofurantoin medications for urinary tract infections interfere with folic acid metabolism. Folic acid deficiencies are unusual, perhaps because the drugs are usually prescribed for less than two weeks. If you need the drug long-term, ask your doctor about supplementation.	**Folic Acid**

References

1. Marcuard, S. P., et al. "Omeprazole Therapy Causes Malabsorption of Cyanocobalamin (vitamin B$_{12}$)." *Ann. Intern. Med.* 1994; 120:211–215.

2. Selhub, Jacob, Paul F. Jacques, et al. "Vitamin Status and Intake as Primary Determinants of Homocysteinemia in an Elderly Population." *JAMA* 1993; 270:2693–2698.

3. Selhub, Jacob, et al. "Association Between Plasma Homocysteine Concentrations and Extracranial Carotid-Artery Stenosis." *N. Engl. J. Med.* 1995; 332:286–291.

4. Stampfer, Meir J., and Walter C. Willett. "Homocysteine and Marginal Vitamin Deficiency: The Importance of Adequate Vitamin Intake." (Editorial) *JAMA* 1993; 270:2726–2727.

5. Kardinaal, A. F. M., F. J. Kok, et al. "Antioxidants in adipose tissue and risk of myocardial infarction: The EURAMIC study." *Lancet* 1993; 342:1379–1384.

6. Spigset, Olav. "Reduced Effect of Warfarin Caused by Ubidecarenone." (Letter) *Lancet* 1994; 344:1372–1373.

7. Kardinaal, op.cit. p. 1382.

8. Leo, M. A., et al. "Interaction of Ethanol with b-Carotene: Delayed Blood Clearance and Enhanced Hepatotoxicity." *Hepatology* 1992; 15:883–891.

References for the Drug/Nutrient Interactions Chart

Campbell, Norman R.C., et al. "Ferrous Sulfate Reduces Thyroxine Efficacy in Patients with Hypothyroidism." *Ann. Intern. Med.* 1992; 117:1010–1013.

Cook, J.D., S.A. Dassenko, and P. Whittaker. "Calcium Supplementation: Effect on Iron Absorption." *Am. J. Clin. Nutr.* 1991 (Jan.); 53:106–111.

Garrison, Robert H., Jr., and Elizabeth Somer. *The Nutrition Desk Reference*, 2nd ed. New Canaan, Conn.: Keats Publishing, 1990, pp. 273–283.

Hansten, Philip D., and John R. Horn, eds. *Drug Interactions & Updates*. Vancouver, Wash.: Applied Therapeutics, 1990.

Olin, Bernie R., ed. *Drug Facts and Comparisons*. St. Louis: Facts & Comparisons, 1991.

Roe, Daphne A. "Diet, Nutrition and Drug Reactions," in *Modern Nutrition in Health and Disease*, 7th ed. Shils, Maurice E., and Vernon R. Young, eds. Philadelphia: Lea & Febiger, 1988, pp. 630–645.

Tatro, David S., ed. *Drug Interaction Facts*. St. Louis: Facts & Comparisons, 1992.

Chapter Six

Prescription Drug/ Over-the-Counter Drug Interactions

Most people perceive nonprescription remedies as wimpy drugs. After all, if the Food and Drug Administration allows everyone access to such products in pharmacies, supermarkets, and convenience stores, surely they must be safe. We hate to burst another bubble, but nothing could be further from the truth.

Over-the-counter (OTC) medications, like all drugs, can cause side effects. Sometimes the complications are merely a minor annoyance, such as drowsiness from an antihistamine. Other times an adverse reaction could land you in the emergency room, as in the case of the man who swallowed a decongestant cold remedy and subsequently couldn't urinate. The label (which he read carefully) did not warn him that if he had an enlarged prostate gland he should avoid this medicine. When his bladder felt like it would burst, he rushed to the hospital (and broke an arm in the process when, in his haste, he slipped on some ice). A catheter had to be inserted to provide him some relief.

The medication this gentleman used was **Sudafed** (pseudoephedrine), an oral decongestant that works by constricting blood vessels. Once upon a time it was available only by prescription. Physicians presumably warned people about complications and interactions to prevent this kind of adverse event from occurring.

When we notified **Sudafed's** manufacturer that its label was inadequate for OTC use, and unreadable at that, there was some initial defensiveness. Fortunately, changes were eventually made and the **Sudafed** label now reads: "Do not take this preparation if you have high blood pressure, heart disease, diabetes, thyroid disease, or difficulty in urination due to enlargement of the prostate gland, except under the advice and supervision of a physician."

Lethal Prescription Drug/OTC Drug Interactions

Unfortunately, many people don't take time to read the cautions and warnings on OTC medications. First, they assume there is no possibility for problems, and second, the print is usually so small you need a magnifying glass to read it, and even when you *can* read it, the precautions are often totally inadequate or nonsensical. Read a little farther on the **Sudafed** box and you will find the words "Drug Interaction Precaution: Do not use this product if you are now taking a prescription monoamine oxidase inhibitor (MAOI) (certain drugs for depression, psychiatric or emotional conditions, or Parkinson's disease)."

Most people wouldn't know if they were taking a pill containing a monoamine oxidase inhibitor. Medical mumbo jumbo may be okay in the *Physicians' Desk Reference*, or *PDR*, but it doesn't belong on OTC labels. In the case of **Sudafed** (and lots of other cold and cough remedies) the monoamine oxidase (MAO) inhibitor warning is serious indeed. If someone were to take pseudoephedrine, ephedrine, phenylephrine, or phenylpropanolamine (PPA) while they were on an antidepressant such as **Nardil** or **Parnate**, blood pressure could soar. Such a hypertensive crisis could lead to a stroke. One person taking **Nardil** experienced a terrible headache, heart palpitations, and an extremely dangerous elevation in blood pressure to 240/120 (normal is 120/80) after downing only 2 teaspoons of an OTC product containing the decongestant phenylephrine.[1] Phenylpropanolamine (a decongestant and appetite suppressant) has also been linked to lethal hypertensive crisis.

Even something as seemingly simple as a cough remedy may produce an extremely hazardous reaction with MAO inhibitor drugs. The combination could bring on symptoms such as nausea, fever, agitation, dizziness, changes in blood pressure, seizures, and coma. A death has been linked with the combination of **Nardil** and two ounces of a dextromethorphan-containing cough remedy.[2] The box below lists the OTC drugs that don't mix with MAO inhibitors.

OTC Drugs That Don't Mix with MAO Inhibitors

(The following is a partial list of OTC drugs containing dextromethorphan, ephedrine, phenylephrine, PPA, or pseudoephedrine.)

Acutrim Late Day Strength
  Appetite Suppressant
Acutrim II Maximum Strength
  Appetite Suppressant
Acutrim 16 Hour Steady Control
  Appetite Suppressant
Actifed Plus
Actifed Sinus Daytime/Nighttime
Actifed Syrup
Advil Cold and Sinus
Afrin Tablets
Alka-Seltzer Plus Cold Medicine
Alka-Seltzer Plus Cough & Cold
  Medicine
Alka-Seltzer Plus Night-Time Cold
  Medicine
Alka-Seltzer Plus Sinus Allergy
  Medicine
Allerest Headache Strength
Allerest Maximum Strength
Allerest No Drowsiness
Allerest Sinus Pain Formula
Allerest 12 Hour
A.R.M. Allergy Relief Medicine
Bayer Select Sinus Pain Relief Formula
BC Cold Powder Multi-Symptom Formula
BC Cold Powder Non-Drowsy Formula
Benadryl Allergy Sinus Headache Formula
Benadryl Cold Nighttime Formula

Benadryl Cold Tablets
Benadryl Decongestant
Benylin Decongestant
Benylin Expectorant
Bronkaid Tablets
Bronkotabs
Cheracol-D Cough Formula
Cheracol Plus Head Cold/Cough Formula
Chlor-Trimeton Allergy Decongestant
Chlor-Trimeton Allergy-Sinus Headache
Comtrex Multi-Symptom Cold Reliever
Contac Continuous Action Decongestant/
  Antihistamine
Contac Day & Night Cold & Flu
Contac Maximum Strength Continuous
  Action Decongestant/Antihistamine
Contac Severe Cold and Flu Formula
Coricidin 'D' Decongestant
Cough Formula Comtrex
Delsym Cough Formula
Dexatrim Maximum Strength Caffeine-Free
Dexatrim Maximum Strength Extended
  Duration Time
Dexatrim Maximum Strength Plus Vitamin C/
  Caffeine-free
Dimetapp Cold & Allergy
Dimetapp Cold & Flu
Dimetapp DM Ellixir
Dimetapp Elixir

cont'd

OTC Drugs That Don't Mix with MAO Inhibitors (cont'd)

Dimetapp Extentabs
Dimetapp Liquid-Gels
Dimetapp Sinus
Dristan Cold
Dristan Cold, Maximum Strength Multi-
  Symptom Formula
Dristan Juice Mix-In
Dristan Sinus
Drixoral Cold and Allergy
Drixoral Sinus
4-Way Cold Tablets
Hold DM Cough Suppressant Lozenge
Maximum Strength Dristan Cold Multi-
  Symptom Formula
Maximum Strength Dristan Cold No
  Drowsiness Formula
Medi-Flu
Primatene Tablets
Robitussin Cough Calmers
Robitussin Maximum Strength
  Cough & Cold
Robitussin Maximum Strength Cough
  Suppressant
Robitussin-CF
Robitussin-DM
Robitussin-PE
Sinarest
Sine-Off Maximum Strength

Sine-Off Sinus Medicine Tablets
Sinus Excedrin Analgesic, Decongestant
Sinutab Sinus Allergy
Sudafed Plus
Sudafed Severe Cold Formula
Sudafed Sinus
Tavist-D
TheraFlu Flu and Cold Medicine
Triaminic Allergy Medicine
Triaminic Cold Medicine
Triaminic Cold, Allergy, Sinus Medicine
Triaminic Multi-Symptom Cold and Cough
  Medicine
Triaminic-12 Maximum Strength 12 Hour
  Relief
Tylenol Allergy Sinus Medication Maximum
  Strength
Tylenol Cold & Flu Hot Medication
Tylenol Cold Medication, Effervescent
Vicks DayQuil
Vicks Formula 44D Cough & Decongestant
  Medicine
Vicks Formula 44E Cough & Expectorant
  Medicine
Vicks Formula 44M Multi-Symptom Cough &
  Cold Medicine
Vicks NyQuil Nighttime Cold/Flu Medicine

Laxatives, Diuretics, and Digoxin

People love laxatives. Goodness only knows why we are so obsessed with bowel function and regularity. Perhaps it's because commercials on television reinforce the notion that we need to make a daily bathroom pit stop to be healthy. Or it may stem from old folk beliefs that one has to rid the body of toxic by-products. A hundred years ago we didn't have very many effective medicines. Most remedies relied on placebo power. But doctors could prescribe a purgative or cathartic and produce a pretty impressive outhouse experience. Patients knew something important was going on and that might have inspired them to believe they were getting better.

Whatever the reason, we are fixated on our bowels. We spend millions of dollars on products such as **Black Draught, Dialose Plus, Doxidan, Dulcolax, Evac-Q-Kwik, Ex-Lax Maximum Relief Formula, Feen-a-mint, Fleet Laxative Tablets, Modane Plus, Nature's Remedy**, and **Senolax**. The occasional use of such stimulant laxatives probably doesn't cause any trouble, though high-fiber foods (such as bran), liquid, and exercise are generally a safer and better solution to constipation.

The real problem occurs when people develop a laxative habit. Regular use of strong laxatives can lead to diarrhea, fluid loss, and serious changes in electrolytes (minerals such as potassium and sodium). A reader of our syndicated newspaper column shared the following story:

> My husband is 73 years old. For the past three or four years he has had problems with his bowels. Either he's constipated or he's taking epsom salts or Ex-Lax. Then he seems to have diarrhea due to his medicating himself. His bowels are so bad he can't control them. There are splatters and messes in his clothes, and the bathroom is one big mess! When we travel I've had to rinse his clothes and head for a laundromat. Then he takes Kaopectate or Pepto-Bismol for the diarrhea, but it doesn't seem to work well. I wish he would go to a doctor but he's embarrassed.

A surprising number of people develop a dependency on laxatives. And we're not just talking about older folks. Young women who are concerned about their weight may get trapped into this kind of regimen. They may also take diuretics to rid themselves of fluid so they can lose a few extra pounds.

Laxative abusers are often afraid to talk to a physician for fear of criticism. But such practices lead to a vicious cycle and can create dangerously low levels of potassium. This can be especially hazardous for people taking certain prescription medications. Diuretics such as **Bumex**, **HydroDIURIL**, **Lasix**, and **Lozol** also deplete potassium from the body. This combination (laxatives and diuretics) could lead to a serious imbalance that could be life threatening, especially if a person were also taking a digitalis-type heart medicine such as **Lanoxin** (see page 321). Irregular heart rhythms or cardiac arrest are real dangers. Bottom line: Avoid regular use of stimulant laxatives if at all possible. And monitor your potassium levels if you also take diuretics (normal values are 3.5 to 5.0 mEq/L).

Laxatives may also alter the absorption and effectiveness of other medications. There is, unfortunately, very little research on this kind of interaction. High-powered investigators probably don't get a whole lot of respect from their colleagues by focusing on laxative complications. But the issues are important because so many people are affected. Some years ago questions were raised about laxatives and oral contraceptives, the fear being that cathartics or harsh laxatives might cause diarrhea, reduce absorption, diminish effectiveness, and increase the risk of an unplanned pregnancy. We have been unable to confirm this rumor, however, and so this is one possible interaction that remains mysterious.

One study has shown that the laxative lactulose (**Cephulac**, **Cholac**, **Chronulac**, **Constilac**, **Constulose**, **Duphalac**, and **Enulose**) could interfere with blood pressure drugs such as **Tenormin** (atenolol) and **HydroDIURIL** (hydrochlorothiazide).[3] Other research has shown that the popular laxative bisacodyl (**Carter's Laxative**, **Dulcogen**, **Dulcolax**, **Fleet Laxative**, etc.) can reduce absorption of the heart medicine **Lanoxin** (digoxin).[4] By the way, bisacodyl should not be swallowed with milk or dairy products. Such food could cause the drug to dissolve in the stomach instead of the small intestine, resulting in a very bad bellyache.

Antacids, Pepto-Bismol, and Broad-Spectrum Antibiotics

People are hard on their stomachs. We vacillate between being dietarily correct—bran, beans, and broccoli—and devilishly decadent—coffee, cookies, and chocolate. No wonder we swallow tons of antacids.

Many people don't think of these products as drugs. One friend won't go anywhere without his roll of **Rolaids**. He pops them down almost out of habit—as if they were candy. And now that calcium is the hottest nutritional supplement, millions of people are relying on antacids such as **Tums** to supply cheap calcium. Some women swallow these OTC remedies religiously and think of them as the nutritional equivalent of a glass of milk or a container of yogurt.

The trouble is that antacids interact with a variety of medications. Broad-spectrum antibiotics called quinolones have become very popular in recent years. They include compounds such as **Cipro** (ciprofloxacin), **Floxin** (ofloxacin), **Maxaquin** (lomefloxacin), **Noroxin** (norfloxacin), and **Penetrex** (enoxacin). These drugs are prescribed for a variety of infections including pneumonia, bronchitis, sinusitis, prostatitis, cervicitis, otitis media, urethritis, pelvic inflammatory disease, and more.

Antacids that contain aluminum, calcium, or magnesium can dramatically interfere with the absorption of these antibiotics. Researchers have demonstrated, for example, that there was a 17-fold reduction in **Cipro** levels in the blood after patients took antacids containing aluminum and magnesium.[5] It would almost be like not taking any medicine. Infections may not be cured if blood levels of antibiotics are inadequate.

Tetracycline is another broad-spectrum antibiotic that is widely prescribed. Dermatologists rely on it as a mainstay in the treatment of acne. It is the drug of choice against *Chlamydia* infection, the most common sexually transmitted disease in women, and deadly Rocky Mountain spotted fever. There are a variety of tetracycline-type antibiotics on the market, including **Achromycin V**, **Declomycin**, **Minocin**, **Panmycin**, **Sumycin**, **Terramycin**, and **Vibramycin**.

Antacids can reduce absorption of such drugs by more than 90 percent. Not only would you be wasting your money on expensive antibiotic therapy, but serious infections might not be cured. (For more details on the interaction between tetracycline and calcium, see page 81.)

So why would anyone even contemplate combining antacids with antibiotics? Clearly no one would ever intentionally sabotage antibiotic therapy. But such antibiotics can cause upset stomach, indigestion, nausea, abdominal pain, and general digestive tract discomfort. Many folks might reach for an antacid without even thinking.

Another easily overlooked problem is **Pepto-Bismol** (bismuth subsalicylate). Because it is not officially an antacid, many people may not realize that this common stomach medicine can also interact with tetracyclines. Since such antibiotics often produce diarrhea and stomach upset, you can imagine how tempted someone might be to reach for the **Pepto** to relieve discomfort. Doing so, however, can reduce absorption of the antibiotic by one third. Levels of tetracycline-like drugs such as **Vibramycin** (doxycycline) can be reduced by over 50 percent—enough to decrease effectiveness.

The take-home message is DO NOT take antacids if your physician prescribes tetracycline or quinolone antibiotics. If you absolutely, positively must seek such stomach relief, do so only with your doctor's awareness. The antacid should be taken at least six hours before or three to four hours after the antibiotic.

Antacids may also interfere with proper absorption of the heart and blood pressure medications **Capoten** (captopril), **Inderal** (propranolol), and **Tenormin** (atenolol); the heart drug **Lanoxin** (digoxin); the ulcer drugs **Zantac** (ranitidine) and **Tagamet** (cimetidine); the antifungal agent **Nizoral** (ketoconazole); the antibacterial **Macrodantin** (nitro-furantoin); the seizure medicine **Dilantin** (phenytoin); and the antistroke compound **Ticlid** (ticlopidine). Although the clinical significance of such interactions remains murky, it only makes sense to avoid such antacids unless they are absolutely essential for health.[6]

Antacids That Affect Antibiotics

aluminum hydroxide gel	Mylanta II
Amitone	Phillips' Milk of Magnesia
Calcium Carbonate	Riopan
Chooz	Riopan Plus Di-Gel
Dicarbosil	Rolaids
Di-Gel Advanced Formula	Rolaids Calcium Rich/
Gas-X	Sodium Free
Gaviscon	Rulox
Gaviscon Cool Mint Flavor	Rulox Plus
Gaviscon ESR	Simaal 2 Gel
Gaviscon-2	Titralac
Gelusil	Titralac Plus
Kudrox	Tums
Maalox HRF	Tums Anti-gas
milk of magnesia	Tums E-X Extra Strength
Mylanta Double Strength	WinGel

The thyroid medicine **Synthroid** (levothyroxine) may also be affected by aluminum-containing antacids. Although this interaction needs better documentation, it would be wise either to stay away from such antacids or to monitor TSH (thyroid-stimulating hormone) levels carefully before and after exposure to antacids.

Activated Charcoal (the Gas-Busters)

It is not a topic for polite company, but flatulence is a fact of life. Everyone passes gas, some more than others. A few of the products sold in pharmacies to fight excess gas contain activated charcoal, the same material found in gas masks and water filters. Charcoal adsorbs all sorts of noxious stuff and is used as an antidote in cases of overdose or poisoning. There is also some research that suggests activated charcoal capsules reduce gaseous emissions. Products that contain activated charcoal include **Charcocaps**, **Charcoal Plus**, and **Flatulex**.

As good as activated charcoal can be at saving people from drug overdoses or sparing them from flatulence, it can also prevent the absorption of medicine. This could reduce effectiveness. Someone who is using a product like **Charcocaps** or **Flatulex** should avoid taking it at least several hours before and after taking medicine.

Drugs Affected by Activated Charcoal

Acetaminophen (**Anacin-3**, **Panadol**, **Tylenol**, etc)
Antidepressants (tricyclic) (**Elavil**, **Pertofrane**, etc.)
Aspirin (**Alka-Seltzer**, **Anacin**, **Ascriptin**, etc.)
Barbiturates (**Fiorinal**, **Nembutal**, etc.)
Carbamazepine (**Tegretol**)
Diabetes drugs (**Diabinese**, **Tolinase**, etc.)
Digoxin (**Lanoxin**)
Furosemide (**Lasix**)
Methotrexate (**Rheumatrex**)
Nizatidine (**Axid**)
Phenothiazines (**Thorazine**, **Mellaril**, etc.)
Phenytoin (**Dilantin**)
Propoxyphene (**Darvon**, **Darvocet-N**, etc.)
Tetracycline (**Achromycin V**, **Sumycin**, etc.)
Theophylline (**Slo-bid**, **Theo-Dur**, etc.)
Valproic acid (**Depakene**, **Depakote**)

Antihistamines

It is almost impossible to find a cold, allergy, cough, or flu remedy these days that doesn't contain an antihistamine as a main ingredient. Check the label on your favorite brand and you are likely to find compounds such as brompheniramine, carbinoxamine, chlorpheniramine, clemastine, diphenhydramine, doxylamine, pyrilamine, tripelennamine, and triprolidine. But these are tongue twisters and most people can't remember such terms.

Brand names are easier to pronounce and recall. Almost everyone has heard of products such as **Actifed**, **Benadryl**, **Benylin**, **Chlor-Trimeton**, **Comtrex**, **Contac 12 Hour**, **Dimetane**, **Dimetapp**, **Nyquil**, **PBZ**, **Sudafed Plus**, **Tavist**, and **TheraFlu Flu Cold & Cough Powder**.

Most over-the-counter antihistamines can make people drowsy, cloudy, fuzzy, or spacey. Many people find these drugs just plain put them to sleep. In fact, ingredients such as diphenhydramine and doxylamine are found in nonprescription sleeping products, including **Compoz**, **Excedrin P.M.**, **Nytol**, **Sleep-Eze 3**, **Sominex**, **Tylenol Extra Strength PM**, and **Unisom Nighttime Sleep Aid**.

It should come as no surprise that such antihistamines interact badly with prescription drugs that also have a sedating potential. People taking anti-anxiety agents such as **Ativan**, **Librium**, **Tranxene**, **Valium**, and **Xanax** should not combine OTC cough, cold, or allergy remedies with their nerve pills. The two drugs could make you a zombie. So could the tension headache pill **Fiorinal**, which contains the barbiturate butalbital. And watch out for traditional tricyclic antidepressants. They too could be a problem. Anticonvulsants, anti-Parkinson's disease drugs, alcohol, prescription pain relievers, and muscle relaxants can also add to the sedative effect. Before taking any antihistamine with a prescription medicine, check with a pharmacist to make sure it won't cause complications. Do not drive if you take antihistamines, even if you think you are unaffected. Reflexes and coordination could be affected.

Pain Relievers

The numbers are mind boggling. Americans toss down almost 30 billion aspirin pills annually. We swallow aspirin to relieve headaches, backaches, muscle sprains and strains, and arthritis. Millions more take a little aspirin every other day to prevent heart attacks and strokes. If preliminary research holds up, lots more will be taking aspirin to prevent a number of common cancers (stomach, colon, rectal, etc.). Now add millions more who casually pop acetaminophen (**Anacin-3, APAP, Bayer Select Maximum Strength Headache, Panadol, Tylenol,** etc.) and ibuprofen (**Advil, Bayer Select Ibuprofen Pain Reliever/Fever Reducer, Excedrin IB, Midol IB, Motrin IB, Nuprin**, etc.) to relieve minor aches and pains.

Analgesics are clearly the most popular pills in the medicine chest. We rely on them so routinely that we hardly think of such products as drugs. And yet aspirin, acetaminophen, and ibuprofen can all interact with a large number of other medications.

Aspirin Versus Capoten and Vasotec

One of the most controversial interactions in this entire book has to do with the combination of aspirin and **Capoten** (captopril) or **Vasotec** (enalapril). Millions of people take these prescription heart and blood pressure medicines. At last count, **Vasotec** was number 8 and **Capoten** was number 13 on the doctor's hit parade of most prescribed drugs.[7] These medications belong to a class referred to as ACE (angiotensin-converting enzyme) inhibitors. Without going into detail, such compounds lower blood pressure and protect against congestive heart failure with relatively few side effects—hence their extraordinary popularity.

It is not surprising that many of the same people who have hypertension or heart problems would also be taking aspirin. After all, this wonder drug saves tens of thousands of lives each year by preventing blood clots. (See *The Aspirin Handbook*, Bantam Books, New York, 1993, by Joe Graedon, Teresa Graedon, and Tom Ferguson, for everything you ever wanted to know about aspirin.)

When we first discovered the possibility that aspirin might partially compromise the effectiveness of ACE inhibitors, we tentatively wrote about it in our newspaper column. We were chastised by the company that makes **Vasotec** for shooting from the lip without adequate documentation. But subsequently we received a fascinating letter:

> A friend told me that you recently had an article in the paper regarding the side effects of aspirin and Vasotec. In December I took four 325 mg Ecotrins a day for three days for back pain. I was on either 5 or 10 mg of Vasotec twice a day when my blood pressure went up to 210/90 and my nose bled profusely.

At this time it is impossible to say whether this increase in blood pressure was caused by the aspirin in **Ecotrin**. But an extraordinary article in the *Journal of the American College of Cardiology* suggests that as little as one aspirin tablet can modify the benefit of **Vasotec** in controlling severe heart failure. These investigators concluded: "Our results indicate that enalapril works better when given without aspirin."[8]

The company that makes **Vasotec** does not specifically warn physicians about this interaction.[9] It may not be cause for concern. Nevertheless, if heart failure is not controlled adequately, this serious health condition could become life threatening. This is the kind of interaction that might sneak up in such a subtle way that no one would even realize that the anticipated benefits of **Vasotec** were not forthcoming. We encourage all physicians who prescribe **Vasotec** and aspirin together to treat heart failure to read Dr. Donald Hall's article in the *Journal of the American College of Cardiology* 1992; 20:1549–1555. Until more research is conducted, caution and vigilance are appropriate watchwords.

What should people with high blood pressure do? Well, they should definitely not stop taking aspirin, especially if it has been prescribed by a physician. Aspirin prevents heart attacks and strokes. But pharmacologist Morton J. Rodman warns that aspirin may partially counteract the blood-pressure-lowering effect of **Capoten**.[10] It may also impact **Vasotec** and other ACE inhibitors.

The answer to this dilemma is to monitor blood pressure carefully before someone starts taking such medicine to get a good baseline. When the ACE inhibitors are started, blood pressure should be recorded before aspirin is introduced. Then blood pressure should be checked once aspirin is added. A careful daily diary should reveal whether aspirin is blunting the benefits of these important medications. If it is, the physician can tailor a program that takes this effect into account. People with hypertension should definitely invest in a home blood pressure monitor so they can track these readings themselves, record them in a diary, and show them to the doctor for supervision.

We have detailed the interactions of ibuprofen together with other arthritis medicines in the Guides to Dangerous Drug Interactions (see pages 255 to 263). On pages 110-115 you will find a table that lists the most common and serious aspirin and acetaminophen interactions. Please refer to this reference material if you rely on any of these pain relievers.

Drugs That Interact with Aspirin

DRUG	INTERACTION WITH ASPIRIN
ACE Blood Pressure Drugs **Capoten** **Vasotec**	The ACE inhibitor drugs, especially **Capoten** (captopril) and **Vasotec** (enalapril), are very widely used, not only to control blood pressure, but also to help ward off congestive heart failure. Current indications suggest they may also delay deterioration of kidney function in diabetics. Aspirin appears capable of interfering with the effectiveness of **Capoten** in lowering blood pressure, although there is little research to document this. It can also reduce the benefit of **Vasotec** in treating congestive heart failure. If you are currently taking aspirin and one of these drugs, *do not stop taking either one.* Aspirin may be essential to your health. Keep track of your blood pressure and check with your doctor on whether you are getting the expected benefit from your blood pressure medicine. The interaction summary in the Guides to Dangerous Drug Interactions on page 329 and the discussion on pages 107-109 have more details.
Activated Charcoal	Activated charcoal, sometimes taken for flatulence, can attach to and reduce the effect of many other drugs, aspirin among them.
Alcohol	Taking aspirin together with an alcoholic drink could easily aggravate stomach irritation. There is also a possibility that blood alcohol levels might end up higher than expected after just one and a half drinks if aspirin is taken an hour beforehand. There is disagreement about the clinical and legal implications of this interaction.
Antacids **Advanced Formula Di-Gel** **Gelusil** **Maalox** Milk of magnesia **Tums** and others	Using antacids regularly can reduce the amount of aspirin circulating in the body. People using anti-inflammatory doses of aspirin should be monitored if they start or stop taking antacids daily.
Anticoagulants **Coumadin** (warfarin) Dicumarol Heparin **Miradon** (anisindione)	Because aspirin also has anticlotting action, any of these prescription blood thinners (including heparin) might work too well in combination with aspirin. The potential exists for dangerous excessive bleeding. Careful monitoring is crucial.

DRUG	INTERACTION WITH ASPIRIN
Arthritis Drugs **Advil** (ibuprofen) **Clinoril** (sulindac) **Feldene** (piroxicam) **Motrin** (ibuprofen) **Naprosyn** (naproxen) and others	Although this interaction is not well established, some people find that these drugs for arthritis, bursitis, tendinitis, and other problems are less effective in combination with aspirin. In addition, stomach irritation may become worse.
Ascorbic Acid Vitamin C	People who take aspirin on a regular basis may have lower levels of this vitamin inside certain cells. It's not clear, though, whether there are any medically significant consequences. The interaction between aspirin and vitamin C is complicated and seems to differ with dietary levels of the vitamin. In one study, aspirin reduced urinary excretion of ascorbic acid when the vitamin was in ample supply; paradoxically, when dietary levels were low, aspirin led to greater excretion of vitamin C. Questions have been raised about whether large doses of vitamin C could make high doses of aspirin more toxic.
Baking Soda	This home remedy for indigestion could make urine alkaline. The result would be more rapid elimination of aspirin from the system.
Beta-Blockers **Blocadren** (timolol) **Cartrol** (carteolol) **Corgard** (nadolol) **Inderal** (propranolol) **Lopressor** (metoprolol) **Sectral** (acebutolol) **Tenormin** (atenolol) **Visken** (pindolol) and others	These medicines used to treat high blood pressure and heart disease may not work as effectively in the presence of aspirin. Research on this issue is not solid, but if you must take aspirin as well as one of the beta-blockers, you and your doctor should monitor your blood pressure response carefully. See the interaction summary on page 340.
Corticosteroids **Cortef** (hydrocortisone) **Decadron** (dexamethasone) **Deltasone** (prednisone) **Medrol** (methylprednisolone)	Aspirin is eliminated more rapidly in the presence of these strong prescription steroids. Physicians should monitor dosing carefully, especially if anti-inflammatory effects are desired.

DRUG	INTERACTION WITH ASPIRIN

Diabetes Drugs
  DiaBeta (glyburide)
  Diabinese (chlorpropamide)
  Glucotrol (glipizide)
  Micronase (glyburide)
  and others
 	
  Insulin
	Type II diabetics should take aspirin only under a doctor's supervision, with careful blood sugar monitoring. Otherwise, blood glucose might drop too low unexpectedly. See the interaction summary on page 289 in the Diabetes Drugs section.

Diuretics
  Bumex (bumetanide)
  Edecrin (ethacrynic acid)
  Lasix (furosemide)
	Aspirin can counteract the effectiveness of these strong "loop" diuretics in people with kidney or liver problems, especially if there is fluid buildup in the abdomen (ascites). This could have serious consequences; consult your physician.

Epilepsy Drugs
  Depakene (valproic acid)
  Dilantin (phenytoin)
	These important anticonvulsant drugs could become more toxic in the presence of aspirin. A person who must take aspirin should be monitored closely for adverse reactions and blood levels of these medicines.

Glaucoma Drugs
  Daranide
   (dichlorphenamide)
  Diamox (acetazolamide)
  Neptazane (methazolamide)
	Aspirin might increase blood levels of these glaucoma medicines to potentially toxic amounts. Elderly patients and people with kidney trouble are at particular risk. Check with your ophthalmologist before adding aspirin.
	    Diamox is also sometimes used to treat mountain sickness in people traveling to high altitudes. Caution should be exercised in mixing this drug with aspirin.

Gout Medicine
  Anturane (sulfinpyrazone)
  Benemid (probenecid)
	Taking aspirin with either of these gout medicines may keep them from controlling the uric acid buildup. In addition, aspirin won't be able to work against gout, either. It takes no more than 700 mg of aspirin to block **Anturane** almost totally.

Methotrexate
  Folex
  Methotrate
  Mexate
  Rheumatrex,
  and others
	This medication, used to treat psoriasis, rheumatoid arthritis, and cancer, could reach surprisingly high levels in the body when combined with aspirin. This is a double-edged action, potentially increasing the power of the drug, but also its toxicity. Don't take any chances. Check with your doctor before taking any aspirin while you are also taking methotrexate.

DRUG	INTERACTION WITH ASPIRIN
Nitroglycerin	In one study, patients who took 1 gram of aspirin (two extra-strength tablets) along with nitroglycerin had lower blood pressure and a faster heart rate than those who took nitroglycerin alone. This could be a beneficial interaction, but it might also result in more nitroglycerin side effects such as headache or dizziness.
Oral Contraceptives	Women using oral contraceptives seem to metabolize aspirin more rapidly and may not get the same effectiveness. If aspirin is being used for minor pain, this is an inconvenience. If it is being used as an anti-inflammatory agent, this interaction might be more of a problem.
Penicillin	In the presence of aspirin, penicillin reaches higher concentrations in the blood and may last longer in the body. No studies have shown whether this makes any practical difference in fighting infection.
Spironolactone **Aldactazide** **Aldactone**	Spironolactone is a potassium-sparing diuretic that helps the body rid itself of sodium. Aspirin can interfere with the sodium-shedding effect, although potassium conservation and blood pressure do not seem to suffer.

Drugs That Interact with Acetaminophen

DRUG	INTERACTION WITH ACETAMINOPHEN
Activated Charcoal	Activated charcoal is sometimes taken for flatulence or other digestive problems. This is also the substance found in gas masks, because it is very efficient at grabbing other chemicals and hanging on to them. It can adsorb acetaminophen and reduce its effectiveness.
Alcohol	Although people often take **Anacin-3**, **Panadol**, or **Tylenol** to treat a hangover, alcohol and acetaminophen is a combination that worries us. Regular drinkers have a much greater risk of liver damage from overuse or overdose of acetaminophen. The danger is greater when a person is not eating much and taking large amounts of either alcohol or the painkiller. Deaths have been reported. Be aware that some medicines, especially cold remedies, contain both ingredients and should not be taken on a regular basis.
Anticoagulants **Coumadin** **Panwarfin** **Sofarin** Warfarin	Acetaminophen is usually safer than aspirin as a pain reliever for a person taking an oral anticoagulant. There is concern, however, that high doses of acetaminophen could increase prothrombin time (PT) and increase the risk of unwanted bleeding. Ask the doctor to monitor PT if you will need to start taking significant doses of acetaminophen.
Anticonvulsants **Dilantin** (phenytoin) **Mesantoin** (mephenytoin) **Peganone** (ethotoin) Phenobarbital **Tegretol** (carbamazepine)	Any of these seizure medicines may reduce the effectiveness of acetaminophen, so that pain relief might be harder to achieve. Don't be tempted to increase the dose of the pain medicine, though; the seizure drugs also make the liver more susceptible to damage from high doses or long-term use of acetaminophen. Please note that any barbiturate taken on a regular basis could interact with this nonprescription pain reliever in a similar way. The headache remedies **Fiorinal** and **Fioricet** both contain a barbiturate, butalbital.
AZT **Retrovir** (zidovudine)	Anyone taking the anti-AIDS drug AZT should consult the doctor before swallowing **Tylenol** or any other acetaminophen pain pill. Acetaminophen speeds elimination of AZT. Just one week of taking 650 mg acetaminophen (two regular-strength pills) with each AZT dose reduced AZT in the body by 33 percent. The clinical significance is unknown, but because **Retrovir** is used for a serious condition, it is probably unwise to interfere with it.

DRUG	INTERACTION WITH ACETAMINOPHIN
Beta-Blockers **Inderal** (propranolol) **Lopressor** (metoprolol) **Tenormin** (atenolol) and others	This interaction is probably no big deal. **Inderal** slows the elimination of acetaminophen slightly, which could lead to higher levels or longer action of the pain reliever. Unless you are taking frequent high doses of acetaminophen, that shouldn't be a problem. Some other beta-blockers may also interact in a similar fashion.
Gout Medicine **Anturane** (sulfinpyrazone)	When **Anturane** is taken on a regular basis, as it normally is in the treatment of gout, it can make the liver more vulnerable to damage. High doses of acetaminophen should be avoided.
Oral Contraceptives **Loestrin** **Lo/Ovral** **Ortho-Novum** and others	Acetaminophen may take a little longer to kick in, and the pain relief may fade a little sooner in women on birth control pills. Overall, however, pain relief shouldn't be much affected. This is not a dangerous interaction.
Parkinson's Disease Drugs **Artane** (trihexyphenidyl) **Cogentin** (benztropine)	These two medications for Parkinson's disease may slow the onset of acetaminophen's action. Overall pain relief should not be greatly affected, however.
Stomach Medicine **Banthine** (methantheline) Belladonna **Bentyl** (dicyclomine) **Pro-Banthine** (propantheline) **Robinul** (glycopyrrolate)	These medications for ulcers and other digestive disorders can delay the onset of pain relief from acetaminophen. The effectiveness is not reduced, however, so patience is in order.
Tuberculosis Drugs **INH** (isoniazid) **Laniazid** (isoniazid) **Nydrazid** (isoniazid)	The tuberculosis drug isoniazid makes the liver more susceptible to potential damage from acetaminophen. High doses or long-term use of the over-the-counter pain reliever should be avoided if at all possible. Discuss this issue with the physician.
Tuberculosis Drugs **Rifadin** (rifampin) **Rimactane** (rifampin)	The tuberculosis medicine rifampin can lower the effectiveness of acetaminophen somewhat. It would, however, be a serious error to increase the dose in a search for better pain relief, because acetaminophen in high doses or over the long term can make the liver more vulnerable to damage from rifampin. Check with the doctor.

Caffeine

Caffeine hardly seems like a drug. After all, many of us rely on that morning cup of coffee to get the day started, not to mention for a midday pick-me-up. Caffeine is a mainstay in many soft drinks including Coke, Pepsi, and Mountain Dew. You will also find caffeine in a surprising number of medications, from pain relievers to daytime stimulants.

Products That Contain Caffeine	
Anacin	Excedrin
Aqua-Ban Plus	Extra-Strength
Bayer Select Maximum	NoDoz
Headache Capsules	Quick Pep
BC Headache Powders	Tirend
Caffedrine	Vanquish Caplets
Vivarin	

Few physicians think to warn their patients about caffeine/drug interactions. Yet a number of prescription medications can boost caffeine levels to the point that someone could be wired for hours. Barry is a photojournalist for a major news magazine. When he developed an ear infection the doctor prescribed **Cipro** (ciprofloxacin). Not a word was mentioned about possible interactions. When Barry had his usual double cappuccino, his nervous system went into overdrive. He was jittery and unable to hold the camera steady. The effect lasted far longer than one might have expected from a strong cup of coffee. Barry had no idea why his normal caffeine hit had left him so uptight.

Cipro, **Noroxin** (norfloxacin), and **Penetrex** (enoxacin) are quinolone antibiotics that can all affect metabolism of caffeine and give it a longer ride in the body. So can the ulcer drug **Tagamet** (cimetidine) and even birth control pills.[11] Women on the Pill may find that they get a bigger jolt from that cup of coffee. Although these interactions are probably not hazardous for most people, the extra caffeine effect can come as a shock to some. Barry certainly wasn't prepared to be wired for hours. Some people may develop serious insomnia from what they think is a modest amount of coffee early in the day. Don't risk it—skip the java.

People with asthma often take theophylline (**Bronkaid Tablets, Bronkodyl, Bronkotabs, Elixophyllin, Primatene Tablets, Slo-bid, Slo-Phyllin, Sustaire, Theo-24, Theobid, Theo-Dur, Theolair, Uniphyl**, etc.). Theophylline can interact with a large number of other medications (see page 264). The chemical structure and pharmacological action of theophylline is very similar to that of caffeine. In fact, if someone were to be caught without his theophylline, and mild symptoms of asthma began to be a problem, several cups of caffeinated coffee might bring relief. But if one were to take theophylline and also drink regular coffee, it would be like getting an overdose of caffeine. That also goes for soft drinks and over-the-counter products that contain this ubiquitous stimulant.

Herbal Remedies

If it is rare for a physician to warn people about interactions between drugs such as caffeine and **Tagamet**, you can imagine how unlikely it would be to get a precaution about herbal products that can interact with drugs. For one thing, few patients are likely even to share with their doctors the fact that they use herbal products. Such products are, after all, considered somewhat flaky by the medical establishment. Yet in recent years alternative remedies—including herbal products available in health food stores and through the mail—have become increasingly popular.

There is, sad to say, very little research on the potential for herbal products to interact with other medications. You won't find many references to such problems in standard interaction references or data bases. That interactions can occur, however, is unquestioned.

Guarana

Guarana is a popular herbal ingredient found in a number of so-called natural products. It has been used as a diet aid and stimulant. One brand name remedy is aptly called **Zoom**. Guarana comes from Central and South America. It is especially popular in Brazil, where natives have used this herb as a treatment for malaria and dysentery. Not surprisingly, they also drink it as a hot beverage, much as we do tea or coffee. Guarana contains a whopping dose of caffeine—3 to 5 percent by dry weight, compared to 1 to 2 percent in coffee beans, by dry weight. Therefore the same warnings that apply to caffeine would also apply to guarana.

Licorice

Many herbal preparations contain licorice (glycyrrhiza). This natural product has been used for centuries in cough and cold remedies and as a digestive aid. It is also employed as a flavoring agent in many natural remedies. But too much licorice (in candy or an herbal product) can deplete the body of potassium. People taking diuretics or digoxin (**Lanoxin**) can get themselves into serious trouble if they also gorge on licorice (see pages 44 and 45 for more details).

Garlic

Garlic, variously nicknamed "stinking rose" and "nectar of the gods," has been used medicinally for thousands of years. Currently garlic extracts are sold in health food stores and pharmacies as a general tonic, but also with the idea that garlic may reduce blood sugar levels, lower blood cholesterol, and help prevent the formation of blood clots that could trigger heart attacks. It may also prove helpful, upon further research, in some intestinal disorders. Experts worry that garlic might interact with diabetes medicines or a blood thinner such as **Coumadin** to increase their activity unexpectedly. No studies have been conducted yet to confirm or refute this possibility of troublesome interactions.

Glucomannan

Also known as konjac, glucomannon is similar in its actions to guar gum, a dietary fiber that is used as a thickening agent in lots of processed foods and pharmaceuticals. Glucomannan is employed as a gentle laxative and has been used in weight loss products to produce a "full feeling." It has also been found to help lower cholesterol levels.

Glucomannan and guar gum can have a major impact on blood sugar. They may lower glucose levels and change insulin requirements. This means that patients with diabetes will have to be especially vigilant about monitoring blood glucose if they take an herbal remedy containing glucomannan or guar gum. Dosage modifications may become necessary for insulin injections or for oral diabetes medicines such as **DiaBeta, Diabinese, Dymelor,**

Glucotrol, Glynase, Micronase, Orinase, Tolamide, and **Tolinase**. Any diabetic considering an herbal remedy containing glucomannon or guar gum must stay in close touch with a physician.

Goldenseal

This plant is found from Arkansas to Vermont. It is also known as yellow root, turmeric root, or orange root. People use it for coughs, menstrual problems, arthritis, and stomach upset. One of the active components in goldenseal, hydrastine, can constrict blood vessels. Although there is little research on drug interactions with goldenseal, we fear that this pharmacological action might raise blood pressure. This could complicate treatment for people taking antihypertensive medication, especially beta-blockers such as **Corgard** (nadolol), **Inderal** (propranolol), **Lopressor** (metoprolol), and **Tenormin** (atenolol).

Feverfew

Feverfew is a European herbal medicine from the Greek tradition. Like many other medicinal herbs, it has recently enjoyed a strong revival of interest. Some people recommend it for the prevention of migraine headaches, and there is research to indicate it is more effective for this purpose than a placebo.[12] There are worrisome reports of a rebound syndrome in those who stop feverfew suddenly, however, and an interaction with anticoagulants such as **Coumadin** is suspected, although it hasn't been studied.

Ubiquinone (Coenzyme Q_{10})

$CoQ_{10,}$ as it is sometimes called, is not an herb, but it is sold in health food stores as a nutrient. It is a very popular alternative treatment for everything from heart failure and gum disease to lowered immunity and lack of energy. Ubiquinone is a natural substance made by the body and is important to many biochemical reactions. While this substance appears to be relatively nontoxic by itself, it may interact in a dangerous way with **Coumadin** (warfarin). Preliminary research suggests that CoQ_{10} may reduce the effectiveness of this anticoagulant and increase the risk of blood clots.[13]

Anyone taking coenzyme Q_{10} must alert a physician and make sure to have frequent blood tests if **Coumadin** is part of the program. In fact, it is probably not a good idea to combine CoQ_{10} and **Coumadin** unless advised to do so by a doctor who is monitoring the situation very carefully.

Chamomile

Chamomile tea is a traditional remedy for stomach upset in many parts of the world. Scientific research backs up this tradition to some extent, suggesting that the principal component of chamomile, bisabolol, may calm intestinal spasms and helps prevent the development of gastric ulcers in rats given ulcer-causing compounds such as indomethacin (a potent arthritis medicine) or alcohol.[14] While this protective effect might potentially be useful for someone who has to take arthritis medicine on a regular basis, the editors of *The Lawrence Review of Natural Products* also warn that chamomile may delay the absorption of medications taken at the same time.[15]

Yohimbine

The bark from the yohimbe tree was a favorite impotence remedy of West African traditional healers, and the compound derived from that bark is being used by many American men for the same purpose. Like many natural remedies, though, yohimbine does have some side effects. It can cause dizziness and a fall in blood pressure. Medical supervision is essential. This compound also appears to block the enzyme monoamine oxidase (MAO) and therefore it should not be taken with a variety of prescription and over-the-counter medications. See pages 47 and 99-100 for lists of foods and drugs that should be avoided.

Valerian

This herb has become very popular as a calming agent. In other words, it may help people relieve minor anxiety and perhaps even get to sleep. Be aware, however, that valerian might interact with alcohol or other tranquilizers or sedatives. This means that someone taking **Valium** (diazepam), **Xanax** (alprazolam), or an antidepressant such as **Elavil** (amitriptyline) that may cause drowsiness should be very cautious about adding valerian.

Herbs are popular these days. People like to think of such remedies as natural and organic, with no side effects or complications. If an over-the-counter remedy or prescription drug doesn't live up to expectations, some folks may decide to self-medicate with an herbal product. Such combinations might lead to serious reactions, however. Caution is called for since your pharmacist may not be able to determine the potential for dangerous interactions.

Conclusion

Over-the-counter medications are not wimpy drugs, and herbal remedies are not necessarily harmless. These products can have side effects and may interact with a wide variety of other compounds. A sensible consumer will learn which precautions apply. As more and more medicines jump the counter (**Aleve**, **Pepcid AC**, and **Tagamet HB** are examples, with **Carafate**, **Feldene**, and **Zantac** under review), you will have greater need than ever to check for interaction potential. The labels on OTC bottles and herbal remedies will likely remain woefully inadequate, so it will be up to you to learn the rules to use such products safely.

References

1. Harrison, W., et al. "MAOIs and Hypertensive Crisis: The Role of OTC Drugs." *J. Clin. Psychiatry* 1989; 50:64.
2. Rivers, N., et al. "Possible Lethal Reaction Between Nardil and Dextromethorphan." *Can. Med. Assoc. J.* 1970; 103:85.
3. Riley, S.A., et al. "Effects of a Non-Absorbable Osmotic Load on Drug Absorption in Healthy Volunteers." *Br. J. Clin. Pharmacol.* 1992; 34:40–46.
4. Wang, D.J. "Drug Interaction Between Digoxin and Bisacodyl." *Taiwan I. Hsueh. Hui. Tsa. Chih.* 1990; 89:915–919.
5. Lomaestro, B.M., et al. "Quinolone-Cation Interactions: A Review." *DICP Ann Pharmacother.* 1991; 25:1249–1258.
6. Holden, Mark D. "Over-the-Counter Medications: Do You Know What Your Patients Are Taking?" *Postgraduate Medicine* 1992; 91(8):191–200.
7. Simonsen, Laura La Piana. "What Are Pharmacists Dispensing Most Often?" *Pharmacy Times* 1993; April: 29–44.
8. Hall, Donald, et al. "Counteraction of the Vasodilator Effects of Enalapril by Aspirin in Severe Heart Failure." *J. Am. Coll. Cardiol.* 1992; 20:1549–1555.
9. Hopkins, Martha, Professional Services. Personal communication, December 21, 1993.
10. Rodman, Morton J. "OTC Interactions: Analgesics and Anti-Inflammatories." *RN* 1993; January: 54–60.
11. Myers, Martin G. "Caffeine, Oral Contraceptives, and Over-the-Counter Drugs." *Arch. Int. Med.* 1989; 149:1217–1222.
12. Murphy, J. J., et al. "Randomised double-blind placebo-controlled trial of feverfew in migraine prevention." *Lancet* 1988; 2:189.
13. Spigset, Olav. "Reduced effect of warfarin caused by ubidecarenone." *Lancet* 1994; 344:1372–1373.
14. Szelenyi, I., et al. "Pharmacological experiments with compounds of chamomile. III. Experimental studies of the ulcer protective effects of chamomile." *Planta Medica* 1979; 35:218.
15. "Chamomile." *Lawrence Review of Natural Products*. St. Louis: Facts & Comparisons, 1991.

References for Aspirin and Acetaminophen Interaction Tables

Graedon, J., et al. *The Aspirin Handbook: A User's Guide to the Breakthrough Drug of the '90s.* New York: Bantam Books, 1993.

Hall, D., et al. "Counteraction of the Vasodilator Effects of Enalapril by Aspirin in Severe Heart Failure." *J. Am. Coll. Cardiol.* 1992; 20:1549–1555.

Holden, M. D. "Over-the-counter Medications." *Postgraduate Medicine* 1992; 91:191–200.

Johansson, U., and B. Akesson. "Interaction Between Ascorbic Acid and Acetylsalicylic Acid and Their Effects on Nutritional Status in Man." *Int. J. Vitam. Nutr. Res.* 1985; 55(2):197–204.

Olin, B.R., editor-in-chief. *Drug Facts and Comparisons.* St. Louis: Facts & Comparisons (A Wolters-Kluwer Company), 1993.

Rodman, M.J. "Analgesics and Anti-inflammatories." *RN* 1993; January: 54–60.

Roine, R., et al. "Aspirin Increases Blood Alcohol Concentrations in Humans after Ingestion of Ethanol." *JAMA* 1990: 264:2406–2408.

Tatro, D. S., ed. *Drug Interaction Facts.* St. Louis: Facts & Comparisons (A Wolters-Kluwer Company), 1993.

Chapter Seven

Drug Interactions That Affect Women, Children, and Older People

Drug Interactions That Affect Women

For centuries women have gotten the short end of the stick. Although they are often called upon to be Dr. Mom, caring for sick children, older parents, and ailing spouses, their own health has often been ignored by medical researchers. Nowhere is this problem more acute than in the world of pharmaceuticals.

There are so many unanswered questions about the relationship between drugs and women's health that it leaves us dazed. For example, estrogen hormones are supposed to help protect women against osteoporosis, heart disease, and ovarian cancer. But they increase the incidence of uterine (endometrial) cancer and possibly even breast cancer (a disease that now strikes one in eight women). Because the research to resolve such an important issue as breast cancer has been delayed for decades, it will be many years before women know if they are trading some benefits for other serious risks.

Investigators running drug studies have traditionally focused their attention on healthy young men. Testing relied on subjects who couldn't become pregnant, didn't suffer from chronic diseases, weren't taking any other medicines, and didn't reflect the real world. Women, children, and older people were pretty much ignored by pharmaceutical researchers.

As a result, we don't really know if women benefit from drug-induced cholesterol reduction. There are unresolved questions about blood pressure treatment in women. We cannot assume that women always react the same way that men do. For example, women appear to lack the enzyme alcohol dehydrogenase in the stomach. There is some preliminary information that suggests this enzyme is responsible for early metabolism of alcohol. Perhaps this explains why some men can seemingly drink more than some women without getting as drunk.

Birth Control Pills

The problem is that there has been little motivation to address many of the health issues that really concern women. Take the Pill. More than ten million women rely on this form of contraception to prevent pregnancy. They have been reassured that this is about as good as it gets, next to sterilization. Many people believe that birth control pills are just about perfect. Yet experts have confided to us that there may be as many as "250,000 pregnancies per year in the U.S. attributed to incorrect use of OCs (oral contraceptives), according to research by the National Academy of Science."[1]

Many of these contraceptive failures are undoubtedly due to mistakes. Instructions are surprisingly confusing. There are now roughly 60 different brands of oral contraceptives on the market. There is an amazing variability in dose and type. And there is conflicting information on the proper use of these pills and what to do if one dose is missed. Since many oral contraceptives now have much lower amounts of estrogen and progestin than they did 30 years ago, there is less room for error. Experts tell us that "being just a few hours late may increase risk for pregnancy."[2]

Drug interactions may also contribute to some of those unwanted pregnancies. Many medications can interfere with the effectiveness of the Pill. Today's low-dose contraceptives are less likely to cause side effects, but they seem more vulnerable to inactivation. Although the package insert on a number of brands mentions drug interaction precautions, this crucial information may be buried amidst the fine print. Anyone who has ever looked at one of these inserts knows that your eyes glaze over pretty fast. We wonder whether physicians read, appreciate, and warn patients about the precaution:

> Reduced efficacy and increased incidence of breakthrough bleeding and menstrual irregularities have been associated with concomitant use of rifampin. A similar association, though less marked, has been suggested with barbiturates, phenylbutazone, phenytoin sodium, and possibly with griseofulvin, ampicillin, and tetracyclines.

The Effect of Barbiturates on Birth Control Pills

The real problem is that good research is lacking. Several years ago the manufacturer of the popular tension headache reliever **Fiorinal** (aspirin, butalbital, caffeine) disputed our warning of women that its product might reduce the effectiveness of the Pill. Our concern seemed justified since the barbiturate butalbital is listed in standard reference books as having the potential to reduce contraceptive effectiveness.[3, 4]

A similar barbiturate comes with the warning "Pretreatment with or concurrent administration of phenobarbital may decrease estradiol by increasing its metabolism. There have been reports of patients treated with antiepileptic drugs (e.g., phenobarbital) who become pregnant while taking oral contraceptives. An alternate contraceptive method might be suggested to women taking phenobarbital."

The company maintained that since they had never heard of accidental pregnancies associated with **Fiorinal** or **Fioricet** (acetaminophen, butalbital, caffeine) and birth control pills, the problem did not exist. Of course, there is no mention of an interaction in the package insert, and many women don't even realize that their headache remedy contains a barbiturate. If they got pregnant it is entirely possible that neither they nor their physicians would make such a connection or report it to the company or the FDA.

There is no good answer to this dilemma. Epidemiological studies are sorely lacking. And don't expect anyone to do quality research anytime soon. There is no incentive for drug companies to look for what they perceive as bad news. As we have stated earlier in this book, there is no scientific system to track, report, or warn about dangerous drug interactions. And make no mistake, an unwanted pregnancy can be dangerous. For some women it is intolerable for health reasons, while for others it may be psychologically devastating. Furthermore, barbiturates themselves may cause birth defects.

We suspect that if there were an effective male contraceptive that could be altered by other medications, a solution would be found swiftly. Unfortunately, the medical establishment is playing catch-up on women's health and many unresolved questions may never be answered.

What we can say with certainty is that there are cases of unintended pregnancy associated with the use of barbiturates and birth control pills. We suggest that common sense would encourage extra contraceptive protection if such an interaction were to occur.

Products Containing Barbiturates

Alurate (aprobarbital)
Amytal (amobarbital)
Anaphen (butalbital)
Anoquan (butalbital)
Axotal (butalbital)
Bancap (butalbital)
Barbased (butabarbital)
Bucet (butalbital)
Butace (butalbital)
Buticaps (butabarbital)
Butisol (butabarbital)
Conten (butalbital)
Dolmar (butalbital)
Esgic (butalbital)
Ezol (butalbital)

Femcet (butalbital)
Fiorgen (butalbital)
Fioricet (butalbital)
Fiorinal (butalbital)
Fiorinal with Codeine
   (butalbital)
Fiormor (butalbital)
Fortabs (butalbital)
Gemonil (metharbital)
Isobutal (butalbital)
Isocet (butalbital)
Isolin (butalbital)
Isollyl (butalbital)
Isopap (butalbital)
Laniroif (butalbital)

Lanorinal (butalbital)
Lotusate (talbutal)
Marnal (butalbital)
Mebaral (mephobarbital)
Medigesic (butalbital)
Mysoline (primidone)
Nembutal (pentobarbital)
Pharmagesic (butalbital)
Phenobarbital
Phrenilin (butalbital)
Sarisol No. 2 (butabarbital)
Seconal (secobarbital)
Tri-Barbs (phenobarbital,
   butabarbital, secobarbital)
Tuinal (amobarbital,
   secobarbital)

The Effect of Antibiotics on Birth Control Pills

Perhaps even more controversial than barbiturate complications is the question of antibiotic interaction with birth control pills. Researchers have been debating the significance of this combination for years. You can understand why. It is not uncommon for a woman to get a urinary tract infection, an ear infection, a reproductive tract infection, or just a common case of acne. The doctor is likely to prescribe an antibiotic for each of these problems.

Check the package insert that comes with oral contraceptives and you will find mention of interaction potential with tetracycline and ampicillin, two of the most commonly prescribed antibiotics. Experts also warn that other penicillin-type antibiotics such as **Amoxil** (amoxicillin), **Prostaphlin** (oxacillin), and **Beepen-VK** (penicillin V) may diminish contraceptive power.[5]

The theory is that these broad-spectrum antibiotics kill bacteria in the digestive tract that play an important role in maintaining adequate blood levels of contraceptive hormones. Researchers have been fighting about the clinical significance of this interaction for years. That there are cases of unintended pregnancy associated with antibiotics and birth control pills seems unequivocal.[6,7] How common this is and what other factors may play a role remain highly controversial.[8,9,10,11,12,13,14] Even the most outspoken British critics of an interaction between antibiotics and birth control pills warn that "practitioners are advised to recommend the use of alternative contraceptive precautions for women receiving broad-spectrum antibiotics concurrently with their OCs [oral contraceptives] preparation."[15] Such advice seems only prudent.

Antibiotics That May Affect Birth Control Pills

Achromycin V (tetracycline)
Ala-Tet (tetracycline)
Amcill (ampicillin)
Amoxil (amoxicillin)
Augmentin (amoxicillin, potassium clavulanate)
Azlin (azlocillin)
Bactocill (oxacillin)
Beepen-VK (penicillin V)
Betapen-VK (penicillin V)
Bikomox (amoxicillin)
Biomox (amoxicillin)
Cloxapen (cloxacillin)
Coactin (aminocillin)
Declomycin (demeclocycline)
Doryx (doxycycline)

cont'd

Antibiotics That May Affect Birth Control Pills (cont'd)

Doxy-Caps (doxycycline)
Doxychel (doxycycline)
Dycill (dicloxacillin)
Dynacin (minocycline)
Dynapen (dicloxacillin)
Geocillin (carbenicillin)
Geopen (carbenicillin)
Ledercillin VK (penicillin V)
Minocin (minocycline)
Monodox (doxycycline)
Nallpen (nafcillin)
Omnipen (ampicillin)
Panmycin (tetracycline)
Pathocil (dicloxacillin)
Pentids (penicillin G)
Pen-V (penicillin V)
Pen-Vee K (penicillin V)
Polycillin (ampicillin)
Polymox (amoxicillin)
Principen (ampicillin)

Prostaphlin (oxacillin)
Robicillin VK (penicillin V)
Robitet (tetracycline)
Spectrobid (bacampicillin)
Staphcillin (methicillin)
Sumycin (tetracycline)
Tegopen (cloxacillin)
Terramycin (oxytetracycline)
Tetracap (tetracycline)
Tetracyn (tetracycline)
Tetralan (tetracycline)
Totacillin (ampicillin)
Trimox (amoxicillin)
Unipen (nafcillin)
Uri-Tet (oxytetracycline)
V-Cillin K (penicillin V)
Veetids (penicillin V)
Vibramycin (doxycycline)
Vibra-Tabs (doxycycline)
Wymox (amoxicillin)

The Effect of Anticonvulsants on Birth Control Pills

There is little doubt that seizure medicine represents a real threat to contraceptive effectiveness. There is near unanimity that epilepsy drugs such as **Dilantin** (phenytoin), **Mesantoin** (mephenytoin), **Mysoline** (primidone), **Peganone** (ethotoin), phenobarbital, and **Tegretol** (carbamazepine) affect the metabolism of birth control pills. According to one source, "In a retrospective analysis of 82 women with seizure disorders receiving oral contraceptives, the risk of pregnancy was 25 times greater in those patients also receiving anticonvulsants than in those patients who were not."[16]

What is so serious about this interaction is that many of these very same drugs may cause birth defects. So a woman with a seizure disorder might well be told by her physician to use a reliable method of contraception while on a drug such as **Dilantin** or phenobarbital. Most women would then conclude that oral contraceptives are the best choice. But, as we have just described, reliability may be far less than anticipated when BC pills are combined with such drugs.

There is one anticonvulsant that does not appear to interact with oral contraceptives. Valproic acid (**Depakene**), and the similar divalproex sodium (**Depakote**) won't change metabolism and shouldn't interfere with effectiveness. There are also new seizure medications coming on line, such as **Neurontin** (gabapentin) and **Lamictal** (lamotrigine), that have fewer side effects than traditional anticonvulsants and do not appear to interact with birth control pills.[17,18] Women need to ask lots of questions and take extra precautions to avoid pregnancy no matter which seizure medicine is prescribed.

The Effect of Antifungal and TB Medicines on Birth Control Pills

Women who rely on oral contraceptives have to watch out for several other kinds of medicine. Drugs that fight fungal infections, such as griseofulvin (**Fulvicin, Grifulvin, Gris-PEG, Grisactin**), may reduce the effectiveness of the Pill. Unintended pregnancies have been reported after this combination. There are alternate antifungal medications on the market that have not been reported to have this interaction potential.

Tuberculosis is back. The current TB epidemic appears to be gaining victims at a rapid pace. The infections are more virulent and harder to treat. It is likely that more and more people will become infected, even some who have otherwise healthy immune systems.

One of the main drugs in the treatment of TB is rifampin (**Rifadin, Rifamate, Rimactane**). This drug increases the metabolism, lowers blood levels, and reduces the effectiveness of contraceptive hormones. Breakthrough bleeding and menstrual disturbances are common consequences of this interaction. It has been estimated that 6 percent of women on such a combination could become pregnant.

The Effect of Vitamin C on Birth Control Pills

A few other interactions with birth control pills concern us. Vitamin C can boost estrogen levels. This obviously won't reduce contraceptive protection but could make the Pill more potent.

In essence this interaction converts a low-dose Pill into a high-dose contraceptive. That could increase the possibility of estrogen side effects, including gallbladder disease, vaginal yeast infections, breast tenderness and enlargement, bloating, nausea, vomiting, cramps, facial skin darkening, hair loss, headaches, migraines, depression, increases in blood sugar, and changes in libido (usually reduction).

Vitamin C may have a similar impact on estrogen replacment therapy. Drugs such as **Estinyl**, **Estrace**, **Estratab**, **Estratest**, **Estrovis**, **Menest**, **Ogen**, **Ovest**, and **Premarin** could also be affected by this common nutrient. What is unclear is the dose of ascorbic acid necessary to produce such an effect. One study found that 1,000 mg could increase estrogen (ethinyl estradiol) levels by almost 50 percent. Whether lower doses (say in the 50- to 100-mg range) have an impact is unknown.

One caution should be noted about stopping vitamin C suddenly. Concern has been expressed that estrogen levels might drop precipitously if this vitamin were discontinued too abruptly. Whether this might cause contraceptive failure has not been researched.

The Effect of Birth Control Pills on Anxiety Drugs and Antidepressants

Benzodiazepines are among the most frequently prescribed medicines for anxiety, panic, agoraphobia, and a host of other conditions that create fear and nervousness. We are talking about drugs such as **Dalmane** (flurazepam), **Doral** (quazepam), **Halcion** (triazolam), **Klonopin** (clonazepam), **Tranxene** (clorazepate), **Valium** (diazepam), and **Xanax** (alprazolam).

Oral contraceptives have been reported to increase blood levels of these medications. Likewise, the Pill appears to boost blood levels of antidepressants such as **Elavil** (amitriptyline). There is confusion about the significance of these interactions. Perhaps someone used to a certain amount of **Valium** or **Xanax** in her system might suddenly experience a greater impact from these anti-anxiety agents if she starts birth control pills. There have been reports of greater "psychomotor impairment" from this kind of combination. That could mean driving or operating machinery would be a greater hazard.

Medicine Containing Theophylline

Accurbron	Sustaire
Aerolate	Theo-Dur
Aquaphyllin	Theobid
Asmalix	Theochron
Bronkodyl	Theoclear
Constant-T	Theolair
Elixomin	Theospan
Elixophyllin	Theostat 80
Lanophyllin	Theo-24
Quibron-T	Theovent
Respbid	T-Phyl
Slo-bid	Uniphyl
Slo-Phyllin	

The Effect of Birth Control Pills on Asthma Medicine

Here is another controversial interaction. The data are hard to interpret. Some studies have shown that oral contraceptives prolong the effects of theophylline in the body. If true, this could lead to symptoms of toxicity, such as nausea, vomiting, stomach pain, diarrhea, nervousness, irritability, muscle twitching, and palpitations. Blood levels of theophylline can be monitored to assess the possibility of an interaction. Be alert for signs of overdose if birth control pills are added to this asthma medication.

The Effect of Birth Control Pills on Caffeine

Don't forget to watch out for caffeine. It is pharmacologically similar to theophylline (see page 53). Someone on oral contraceptives could get an extra jolt from her java. Studies have shown that the effects of caffeine are prolonged and possibly even intensified. This could lead to nervousness, insomnia, and a generally wired feeling. Women on the Pill should probably be moderate in caffeine intake, especially late in the day, until they find out if they are affected by such an interaction.

The Effect of Smoking on Birth Control Pills

We have saved the scariest interaction for last. This one is definitely verboten. DON'T DO IT. Smoking and oral contraceptives just plain do not mix. The package insert has a bold, boxed warning that says:

> Cigarette smoking increases the risk of serious cardiovascular side effects from oral contraceptive use. This risk increases with age and with heavy smoking (15 or more cigarettes per day) and is quite marked in women over 35 years of age. Women who use oral contraceptives should be strongly advised not to smoke.

This combination increases the possibility of stroke, heart attack, pulmonary embolism (blood clots in the lungs), and other vascular problems. Women can die from this interaction.

Drug Interactions That Affect Children

Nothing is harder on a parent than a sick child. We feel so inadequate when that vulnerable person we love comes down with a high fever, a terrible cough, or an asthma attack. Giving medicine seems like such a caring thing to do. But watch out: There are thousands of products on drugstore shelves that are inappropriate and possibly even dangerous for children.

Children are not just smaller versions of adults. They react differently to medicine than adults because their nervous systems are not yet fully developed, their metabolism is different, and they are far smaller. That makes them far more susceptible to drug dangers. When a well-meaning adult tells a trusting toddler to swallow an irrational mixture of ingredients, we get angry. And believe us when we tell you that there are illogical products in pharmacies these days.

Cold and Cough Remedies

Let's start with cold remedies. When a child starts sniffling and sneezing, most parents go on alert. A runny nose and a horrible hack really get their attention. With so many products advertising instant relief, the temptation is great to start pumping medicine. And because so many products come in liquid formulas, it's tempting to reach for whatever is lurking in the medicine chest.

Don't do it, Dr. Mom. First, be especially wary of antihistamines. They are everywhere. In fact, it is hard to find a remedy that *doesn't* have an antihistamine on board. Although there is real doubt that they do anything for colds even in adults (they do provide some relief for allergies), in children they may cause more harm than good. See page 106 for a list of antihistamines common in over-the-counter cough and cold remedies.

Adults know that antihistamines make them drowsy. They assume the same thing happens to kids. Wrong! For reasons that are not entirely clear, many children react paradoxically to antihistamines. Such drugs can cause irritability, jitteriness, and insomnia.

Imagine the following scenario. Little Jimmy is snuffling and sneezing and has a nasty cough. It's bedtime and dear old dad thinks that a little of that leftover **NyQuil Adult Nighttime Cold/ Flu Medicine, Cherry Flavor** would be just the thing. Big mistake. The antihistamine could have Jimmy wired for hours. Not only that, here is a remedy that also contains a decongestant (pseudoephedrine) that may also produce hyperactivity. There are even reports that some children have experienced terrifying visual hallucinations—most of which involved insects or spiders— after having taken a cold medicine containing both an antihistamine and a decongestant. **NyQuil** also contains 25 percent alcohol (50 proof). What parent would intentionally give a child a shot of booze? But that is about what happens when you administer adult-formula **Nyquil**. (See page 154 for other medications that contain alcohol.)

The problem parents face is that many of these over-the-counter products come with a drug interaction potential built in. These multi-symptom remedies often contain three, four, or five ingredients. It's like the proverbial kitchen sink. Even so-called pediatric formulas may have antihistamines and decongestants that could make a sick child feel worse.

The American Academy of Pediatrics has recommended single-ingredient cough preparations if your child has a hack that keeps her awake. Small doses of codeine are extremely effective. Dextromethorphan is also helpful. Look for **Robitussin Pediatric Cough Suppressant** or **St. Joseph Cough Suppressant for Children**.

Antibiotics

Ask pediatricians what kind of prescriptions they write most often and the answer will be antibiotics. Children come down with all sorts of bugs—from strep throat and ear infections to bronchitis and cystitis. Out comes a prescription for **Amoxil** (amoxicillin), **Augmentin** (amoxicillin plus potassium clavulanate), **Bactrim** or **Septra** (co-trimoxazole), **Ceclor** (cefaclor), **Ceftin** (cefuroxime), **Cefzil** (cefprozil), **Duricef** (cefadroxil), **Lorabid** (loracarbef), **Pediazole** (erythromycin ethylsuccinate and sulfisoxazole), **Polycillin** (ampicillin), or **Suprax** (cefixime).

Although some of these medicines can interact with other prescription drugs, the good news is that children are unlikely to be taking many other conflicting compounds. Anticoagulants, for example, are usually taken only by older people at risk for blood clots. Oral contraceptives are not likely to be an issue, except for some female adolescents.

The one interaction that we really do worry about, though, has to do with the antibiotic erythromycin. It is found in various formulations including **E.E.S., ERYC, E-Mycin, EryPed, EryTab, Eryzole, Ilosone**, PCE, and **Pediazole**. The nonsedating antihistamines **Seldane** and **Hismanal** may interact with erythromycin to produce life-threatening irregular heart rhythms.

This combination could be especially problematic for children, since a dermatologist could prescribe the antibiotic for acne, and an allergist could write a prescription for the antihistamine to relieve congestion. Neither might realize what the other had done. Such a combination could be a disaster. Please see pages 33-34 for other important erythromycin interactions, and talk to the pediatrician about these issues if she prescribes this common medicine.

Ritalin (methylphenidate)

This is probably the single most controversial medicine for children. These days it seems as if every fifth kid is on this drug for ADHD (attention deficit hyperactivity disorder). Children with ADHD have a hard time focusing or concentrating. Some also have a hard time sitting still and can become behavior problems as well.

We won't enter the battle of whether **Ritalin** is a good drug or a bad drug. No one really understands exactly how it works to help children stay on task. It is a stimulant, pharmacologically similar to amphetamine. Such drugs can make an adult hyper, but they tend to calm overactive children and allow them to focus. Some physicians and parents think **Ritalin** is evil incarnate. Others believe it is heaven-sent. No matter what your philosophy, **Ritalin** should be used only as part of a total treatment program, with behavioral modification and lots of support.

Ritalin has the potential to cause side effects such as irritability, jitteriness, skin rash, loss of appetite, stomach pain, weight loss, palpitations, mood swings, insomnia, and growth delay. Most children, however, do not experience such problems, especially if the dose is kept under control and the last pill is not taken late in the day. What concerns us more is the potential for dangerous interactions with drugs such as clonidine, **Tofranil,** and **Dilantin**.

Although we find it hard to understand, some physicians prescribe tricyclic antidepressants to children who have problems with bed-wetting. **Tofranil** (imipramine) and other drugs in this class have side effects such as urinary retention and delayed urination. Physicians have tried to employ this adverse reaction to prevent the condition they call enuresis (bed-wetting). While it may help some children, we find this to be a heavy-duty drug with a number of worrisome side effects including nervousness, tiredness, sleep problems, digestive upset, constipation, palpitations, and emotional instability. In overdose, tricyclic antidepressants can kill.

The problem occurs when you combine **Ritalin** and drugs such as **Tofranil**. This interaction may lead to increased levels of the tricyclic antidepressant in the bloodstream. There is a report that two adolescents developed dysfunctional behavior (including violence) and depression when put on this combination. While cause and effect has not been clearly established, we think the potential for such an interaction is strong enough to demand great caution.

The other interaction with **Ritalin** that concerns us involves the anticonvulsant drug **Dilantin** (phenytoin). Children with seizure disorders are frequently prescribed this medication. But anecdotal reports suggest that **Ritalin** could increase blood levels of **Dilantin** and possibly produce side effects such as dizziness, nausea, and headaches. If such a drug combination is contemplated, blood levels of phenytoin should be monitored very carefully. Side effects of **Dilantin** to watch out for include incoordination, confusion, dizziness, slurred speech, difficulty sleeping, muscle twitches, double vision, tiredness, tremor, nervousness, depression, bellyaches, headaches, diarrhea, and rashes.

How to Protect Your Children from Drug Interactions

Whenever you receive a prescription for a child, ask some important questions. First, always find out exactly what the medicine is, why it is being prescribed, how it should be taken (with food or on an empty stomach), and what side effects to watch out for. We will never forget the tragic story we heard from a grandmother who lost her grandchild because of a terrible skin side effect (Stevens-Johnson syndrome) brought on by an antibiotic. Neither the parents nor the physician realized this adverse reaction was caused by the medicine until it was too late. And always ask about interaction precautions. While children rarely receive more than one medicine at a time, it is better to be informed than ignorant.

Finally, be supercautious about giving children over-the-counter remedies. Never administer an adult drug to a child, and always check with your pediatrician to make sure what you are doing is appropriate. Children cannot defend themselves against adult ignorance. They trust us when we insist that the medicine is good for them. Such faith may be unwarranted. We all want our children to get better as quickly as possible, but don't let the cure become worse than the disease.

Drug Interactions That Affect Older People

In a very real sense this book is dedicated to people over 50. Just like a car that has accumulated more than 100,000 miles and may need some extra love and attention, an older person deserves admiration, support, and respect for surviving in what is often a cruel world.

Nowhere is the environment fraught with greater danger than in this crazy world of drug interactions. Here is a place where, as Lewis Carroll once wrote,

"The time has come," the Walrus said,
"To talk of many things:
Of shoes—and ships—and sealing wax—
Of cabbages—and kings—
And why the sea is boiling hot—
And whether pigs have wings."

Standard rules fall apart in this pharmacological wonderland. Because older people often see so many different kinds of physicians for a variety of ills, they are the ones most likely to suffer interaction misadventures. The rheumatologist may prescribe an arthritis medicine, the cardiologist could add a high blood pressure pill, something for heart palpitations, and aspirin to prevent blood clots. The gastroenterologist must deal with the stomach upset and possible ulceration so he adds several more prescriptions to the mix. A case of seborrheic dermatitis could send this patient to the dermatologist for more medicine. Oh, and let's not forget the urologist. As we age the plumbing tends to break down too.

As you can see, older people are the most likely targets for dangerous or deadly drug interactions. The nervous system can become more sensitive to a variety of medications, making us vulnerable to dizziness, drowsiness, or slowed reflexes. Now add to this the fact that liver and kidney function may gradually diminish as we age and you have a volatile mixture.

There is only one answer—vigilance. Become an active participant in your own health care. Ask questions and demand answers. Do not try to be a "good" patient if that means passivity. The meek may inherit the earth, but they may also die prematurely from deadly drug interactions. Ask your physician and pharmacist to check periodically on the compatibility of all your medicines, including over-the-counter remedies and even vitamins and minerals.

Look out for your friends, neighbors, and loved ones; they may not always be able to protect themselves. Why not loan them this book so they can do some checking of their own? Remember, good health is your most valuable possession. Fame and fortune fade very quickly in the face of illness and death.

References

1. Reid, Dee, Managing Editor, Publications, Family Health International. Personal letter, November 14, 1990.
2. Ibid.
3. *The Johns Hopkins Handbook of Drugs*. Margolis, Simeon, ed. New York: Rebus (Distributed by Random House), 1993.
4. *Drug Interaction Facts*. Tatro, David S., ed. St. Louis: Facts and Comparisons (A Wolters Kluwer Company), 1995.
5. Ibid.
6. Fleissig, A. "Unintended Pregnancies and the Use of Contraception: Changes from 1984 to 1989." *British Med. J.* 1991; 302:147
7. Orme, Michael L.E., and David J. Black, "Pharmacokinetics of Oral Contraceptive Steroids and Drug Interactions: Factors Affecting the Enterohepatic Circulation of Oral Contraceptive Steroids." *Am. J. Obs. Gyn.* 1990; 163(6S):2146–2152.
8. Orme, Michael, and David J. Black. "Unintended Pregnancies and Contraceptive Use." *British Med. J.* 1991; 302:789.
9. Guengerich, F. Peter. "Pharmacokinetics of Oral Contraceptive Steroids and Drug Interaction: Inhibition of Oral Contraceptive Steroid-Metabolizing Enzymes by Steroids and Drugs." *Am. J. Obs. Gyn.* 1990; 163(6S):2159–2163.
10. Fotherby, Kenneth. "Pharmacokinetics of Oral Contraceptive Steroids and Drug Interaction: Interactions with Oral Contraceptives." *Am. J. Obs. Gyn.* 1990; 163(6S):2153–2159.
11. Zachariasen, R.D. "Effect of Antibiotics on Oral Contraceptive Efficacy." *J. Dent. Hyg.* 1991; 65:334–338.
12. Fazio, A. "Oral Contraceptive Drug Interactions: Important Considerations." *South. Med. J.* 1991; 84:997–1002.
13. Shenfikeld, G.M., and J.M. Griffin. "Clinical Pharmacokinetics of Contraceptive Steroids. An Update." *Clin. Pharmacokinet.* 1991; 20:15–37.
14. Willis, Judith. "'The Pill' May Not Mix Well with Other Drugs." *FDA Consumer* 1987; 21(March):26.
15. Orme, Michael, and David J. Black. "Oral Contraceptive Steroids— Pharmacological Issues of Interest to the Prescribing Physician." *Adv. Contracept.* 1991; 7:325–331.
16. *Drug Interaction Facts*. Tatro, David S., ed. St. Louis: Facts & Comparisons (A Wolters Kluwer Company), 1995.
17. Welling, Peter, Parke-Davis/Warner Lambert. Personal Communication, December 22, 1993.
18. Brodie, Martin J. "Lamotrigine (Drug Profiles)" *Lancet* 1992; 339:1397–1401.

Chapter Eight

Drug/Alcohol Interactions

Alcohol is so much a part of our daily lives that most of us don't think of it as a drug. We have a glass of wine at lunch, a beer at the ball park, or a cocktail before dinner without a moment's hesitation; yet alcohol was one of the first drugs discovered by humans. Use of fermented beverages probably dates back to earliest civilization. If you can make bread, you can make beer.

Putting aside issues of alcohol abuse, we are most concerned with the very serious potential for this substance that is so much a part of our behavior to interact with other medications we may take. People rarely volunteer to their physicians that they occasionally indulge in a nightcap. It may seem too trivial a detail. And yet an amazing number of drugs can create unexpected and hazardous combinations with alcohol.

As we described in the introduction, sailors were among the first guinea pigs of drug and alcohol interaction. Captains of sailing ships often needed extra crew members at the last minute. Knowing that it might be hard to round up voluntary recruits, they sometimes made a deal with scurrilous bartenders. A likely prospect would be slipped some chloral hydrate (a tranquilizer that was a forerunner of barbiturates) in the rum or grog. The chloral hydrate produced a supra-additive effect. By delaying and modifying alcohol metabolism and adding a sedative action all its own, the drug would knock the sailor out cold. By the time he awoke, he could be far out at sea.

Many medicines can add to alcohol's wallop. Anti-anxiety agents such as **Librium**, **Tranxene**, **Valium**, or **Xanax** should never be combined with alcohol (even a beer) since reflexes can be slowed and mental function impaired at very low doses.

Antidepressants are a no-no for the same reason. Even a tension headache reliever such as **Fiorinal** or **Fioricet** (which contain the barbiturate butalbital) could get people into trouble if they also drink. Antihistamines are another danger. They are found in hundreds of allergy, cold, cough, and flu remedies. Always read labels, ask the pharmacist, and be cautious with OTC remedies.

Ulcer Drug/Alcohol Interactions

The most controversial drug/alcohol interactions involve drugs that may raise blood alcohol levels. Researchers have been fighting over this one for years, and the Food and Drug Administration has tried to make sense out of confusion. Because profits are at stake, pharmaceutical manufacturers have been battling to prove there is no problem. We are still undecided and await further research.

The controversy erupted when one of this country's leading alcohol investigators, Dr. Charles Lieber, reported that a number of common drugs could boost blood alcohol levels unexpectedly. What Dr. Lieber discovered was an enzyme in the stomach called alcohol dehydrogenase (ADH). According to his team of researchers, this enzyme breaks down some of the alcohol from a drink even before it is absorbed into the blood stream.[1,2] ADH in the stomach diminishes with age and regular alcohol intake, and is present only at low levels in women. Perhaps this is why it is believed that some women seem to get drunk more easily than men after less alcohol.[3]

This esoteric enzyme would be of interest only to a few scientists except for one thing: a number of medicines can deactivate it. Dr. Lieber believes that these drugs could lead to higher blood alcohol levels and a longer period of elevated alcohol concentrations. His work has shown that aspirin (two extra-strength tablets) taken an hour before drinking interferes with ADH activity enough to cause a measurable increase of alcohol in the bloodstream.[4] There is preliminary evidence that some other drugs may also affect this enzyme, including acetaminophen and propranolol.

What really got the drug companies' attention, though, was the report that ranitidine (**Zantac**) and cimetidine (**Tagamet**) could also affect blood alcohol.[5,6] **Zantac** is one of the most successful drugs in the history of the pharmaceutical industry. Last year alone it earned roughly three billion dollars. **Tagamet** is not far behind. These drugs are prescribed for ulcers and bad heartburn (reflex esophagitis). Since drinkers often tend to have stomach trouble, you can see that they might be prime candidates for these medications.

Dr. Lieber and his colleagues concluded:

> "Thus our study revealed that ranitidine and cimetidine (but not famotidine) lead to substantial increases in blood alcohol levels after consumption of an amount of ethanol that corresponds to common social drinking. The blood alcohol levels achieved have been clearly shown to impair tasks that require a high degree of attention and motor coordination. Therefore, the possibility exists that some patients who are receiving treatment with these H_2-receptor antagonists may suffer unexpected impairment . . . a warning may be appropriate when these drugs are prescribed, especially in social drinkers who may drive vehicles or operate other machinery that require a high degree of attention and/or coordination."[7]

The article in which these findings were reported, published in *The Journal of the American Medical Association*, created a firestorm of controversy. The companies complained that the conclusions were not justified, that the results were inaccurate, that the studies were conducted incorrectly, that there was no clinical significance to the reaction, and that no warning or label change was necessary. Additional research has shown that Dr. Lieber's results are still debatable. Dr. M. D. Levitt reviewed all available data and concluded "very little, if any, metabolism of ethanol is likely to occur in the gastric mucosa, and the interaction between

H_2-antagonists and ethanol is clinically insignificant."[8]

An expert committee for the Food and Drug Administration concluded in 1993 that although blood alcohol levels do go up, "H_2 blockers' interaction with alcohol has not been shown to be clinically significant."[9] So why have we belabored this issue if there is no problem? We are not yet convinced the final chapter has been written on this fascinating and controversial interaction. There is still disagreement among researchers, and Dr. Lieber believes that caution is appropriate. The FDA committee has called for more data to determine if there could be an effect on coordination, reflexes, or behavior. Until that work is completed, we urge people who take such drugs and drink alcohol to take care to be moderate in consumption and be vigilant for unexpected impairment.

Verapamil (Calan, Isoptin, Verelan)/Alcohol Interactions

This is one of the most popular heart and high blood pressure medications on the market. It is far less likely to cause side effects when compared to drugs that used to be prescribed for hypertension. Millions of people rely on these pills to prevent heart disease, stroke, irregular heart rhythm, and chest pain.

We can claim with some assurance that verapamil does not mix well with alcohol. This medicine raises blood alcohol levels and prolongs the effect in the body. The subjects of this experiment were young healthy men and they felt inebriated longer. Goodness knows how older people taking other multiple prescriptions would be affected. The investigators concluded: "The findings of our study suggest that verapamil significantly inhibits ethanol elimination, resulting in elevated blood ethanol concentrations that prolong the intoxicating effects of alcohol."[10]

Beta Carotene/Alcohol Interactions

Beta carotene is one of the hottest nutrients in the health food store. It is a precursor to vitamin A, and people are swallowing these little orange pills with great enthusiasm. You can get beta carotene from carrots, other orange fruits and vegetables, and green leafy vegetables such as spinach, chard, and kale.

The excitement about beta carotene surrounds its antioxidant properties. This pharmacological action may help prevent heart disease and even certain cancers. But heavy drinkers, beware. Researchers at the Bronx Veterans Administration Hospital have found that the combination of booze and beta carotene could be hard on the liver. The preliminary studies have been done only on baboons. What they found was that the combination of alcohol and beta carotene led to more liver damage than that produced by alcohol exposure alone.[11] Although this work needs to be confirmed with further research on humans, the warning flags are flying. People who drink regularly and use beta carotene should discuss this interaction with their physician. Maybe some liver enzyme tests would be in order.

Conclusion

Alcohol is a drug, one of the most widely used in the world. Like any chemical compound it can interact with other medications. Please protect yourself and those around you from a dangerous combination. Too many people die on our highways because of the effects of alcohol. Check the following table for detailed information on the most common and dangerous drug/alcohol interactions.

Drug/Alcohol Interactions

DRUG	INTERACTION WITH ALCOHOL
Acetaminophen	The risk that this over-the-counter pain reliever might cause higher blood alcohol levels from modest amounts of alcohol is still uncertain and may not turn out to be terribly important. The real trouble comes when someone uses both acetaminophen and alcohol on a regular basis. This can put quite a strain on the liver, which metabolizes both drugs. You don't have to be an "alcoholic" to get into trouble. If you have a drink every day, don't make a habit of using medicines containing acetaminophen. Not only might you risk serious liver damage, but also you might find that ordinary doses are less effective than expected and be tempted to take extra.
	Be alert for acetaminophen in many other products besides nonprescription pain relievers. It is an ingredient in many cold, allergy, or sinus formulas, menstrual cramp remedies, and even a number of prescription pain relievers (for example, **Darvocet-N** and **Tylox**). Be sure to read the label of any medication if you need to watch for this interaction.
Antabuse	This interaction is almost too obvious to mention. It can, however, be extremely hazardous. **Antabuse** (disulfiram) is prescribed for alcoholics who need chemical assistance to reinforce their resolve to abstain. In combination with alcohol, even the small amounts found in cough syrup or cold remedies, this medication produces violent illness. The symptoms are nausea, vomiting, stomach cramps, palpitations, flushing, low blood pressure, blurred vision, breathing problems, and headache. In some cases, the reaction could be lethal, so anyone on **Antabuse** really needs to watch out for alcohol.
Anticoagulants **Coumadin** warfarin	Moderate to heavy drinkers (at least two or three drinks daily) may metabolize blood thinners such as **Coumadin** (warfarin) more rapidly. This could be a problem if a person suddenly changed drinking habits dramatically. The dose of the medicine might need adjustment. For most people an occasional beer or cocktail is not likely to interfere with anticoagulant medication.

DRUG	**INTERACTION WITH ALCOHOL**
Antidepressants amitriptyline **Norpramin** desipramine **Pertofrane** **Desyrel** **Sinequan** doxepin **Surmontil** **Elavil** **Tofranil** **Endep** **Triavil**	Beware! Some antidepressants can make people feel drowsy or "spaced out." They may have trouble paying attention. Alcohol in addition could make matters worse and affect coordination. A drink or two can also slow metabolism of amitriptyline and possibly other antidepressants. Driving or operating machines may become far more dangerous with the double whammy of alcohol and medicine.
Antidepressants **Wellbutrin**	The antidepressant **Wellbutrin** (bupropion) can cause trouble when combined with alcohol. Susceptibility to seizures may increase when people change drinking patterns. Abstinence is recommended.
Antihistamines	Most antihistamines, except for **Claritin**, **Hismanal**, and **Seldane**, tend to make people feel groggy and less than completely alert. In fact, a person taking a sedating nonprescription antihistamine such as **Benadryl**, for example, might be just as dangerous behind the wheel as someone who is legally drunk. Alcohol can intensify this common reaction. Remember, cold medicines as well as allergy pills may contain antihistamines. Do not drive or do anything else requiring attention if you have had alcohol together with such medication. Reflexes and coordination could be seriously impaired.
Anxiety Pills **Ativan** diazepam **Klonopin** **Librium** meprobamate **Paxipam** **Serax** **Tranxene** **Valium** **Xanax**	We worry more about this drug alcohol interaction than most others because it is so common. People swallow tons of anti-anxiety agents and often seem to take these drugs for granted. But many of these compounds, both the popular benzodiazepines such as **Xanax** and the much older meprobamate (**Equanil** or **Miltown**), can alter reaction time and interfere with driving ability. Adding alcohol can lead to severe impairment of coordination and concentration, worse than with alcohol alone. Do not try to drive or engage in work that requires hand–eye coordination if you take one of these drugs and have anything to drink.

DRUG	INTERACTION WITH ALCOHOL

Aspirin and Salicylates
Alka-Seltzer
Anacin
Ascriptin
aspirin
Bayer Aspirin
Bufferin
Excedrin caplets
Pepto-Bismol
and others

Many people pop a few aspirin tablets before going out for a big night on the town in the hope of heading off a hangover. New research suggests this might be a bad idea. Not only could it increase stomach irritation, but also it could make someone more impaired because of higher blood alcohol levels.

One study found that aspirin taken an hour before drinking a modest amount of alcohol (one and a half drinks) raised levels in the bloodstream 26 percent. The authors caution that this could be enough to "impair some complex forms of human behavior." Be careful.

Barbiturates

Amytal	**Nembutal**
Butisol	phenobarbital
Fiorinal	**Seconal**
Gemonil	**Tuinal**
Mysoline	and others

Barbiturates don't mix well with alcohol at all. The interaction is actually rather complicated, because it differs if people are regular drinkers or go on a binge. Those who imbibe every day or several times a week metabolize these medicines more rapidly. The medicine may not work as it should. In some cases, that could lead to seizures. Both barbiturates and alcohol can put a strain on the liver.

People who don't usually drink and then have a couple of stiff ones also get into big trouble. They may become incapable of doing complicated things such as driving, walking, or even breathing. If you are taking one of these medicines, play it safe and steer clear of alcohol in any guise, including medicines. See the list on page 154.

Beta-Blockers

atenolol	**Lopressor**
Blocadren	propranolol
Cartrol	**Tenormin**
Corgard	timolol
Inderal	and others

Heart and blood pressure medicines such as **Corgard**, **Inderal**, **Lopressor**, **Tenormin**, and others like them may be affected by alcohol. Beta-blockers like these can increase the impact alcohol has on reflexes and coordination. Current research suggests this is not usually a serious interaction unless you are driving, but you might want to be judicious in your alcohol intake.

Beta Carotene

Beta carotene, a building block for vitamin A, may help reduce the risk of heart disease or even some types of cancer. This supplement may be harmful, however, to people who are regular or heavy drinkers. In studies on baboons, the combination of alcohol and beta carotene led to more liver damage than that produced by alcohol exposure alone. This work needs to be confirmed with further research on humans. See page 144 for further details.

DRUG	INTERACTION WITH ALCOHOL
Cephalosporin Antibiotics Cefobid Cefotan Mandol Moxam	Some of these high-powered antibiotics for injection can trigger an **Antabuse**-like reaction. **Cefobid, Cefotan, Mandol,** and **Moxam** are all reported to cause flushing, wheezing and breathing difficulties, nausea and vomiting, sweating, and rapid heart beat after alcohol ingestion. These medicines would normally be given in the hospital, but the effect can last up to two or three days after stopping the antibiotic. Celebrating a hospital discharge prematurely could land you back there! **Monocid** or **Precef** might interact in a very similar way. It would be wise to avoid medicines containing alcohol. See the table on page 154.
Diabetes Drugs DiaBeta Diabinese Dymelor Glucotrol Micronase Orinase Tolinase	Oral diabetes medicines interact in peculiar ways with alcohol. People on **Glucotrol** may find that their blood sugar stays low longer after a drink or two, but drinkers on **Orinase** might discover that its effectiveness starts wearing off more quickly. In other words, more than a single drink from time to time could make blood sugar harder to control. **Diabinese** is reported to interact with alcohol much as **Antabuse** does, producing flushing, headache, nausea, a burning sensation, and rapid heart beat. This unpleasant experience is more likely with moderate or heavy alcohol intake. Even people on other diabetes pills, such as **DiaBeta, Dymelor, Micronase,** and **Tolinase,** would be wise to exercise caution.
Ibuprofen Advil Ibuprin Medipren Motrin IB Nuprin and others	This popular pain reliever may interact with alcohol in several ways. For one thing, both ibuprofen and alcohol can have a negative effect on the digestive tract. Regular use could increase the risk of indigestion, heartburn, and even ulceration. There is also the possibility that ibuprofen may prolong the effects of alcohol within the system. Although this interaction is not yet well documented, it would be wise to use caution in drinking if you are relying on ibuprofen for pain relief.

DRUG	INTERACTION WITH ALCOHOL

Indomethacin
Indocin

Indomethacin and alcohol are both irritating to the digestive tract and should not be ingested together. Equally dangerous is their combined effect on the brain. **Indocin** can cause dizziness, drowsiness, and incoordination. Combined with alcohol, this complication could be aggravated.

Most other anti-inflammatory agents can cause stomach upset, and many can produce some degree of sedation. People taking **Anaprox**, **Ansaid**, **Clinoril**, **Feldene**, **Lodine**, **Meclomen**, **Motrin**, **Nalfon**, **Naprosyn**, **Orudis**, **Tolectin**, and **Voltaren** should also be prudent and avoid alcoholic beverages.

Ketoconazole
Nizoral

Nizoral (ketoconazole) is a very effective antifungal drug. It can, however, cause liver toxicity and requires periodic monitoring with blood tests. Regular drinking might increase the risk of liver problems.

There are also reports that some individuals may react to the combination of alcohol and **Nizoral** with symptoms of nausea, headache, flushing, and discomfort, apparently similar to an **Antabuse** reaction. Watch out for medicines that contain alcohol, page 154.

Major Tranquilizers
chlorpromazine **Sparine**
Compazine **Stelazine**
Mellaril **Temaril**
Permitil **Thorazine**
Phenergan **Tindal**
Prolixin **Trilafon**
Serentil **Vesprin**

Many of the medicines used to treat serious mental disturbances can make people feel "spaced out" or interfere with their alertness. Add alcohol, and you have a situation in which dizziness, drowsiness, and lack of coordination could become downright dangerous. Muscle twitching and uncontrolled movements can be triggered with such a combination.

No one taking a major tranquilizer should be drinking. Driving is dangerous with these medicines all by themselves. If someone were foolish enough to add even one glass of wine, he could be a major hazard on the highways. Don't do it!

Methotrexate
Methotrate
Rheumatrex

Methotrexate is a potent medication used to treat cancer, severe arthritis, and psoriasis. It can cause liver toxicity and requires very careful monitoring. Since alcohol can also injure the liver, it is probably a good idea to avoid drinking alcoholic beverages while on methotrexate.

DRUG	INTERACTION WITH ALCOHOL
Metoclopramide **Reglan**	Few people would suspect that their medicine for heartburn can interact with a beer or cocktail. But **Reglan** can cause drowsiness, involuntary muscle movements, and dizziness. Alcohol could make such reactions worse. It would be prudent to avoid alcoholic beverages.

Metronidazole
  Femizole
  Flagyl
  Metizol
  Metryl
  Protostat
	This medication is useful for fighting a number of infections. It can cause dizziness, unsteadiness, and incoordination all by itself. These side effects may be aggravated by alcohol. In addition, some people experience nausea, vomiting, stomach cramps, flushing, and headaches when they consume alcohol together with metronidazole. Best to avoid drinking while on this drug.

Narcotics
  codeine **Percodan**
  Darvocet propoxyphene
  Darvon **Talwin**
  Demerol **Tylenol**
  Empirin **w/ Codeine**
   w/ Codeine Tylox
  Percocet **Vicodin**
	Heavy-duty pain relievers can themselves interfere with alertness and coordination. In combination with alcohol, any of them could make a person feel like a zombie. Driving or doing anything that requires concentration would be a big mistake. Medical examiners see far too many overdose deaths associated with this combination of drugs. Stay alive–don't imbibe.

Nitroglycerin
  Nitro-Bid
  Nitro-Dur
  Nitrostat
  Transderm-Nitro,
  and others
	Nitroglycerin comes in many formulations. There are pills (**Nitro-Bid**, **Nitrong**, **Nitrostat**), ointments (**Nitrol**), and transdermal patches (**Minitran**, **Nitrodisc**, **Nitro-Dur,** and **Transderm-Nitro**). No matter how you use nitro, though, you should avoid alcohol, as it may lower your blood pressure and make you dizzy and vulnerable to fainting and falls.

Oral Contraceptives	This interaction isn't well documented so it may not be a problem for all women. In one study, alcohol was metabolized more slowly by women on estrogen-containing birth control pills. One or two glasses of wine might not cause trouble. Heavier drinking may produce longer-lasting intoxication.
Parlodel bromocriptine	**Parlodel** (bromocriptine) may produce more severe side effects if alcohol is taken at the same time. Watch out for nausea, stomach pain, and dizziness.

DRUG	INTERACTION WITH ALCOHOL

Sleeping Pills
  Dalmane
  Doral
  Doriden
  Halcion
  ProSom
  Restoril
	This drug/alcohol interaction is, unfortunately, all too common. A lot of people take sleeping pills, and often take these drugs for granted. But many of these compounds can cause drowsiness, incoordination, and slow reaction time. In combination with a nightcap, coordination and concentration could be severely impaired. This is true of both the old-fashioned sleeping pills such as **Doriden** and the benzodiazepines.
	
	A long-acting sleeping pill such as **Dalmane** taken the night before can even interact badly with a drink or two the next afternoon. If you need sleeping pills, it is better to avoid alcohol.

Time Capsules
  Compazine Spansule
  Dexedrine Spansule
  Isoclor Timesule
  Nicobid Tempule
  Ornade Spansule
  Tuss-Ornade Spansule
	This interaction is controversial, but if you use one of these timed-release medicines, you may want to keep it in mind. The fear is that alcohol might dissolve the protective coating that would normally slow absorption and spread it out over several hours. Once this coating is gone, the active ingredients can quickly end up in the bloodstream, and instead of 12-hour action you might end up getting too much medicine too fast. Play it safe and avoid alcohol when taking any slow-release time capsules.

Tuberculosis Drug
  INH
  Laniazid
  Nydrazid
	Isoniazid, a medication often used in combination with others to treat tuberculosis, has the potential to be harmful to the liver. Regular intake of alcohol (drinking every day or several times a week) increases the risk of drug-induced hepatitis. This is a nasty possibility and is better avoided.

DRUG	INTERACTION WITH ALCOHOL
Ulcer Drugs **Tagamet** **Zantac**	There is controversy over the clinical significance of this interaction. Research has shown that **Tagamet**, **Zantac**, and possibly **Axid** can interfere with the activity of the stomach enzyme called alcohol dehydrogenase. Since some alcohol may be metabolized by this enzyme even before it gets into the bloodstream, drinking while on one of these ulcer medications could lead to higher blood alcohol levels. The manufacturers of **Zantac** and **Tagamet** insist that this interaction is unimportant in the real world, as investigations showed the biggest effect in men who drink modestly, just about one and a half or two drinks, after eating. Although in such a situation a man might be more impaired than he realized, he might not be legally drunk. We agree with the researchers, who concluded, "A warning may be appropriate when these drugs are prescribed, especially in social drinkers who may drive vehicles or operate other machinery that require a high degree of attention and/or coordination." [7]
Verapamil **Calan** **Isoptin** **Verelan**	A careful study has shown that a standard amount of alcohol results in higher blood alcohol levels that last longer in the body when a person is taking verapamil. This could interfere with the judgment and coordination needed to drive or do other complex tasks. A person who had not been warned about this interaction might not realize how much more impaired he or she would become.
Vitamin C	Here's a twist. In one study, the volunteers who took 1 gram of ascorbic acid (vitamin C) every day for two weeks got the alcohol out of their bloodstream slightly more quickly. Perhaps they revved up their alcohol dehydrogenase this way; no one is quite sure. This doesn't offer license to go out and drink heavily, but it shows it's hard to go wrong with vitamin C.

Medicines Containing Alcohol

Alcohol is an ingredient in many over-the-counter and even some prescription medicines. The amounts are modest in most cases, but a few reach concentrations of 40 or 50 proof. Cough and cold elixirs are the most likely sources, but some vitamin "tonics" and laxatives also contain alcohol.

For most people, the amount of alcohol in a spoonful of cough syrup is negligible. Anyone taking a medicine that reacts with alcohol the same way **Antabuse** does needs to be especially cautious. Some alcohol-containing medicines are listed below. Careful label reading is also advised.

Ambenyl-D Decongestant
Benadryl Plus Nighttime
Benylin Decongestant
Black-Draught
Cheracol Plus Head Cold/
    Cough Formula
Comtrex Liquid
Contac Nighttime Cold
    Medicine Liquid
Entex Liquid
Geravite Elixir
Geriplex-FS Liquid
Gevrabon Liquid
Hycotuss Expectorant
Lomotil Liquid
Medi-Flu Liquid
Novahistine Elixir

NyQuil Nighttime Cold
Peri-Colace
Pertussin PM Liquid
Phenergan VC Syrup
Senokot Syrup
Triaminic Expectorant
    with Codeine
Trind Liquid
Tussar SF Syrup
Tuss-Ornade Liquid
Tylenol Cold Night Time
Vicks Formula 44
    (D or M) Liquid
Vigortol Liquid
Vitamin B
    Complex Elixir
Zantac Syrup

References

1. Caballeria, J., et al. "The Contribution of the Stomach to Ethanol Oxidation in the Rat." *Life Sci.* 1987; 41:1021–1027.
2. Caballeria, J., et al. "Gastric Origin of the First-Pass Metabolism of Ethanol in Humans: Effects of Gastrectomy." *Gastroenterology* 1989; 97:1205–1209.
3. Frezza, C., et al. "High Blood Alcohol Levels in Women. The Role of Decreased Gastric Alcohol Dehydrogenase Activity and Blood Ethanol Levels. *N. Engl. J. Med.* 1990; 322:95–99.
4. Roine, Risto, et al. "Aspirin Increases Blood Alcohol Concentrations in Humans after Ingestion of Ethanol." *JAMA* 1990; 264:2406–2408.
5. DiPadova, Carlo, et al. "Effects of Ranitidine on Blood Alcohol Levels after Ethanol Ingestion." *JAMA* 1992; 267:83–86.
6. Caballeria J., et al. "Effects of Cimetidine on Gastric Alcohol Dehydrogenase Activity and Blood Ethanol Levels." *Gastroenterology* 1989; 96:388–392.
7. DiPadova, op. cit.
8. Levitt, M.D. "Review Article: Lack of Clinical Significance of the Interaction Between H_2-receptor Antagonists and Ethanol." *Aliment. Pharmacol. Ther.* 1993; 7:131–138.
9. F.D.C Reports: "The Pink Sheet." March 22, 1993, pp. 10–11.
10. Bauer, L.A., et al. "Verapamil Inhibits Ethanol Elimination and Prolongs the Perception of Intoxication." *Clin. Pharmacol. Ther.* 1992; 52:6–10.
11. Leo, M.A.: "Interaction of Ethanol with B-Carotene: Delayed Blood Clearance and Enhanced Hepatotoxicity." *Hepatology* 1992; 15:883–891.

References for the Drug/Alcohol Interactions Table

DiPadova, C., et al. "Effects of Ranitidine on Blood Alcohol Levels after Ethanol Ingestion." *JAMA* 1992; 267:83–86.

Graedon, J. *The People's Pharmacy-2.* New York: Avon, 1980.

Graedon, J., and T. Graedon. *The People's Pharmacy (Totally New & Revised).* New York: St. Martin's Press, 1985.

Hansten, P. D., and J.R. Horn, eds. *Drug Interactions and Updates.* Vancouver, Wash.: Applied Therapeutics, 1993.

Holford, N. "Clinical Pharmacokinetics of Ethanol." *Clin. Pharmacokinet.* 1987; 13:273–292.

Leo, M.A., et al. "Interaction of Ethanol with ß-Carotene: Delayed Blood Clearance and Enhanced Hepatotoxicity." *Hepatology* 1992; 15:883–891.

Palmer, R.H., et al. "Effects of Various Concomitant Medications on Gastric Alcohol Dehydrogenase and the First-Pass Metabolism of Ethanol." *Am J. Gastroenterology* 1991; 86:1749–1755.

Roine, R., et al. "Aspirin Increases Blood Alcohol Concentrations in Humans after Ingestion of Ethanol." *JAMA* 1990; 264:2406–2408.

Tatro, D., ed. *Drug Interaction Facts*. St.Louis: Facts & Comparisons (A Wolters Kluwer Company), 1993.

Yamanaka-Yuen, N. "Ethanol and Drug Interactions." *Drug Interactions Newsletter* 1985; 5:45–58.

Guides to Dangerous Drug Interactions

ATTENTION

These guides are not intended as a substitute for the medical advice of physicians. Due to space limitations, the charts do not include every serious or even potentially deadly drug interaction that has been reported in the medical literature.

This is a constantly changing field. After we completed the book, controversial interactions continued to come to our attention. For example, there is a possibility that **Prozac** (fluoxetine) may interact with **Seldane** (terfenadine) to increase the risk of heart problems. In addition, **Luvox** (fluvoxamine), a **Prozac**-like drug that is prescribed for obsessive-compulsive disorder, has the potential for very dangerous interactions with **Anafranil** (clomipramine), **Elavil** (amitriptyline), **Eldepryl** (selegiline), **Hismanal** (astemizole), **Nardil** (phenelzine), **Parnate** (tranylcypromine), **Seldane**, **Surmontil** (trimipramine), and **Tofranil** (imipramine). Doubtless other serious interactions will come to light.

Please remember that certain drugs with potentially lethal interactions can be successfully used together if appropriate monitoring and other precautions are undertaken. To better use these guides, take a moment to review the explanation on pages 12 to 17. Anyone who discovers an interaction in this book that is of concern must consult a physician before making any changes in drug therapy. **Every reader must consult with his or her physician before starting or stopping any medication.** Any side effects should be reported promptly to a physician.

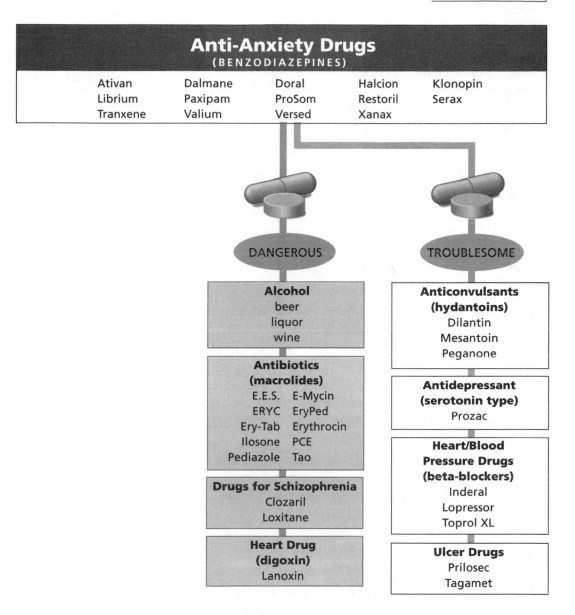

Anti-Anxiety Drugs
(BENZODIAZEPINES)

Ativan	Dalmane	Doral	Halcion	Klonopin
Librium	Paxipam	ProSom	Restoril	Serax
Tranxene	Valium	Versed	Xanax	

DANGEROUS

TROUBLESOME

Alcohol
beer
liquor
wine

**Antibiotics
(macrolides)**
E.E.S.   E-Mycin
ERYC   EryPed
Ery-Tab   Erythrocin
Ilosone   PCE
Pediazole   Tao

Drugs for Schizophrenia
Clozaril
Loxitane

**Heart Drug
(digoxin)**
Lanoxin

**Anticonvulsants
(hydantoins)**
Dilantin
Mesantoin
Peganone

**Antidepressant
(serotonin type)**
Prozac

**Heart/Blood
Pressure Drugs
(beta-blockers)**
Inderal
Lopressor
Toprol XL

Ulcer Drugs
Prilosec
Tagamet

Not every benzodiazepine drug interacts with each drug listed on this tree. See individual descriptions for details. Be sure to check with your physician and pharmacist if you must take any other drugs in combination with a benzodiazepine.

LEVELS OF HAZARD: LIFE THREATENING   DANGEROUS   TROUBLESOME

Anti-Anxiety Drugs

(BENZODIAZEPINES)

Alcohol

BRAND NAME	GENERIC NAME
Ativan	lorazepam
Dalmane	flurazepam
Doral	quazepam
Halcion	triazolam
Klonopin	clonazepam
Librium	chlordiazepoxide
Paxipam	halazepam
ProSom	estazolam
Restoril	temazepam
Serax	oxazepam
Tranxene	clorazepate
Valium	diazepam
Versed	midazolam
Xanax	alprazolam

DESCRIPTION

Benzodiazepines are used primarily to treat anxiety disorders and insomnia. Some have also been employed to relieve panic attacks, seizures, muscle cramps, and contractions. Anesthesiologists often use such medications before certain surgical procedures.

Prolonged use may lead to dependence. Sudden withdrawal can produce unpleasant side effects and should always be supervised by a physician.

INSTRUCTIONS

These drugs may be taken with food, especially if they upset the digestive tract.

NAME

beer
liquor
wine
medicines that contain alcohol

DESCRIPTION

Alcohol comes in many guises. The obvious ones are liquor, beer, and wine. But you can also find substantial amounts of alcohol in certain medicines. Over-the-counter cough and cold products can contain up to 40 or 50 proof (20 to 25 percent by volume), which is a higher alcohol content than you would find in beer or wine. "Nighttime" remedies such as NyQuil, Nytcold Medicine, and Pertussin PM Liquid are all 50 proof. This may not be a problem if all you take is a spoonful before bedtime, but some drugs may interact poorly with even modest amounts of alcohol.

INSTRUCTIONS

The absorption and effects of alcohol are magnified if you drink on an empty stomach. Fatty food can delay alcohol absorption. If you drink, do so in moderation, and never drive.

INTERACTION

Benzodiazepines such as Valium, Librium, and Xanax can make people more relaxed, uncoordinated, confused, sedated, and unsteady. Reflexes and judgment may also be affected. Alcohol can cause many of the same effects. Combine alcohol with an anti-anxiety agent and driving becomes extremely hazardous, as does any task that requires alertness, good reflexes, and judgment. Older people may be more likely to fall. That could lead to a hip fracture, which can be devastating or lethal. Be safe; don't mix alcohol with sedating drugs.

Symptoms of Alcohol or Benzodiazepine Overdose

This interaction could lead to symptoms of overdose such as disorientation, unsteadiness, confusion, slurred speech, drowsiness, dizziness, or loss of motor coordination. Driving or operating machinery would be a mistake. Contact your physician if such symptoms occur.

Never take or stop medication without your doctor's advice.

INTERACTION

DANGEROUS

Anti-Anxiety Drugs

(BENZODIAZEPINES)

Antibiotics

(MACROLIDES)

BRAND NAME	GENERIC NAME
Halcion	triazolam
Versed	midazolam

(other benzodiazepines may also be affected)

BRAND NAME	GENERIC NAME
E.E.S.	erythromycin
E-Mycin	erythromycin
ERYC	erythromycin
EryPed	erythromycin
Ery-Tab	erythromycin
Erythrocin	erythromycin
Ilosone	erythromycin
PCE	erythromycin
Pediazole	erythromycin
Tao	troleandomycin

DESCRIPTION

The benzodiazepines have been used primarily to treat anxiety disorders. Halcion is very short acting and is employed to relieve insomnia. Anesthesiologists often give Versed just prior to surgery to produce sedation. It is sometimes injected by itself or with a narcotic pain reliever for short diagnostic procedures (endoscopy) or for minor surgery.

Prolonged use of Halcion may lead to dependence. Sudden withdrawal can produce unpleasant side effects including rebound insomnia, anxiety, panic attacks, and disorientation and should always be supervised by a physician.

DESCRIPTION

These broad-spectrum antibiotics are widely prescribed for respiratory tract, sinus, ear, and skin infections. They are also effective against *Chlamydia* and certain other infections of the reproductive tract.

INSTRUCTIONS

Halcion may be taken with food, especially if it upsets the digestive tract. It should be taken just before bedtime.

INSTRUCTIONS

Some forms of erythromycin must be taken on an empty stomach; others may be taken with food See the table of Food and Drug Compatibility on pages 59-73 for specifics.

INTERACTION

Erythromycin and Tao appear to have a profound effect on the metabolism of certain benzodiazepines. Blood levels of Halcion could be doubled by erythromycin. Tao has increased blood levels of Halcion by over 100 percent and has prolonged the action of the drug in the body. Elevated levels of Halcion can lead to cognitive impairment and amnesia.

Erythromycin may also have an important impact on Versed, and can cause blood levels of this preanesthetic to climb. This could create increased sedation during or after surgery. Anyone taking such antibiotics must alert the surgeon and anesthesiologist before surgery so that they can anticipate any potential problems due to this interaction.

Symptoms of Benzodiazepine Overdose

This interaction could lead to symptoms of overdose such as disorientation, unsteadiness, confusion, slurred speech, drowsiness, dizziness, amnesia, and loss of motor coordination. Some other benzodiazepines may also be affected by these antibiotics. Contact your physician if such symptoms occur.

Never take or stop medication without your doctor's advice.

INTERACTION

DANGEROUS

Anti-Anxiety Drugs
(BENZODIAZEPINES)

Drugs for Schizophrenia

BRAND NAME	GENERIC NAME
Ativan	lorazepam
Valium	diazepam

BRAND NAME	GENERIC NAME
Clozaril	clozapine
Loxitane	loxapine

DESCRIPTION

Benzodiazepines are used primarily to treat anxiety disorders and insomnia. Some have also been employed to relieve panic attacks, seizures, muscle cramps, and contractions. Anesthesiologists often use such medications before certain surgical procedures. Ativan is also used with cancer chemotherapy to ease symptoms of nausea and vomiting.

Prolonged use may lead to dependence. Sudden withdrawal can produce unpleasant side effects and should always be supervised by a physician.

DESCRIPTION

Clozaril and Loxitane are prescribed to treat schizophrenia. While chemically different from such major tranquilizers as Thorazine, Stelazine, Mellaril, and Haldol, they produce many of the same effects. These medications can cause uncontrollable muscle movements called tardive dyskinesia. Even if the drugs are stopped, the symptoms may sometimes persist. Clozaril may be more easily tolerated, but it can cause a dangerous blood disorder. Check with the physician and pharmacist before taking any other drugs.

INSTRUCTIONS

Ativan and Valium may be taken with food, especially if they upset the digestive tract.

INSTRUCTIONS

The dose should be individualized. Driving is dangerous. Those on Loxitane should avoid sunlight (unless adequately protected) because it may cause a bad sunburn. Clozaril patients require weekly blood tests. They should notify the doctor promptly of fever above 100.4°F.

INTERACTION

A number of cases in the medical literature point to an interaction between loxapine and lorazepam, as well as between Clozaril and Valium or Ativan. These patients, treated with both drugs, developed difficulty breathing and very low blood pressure. In some instances respiration slowed to between four and eight breaths a minute. One patient died, although it is unclear whether the interaction was responsible. Many patients fell deeply asleep and could not be roused. The stupor lasted a number of hours.

Research on this interaction is incomplete and many patients do well with a benzodiazepine and one of these schizophrenia medicines. Because there is potential for a dangerous interaction, though, it would seem prudent to try to avoid such a combination if possible. If these drugs are prescribed simultaneously, patients should have vital signs monitored closely! *Symptoms of an Adverse Lorazepam/Loxapine or Diazepam/Clozapine Reaction* Dizziness, drowsiness, and fatigue may occur quickly and lead to delirium or stupor, low blood pressure, and very slow breathing. Blue fingernails and lips are a danger sign. Careful monitoring of respiration and blood pressure are essential. Notify the physician immediately of any such symptoms of an adverse interaction.

INTERACTION

DANGEROUS

Anti-Anxiety Drugs

(BENZODIAZEPINES)

Heart Drug

(DIGOXIN)

BRAND NAME	GENERIC NAME
Ativan	lorazepam
Dalmane	flurazepam
Doral	quazepam
Halcion	triazolam
Klonopin	clonazepam
Librium	chlordiazepoxide
Paxipam	halazepam
ProSom	estazolam
Restoril	temazepam
Serax	oxazepam
Tranxene	clorazepate
Valium	diazepam
Versed	midazolam
Xanax	alprazolam

DESCRIPTION

Benzodiazepines are used to treat anxiety disorders and insomnia. Some are employed to relieve panic attacks, seizures, and muscle cramps. Anesthesiologists use such medications before certain surgical procedures.

Prolonged use may lead to dependence. Withdrawal should always be supervised by a physician.

INSTRUCTIONS

These drugs may be taken with food, especially if they upset the digestive tract.

BRAND NAME	GENERIC NAME
Lanoxin	digoxin

DESCRIPTION

Digoxin is a heart drug that is often very helpful in treating congestive heart failure. It is also prescribed for certain heart rhythm changes, especially atrial fibrillation, atrial flutter, and paroxysmal atrial tachycardia (PAT). The doctor must monitor digoxin dose carefully, because the effective dose is not far below the toxic dose. Older people may need dose adjustment.

INSTRUCTIONS

Digoxin should be taken in a consistent fashion, preferably with food but not with a meal high in fiber. Bran may limit the absorption of this drug.

Do not stop this medicine unless your doctor so directs.

INTERACTION

Valium (diazepam) has been shown to raise the blood levels of digoxin. One woman had a dramatic jump in digoxin after she started taking Xanax at bedtime for insomnia. She experienced symptoms of digoxin toxicity, including digestive tract upset, fatigue, and "head pressure." This Xanax and digoxin interaction remains unconfirmed in a more scientific study, however. Other benzodiazepines have not be adequately tested. Until such research is completed, people should have their digoxin levels monitored frequently if they need to take a benzodiazepine-type drug simultaneously.

Symptoms of Digoxin Toxicity

Nausea, vomiting, loss of appetite, diarrhea, stomach pain, visual disturbances (green or yellow tint and a halo around lights), weakness, drowsiness, depression, confusion, palpitations, rash, headaches, and hallucinations. Notify the doctor immediately if you experience any of these symptoms.

INTERACTION

DANGEROUS

Anti-Anxiety Drugs

(BENZODIAZEPINES)

Anticonvulsants

(HYDANTOINS)

BRAND NAME	GENERIC NAME
Ativan	lorazepam
Dalmane	flurazepam
Doral	quazepam
Halcion	triazolam
Librium	chlordiazepoxide
Paxipam	halazepam
ProSom	estazolam
Restoril	temazepam
Serax	oxazepam
Tranxene	clorazepate
Valium	diazepam
Xanax	alprazolam

DESCRIPTION

Benzodiazepines are used primarily to treat anxiety disorders and insomnia. Some have also been employed to relieve panic attacks, seizures, muscle cramps, and contractions. Anesthesiologists often use such medications before certain surgical procedures.

Prolonged use may lead to dependence. Sudden withdrawal can produce unpleasant side effects and should always be supervised by a physician.

INSTRUCTIONS

These drugs may be taken with food, especially if they upset the digestive tract.

BRAND NAME	GENERIC NAME
Dilantin	phenytoin
Mesantoin	mephenytoin
Peganone	ethotoin

DESCRIPTION

These anticonvulsants are used to prevent epileptic seizures or seizures associated with brain surgery. Occasionally they may be prescribed to treat severe stabbing facial pain (trigeminal neuralgia). Tests may be needed to check blood cells, blood levels of the drug, liver function, and blood sugar. Special attention to oral hygiene is needed to prevent gum problems often associated with taking these anticonvulsants. Hydantoin anticonvulsants interact with many other drugs as well as alcohol, so check carefully with your physician and pharmacist before taking any other medication.

INSTRUCTIONS

Any of these medicines could upset the stomach. This is less likely if they are taken with food. All of them can cause drowsiness or blurred vision and could make driving dangerous.

INTERACTION

This is a confusing interaction. The data are contradictory and no firm conclusions can be drawn. Nevertheless, there is some concern that Dilantin (phenytoin) levels may be increased by Valium or Librium. Some patients have apparently experienced symptoms of phenytoin toxicity as a result of this combination. Experts suggest that if patients need a benzodiazepine in addition to Dilantin, their blood phenytoin levels be monitored carefully, especially when starting or stopping the benzodiazepine. Although there is no information about anti-anxiety drugs other than Valium and Librium, the possibility exists that other benzodiazepines might interact as well.

Symptoms of Phenytoin Toxicity

Uncontrollable eye movements (nystagmus), unsteadiness, difficulty speaking clearly, dizziness, and stupor. Notify your physician immediately of any of these symptoms.

INTERACTION

TROUBLESOME

Anti-Anxiety Drugs

(BENZODIAZEPINES)

Antidepressant

(SEROTONIN-BASED)

BRAND NAME	GENERIC NAME
Valium	diazepam
Xanax	alprazolam

DESCRIPTION

The benzodiazepines have been used primarily to treat anxiety disorders and insomnia. Some have also been employed to relieve panic attacks, seizures, muscle cramps, and contractions. Anesthesiologists often give such medications prior to certain surgical procedures. Xanax has also been prescribed for agoraphobia (fear of crowds or open spaces), premenstrual tension, and psychological depression.

Prolonged use may lead to dependence. Sudden withdrawal can produce unpleasant side effects and should always be supervised by a physician.

INSTRUCTIONS

These drugs may be taken with food, especially if they upset the digestive tract.

BRAND NAME	GENERIC NAME
Prozac	fluoxetine

DESCRIPTION

This antidepressant works by blocking the reuptake into brain cells of serotonin, a chemical messenger. Because it works differently from the older cyclic-type antidepressants, it has a different set of side effects and has become more popular. It may also work against a different array of problems, for instance, bulimia or obsessive-compulsive disorder. Older people and those with kidney or liver problems may need reduced doses. Prozac is cleared from the body very slowly and may linger weeks after discontinuation.

INSTRUCTIONS

Prozac is taken in the morning, or, if a higher dose has been prescribed, in the morning and at noon. It may be taken without regard to meals. Taking it with food may reduce stomach upset. A few patients experience serious weight loss on this medication. If this occurs, the doctor should be notified.

INTERACTION

This is not a particularly worrisome interaction. In fact, physicians may often prescribe drugs such as Valium or Xanax to counteract the jittery feelings and insomnia that are sometime associated with Prozac. If this combination is contemplated, however, there should be some consideration for the potential of these drugs to interact. Reports have surfaced linking Prozac to slightly higher blood levels of diazepam. Diazepam lasted longer in the body when people were also taking Prozac. The clinical significance of this interaction is unclear. Data on Xanax and Prozac are contradictory. One study demonstrated a slight effect while another showed no impact. There may be no cause for concern, but until further research is done people should be alert for increased effects from Valium or Xanax. Tasks that require coordination and attentiveness, like driving, could be affected.

Symptoms of Benzodiazepine Overdose

Disorientation, unsteadiness, confusion, slurred speech, drowsiness, dizziness, amnesia, and loss of motor coordination are tipoffs to overdose. Driving is hazardous! Contact the physician immediately if any such signs of overdose appear.

INTERACTION

TROUBLESOME

Anti-Anxiety Drugs
(BENZODIAZEPINES)

Heart/Blood Pressure Drugs
(BETA-BLOCKERS)

BRAND NAME	GENERIC NAME
Dalmane	flurazepam
Halcion	triazolam
Librium	chlordiazepoxide
Tranxene	clorazepate
Valium	diazepam
Xanax	alprazolam

DESCRIPTION

Benzodiazepines are used primarily to treat anxiety disorders and insomnia. Some have also been employed to relieve panic attacks, seizures, muscle cramps, and contractions. Anesthesiologists often use such medications before certain surgical procedures. Xanax has also been prescribed for agoraphobia (fear of crowds or open spaces), premenstrual tension, and psychological depression.

Prolonged use may lead to dependence. Sudden withdrawal can produce unpleasant side effects and should always be supervised by a physician.

INSTRUCTIONS

These drugs may be taken with food, especially if they upset the digestive tract.

BRAND NAME	GENERIC NAME
Inderal	propranolol
Lopressor	metoprolol
Toprol XL	metoprolol

DESCRIPTION

Beta-blockers such as these are often used to lower blood pressure, stabilize irregular heartbeats, relieve angina, or prevent migraines. Despite the great usefulness and versatility of these medicines, in general they are not appropriate for people with chronic breathing problems because they can trigger airway tightening. Other side effects include changes in heart rate, cold hands and feet, and depression.

INSTRUCTIONS

Propranolol and metoprolol are best absorbed with meals, but consistency is the most important factor. These drugs should be taken at about the same time every day. Do not stop any of these medicines suddenly except on doctor's orders. Serious side effects could result.

INTERACTION

Blood levels of diazepam may be slightly increased by beta-blockers such as metoprolol or propranolol. The anti-anxiety agent also appears to persist longer in the body. People may find they are less alert when on such a combination and their visual acuity and reaction time might be affected. Serax does not seem to be impacted by propranolol. Be sensitive for any change in consciousness.

Symptoms of Benzodiazepine Overdose

This interaction could lead to symptoms of overdose such as disorientation, unsteadiness, confusion, slurred speech, drowsiness, dizziness, amnesia, or loss of motor coordination. Some other benzodiazepines may also be affected by these beta-blockers. Contact your physician if such symptoms occur.

INTERACTION

TROUBLESOME

Anti-Anxiety Drugs

(BENZODIAZEPINES)

Ulcer Drugs

BRAND NAME	GENERIC NAME
Ativan	lorazepam
Dalmane	flurazepam
Doral	quazepam
Halcion	triazolam
Klonopin	clonazepam
Librium	chlordiazepoxide
Paxipam	halazepam
ProSom	estazolam
Restoril	temazepam
Serax	oxazepam
Tranxene	clorazepate
Valium	diazepam
Versed	midazolam
Xanax	alprazolam

DESCRIPTION

Benzodiazepines are used primarily to treat anxiety disorders and insomnia. Some have also been employed to relieve panic attacks, seizures, and muscle cramps. Anesthesiologists often give such medications before certain surgical procedures. Prolonged use may lead to dependence. Sudden withdrawal can produce unpleasant side effects and should always be supervised by a physician.

INSTRUCTIONS

These drugs may be taken with food, especially if they upset the digestive tract.

BRAND NAME	GENERIC NAME
Prilosec	omeprazole
Tagamet	cimetidine

DESCRIPTION

Tagamet treats ulcers and serious heartburn by blocking special receptors, thereby reducing the acid environment of the stomach. Cimetidine usually has few side effects, although headaches, dizziness, and mild diarrhea are potential reactions. Antitestosterone effects at higher doses may lead to enlarged breasts or sexual problems for men. The elderly and the ill may experience depression, confusion, or disorientation, requiring a dose adjustment. Tagamet may modify the metabolism of a number of medications, so check with your doctor and pharmacist if you take cimetidine with another medicine.

Prilosec is a powerful acid suppressor that works through an entirely different mechanism. It too is effective for ulcers and severe heartburn.

INSTRUCTIONS

Tagamet is usually taken with meals and/or at bedtime. Antacids may reduce absorption of Tagamet; do not take one for at least two hours after taking Tagamet. Prilosec should be taken just before eating, preferably in the morning.

INTERACTION

Tagamet can increase blood levels of benzodiazepines and prolong their stay in the body. Sedation and impairment could result, especially for older people. This interaction remains controversial since the data are contradictory. Be vigilant for any drowsiness or incoordination. Prilosec may have even more potential to increase blood levels of drugs such as diazepam and prolong their action. Sleeping pills such as Dalmane and Halcion may be affected by Prilosec. Unsteadiness is a possible complication.

Symptoms of Benzodiazepine Overdose

This interaction could lead to symptoms of overdose such as disorientation, unsteadiness, confusion, slurred speech, drowsiness, dizziness, amnesia, and loss of motor coordination. Some other benzodiazepines may also be affected by these ulcer drugs. Contact your physician if such symptoms occur.

INTERACTION

TROUBLESOME

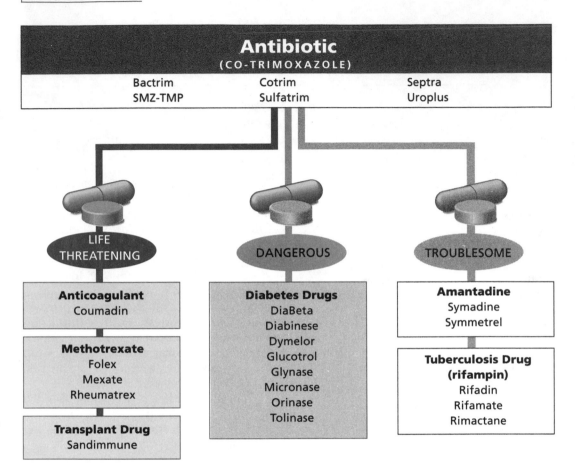

Antibiotic
(CO-TRIMOXAZOLE)

Bactrim	Cotrim	Septra
SMZ-TMP	Sulfatrim	Uroplus

LIFE THREATENING

DANGEROUS

TROUBLESOME

Anticoagulant
Coumadin

Methotrexate
Folex
Mexate
Rheumatrex

Transplant Drug
Sandimmune

Diabetes Drugs
DiaBeta
Diabinese
Dymelor
Glucotrol
Glynase
Micronase
Orinase
Tolinase

Amantadine
Symadine
Symmetrel

**Tuberculosis Drug
(rifampin)**
Rifadin
Rifamate
Rimactane

Interactions listed on this overview tree are the most important but not the only medicines with which co-trimoxazole interacts. See individual descriptions for details. Be sure to check with your physician and pharmacist if you must take any other drugs in combination with this antibiotic.

LEVELS OF HAZARD: LIFE THREATENING DANGEROUS TROUBLESOME

Antibiotic

(CO-TRIMOXAZOLE)

Anticoagulant

(WARFARIN)

BRAND NAME

Bactrim   Cotrim   Septra
SMZ-TMP   Sulfatrim   Uroplus
(All co-trimoxazole, formerly known as trimethoprim-sulfamethoxazole)

DESCRIPTION

Bactrim, Septra, and other brands of co-trimoxazole are often prescribed for urinary tract infections or ear infections. They may also be useful in treating traveler's diarrhea and certain types of bronchitis and pneumonia. Occasionally such antibiotics may result in superinfection that must be treated with a different drug. Some people become more sensitive to sunlight—and more susceptible to sunburn—when taking one of these drugs. Side effects may include gastrointestinal upset, headache, rash, and yellow skin and eyes.

INSTRUCTIONS

This drug is best absorbed when taken on an empty stomach, at least one hour before or two hours after a meal. It may be taken with food if it upsets the stomach. Drink at least eight cups of water a day to help keep the drug from crystallizing in the kidneys, and avoid large doses of vitamin C.

BRAND NAME   GENERIC NAME

Coumadin   warfarin

DESCRIPTION

Warfarin slows the liver's production of factors essential for the formation of blood clots. It is prescribed when there is a risk that a dangerous clot could form in a deep vein or a blood vessel leading to the lungs, heart, or brain. The most serious complication of anticoagulant treatment is excessive bleeding. The dosage must be individually adjusted, requiring daily blood tests at first, then tests every four to six weeks. Other side effects may include nausea, loss of appetite, rash, fever, yellow eyes and skin, prolonged painful erection, and hair loss.

INSTRUCTIONS

Warfarin tablets can be swallowed with food or on an empty stomach. Try to avoid large variations in the quantity of vitamin-K–containing vegetables—such as broccoli, cabbage, or spinach—that you eat each day. Consuming much more or less than usual could change the action of the drug.

INTERACTION

Sulfa antibiotics such as Bactrim can substantially increase the effects of warfarin. *This interaction could trigger life-threatening bleeding.*

Apparently, co-trimoxazole interferes with the metabolism of warfarin in the liver, leading to higher blood levels of the anticoagulant. When this combination of medications is required, the doctor will order frequent blood tests to check prothrombin (clotting) time.

Symptoms of Warfarin Overdose

There may be no early warning signs of danger. Blood tests are essential. Symptoms include any unusual bleeding, including rectal or urinary tract bleeding, excessive menstrual bleeding, nosebleeds, bleeding around gums, bruising, red or tar-black stools, vomiting blood, red or dark-brown urine. Notify your doctor immediately if you suspect a problem.

Never take or stop medication without your doctor's advice.

INTERACTION

LIFE THREATENING

Antibiotic

(CO-TRIMOXAZOLE)

Methotrexate

BRAND NAME

**Bactrim   Cotrim   Septra
SMZ-TMP   Sulfatrim   Uroplus**
(All co-trimoxazole, formerly known as
trimethoprim-sulfamethoxazole)

DESCRIPTION

Bactrim, Septra, and other brands of co-trimoxazole are often prescribed for urinary tract infections or ear infections. They may also be useful in treating traveler's diarrhea and certain types of bronchitis and pneumonia. Occasionally such antibiotics may result in superinfection that must be treated with a different drug. Some people become more sensitive to sunlight—and more susceptible to sunburn—when taking one of these drugs. Side effects may include gastrointestinal upset, headache, rash, and yellow skin and eyes.

INSTRUCTIONS

This drug is best absorbed when taken on an empty stomach, at least one hour before or two hours after a meal. It may be taken with food if it upsets the stomach. Drink at least eight cups of water a day to help keep the drug from crystallizing in the kidneys, and avoid large doses of vitamin C.

BRAND NAME

Folex   Mexate   Rheumatrex

DESCRIPTION

Methotrexate interferes with folic acid metabolism in rapidly growing cells, making it a useful agent for treating certain cancers and for severe psoriasis, another condition characterized by too-rapid cell division. It is also prescribed for rheumatoid arthritis. Methotrexate is a heavy-duty drug with potentially serious side effects, particularly for the liver. Frequent blood and urine tests will be needed to monitor lung, blood, liver, and kidney function. Let your doctor know if you have trouble with nausea, vomiting, loss of appetite, rash, hair loss, boils, or acne. Because methotrexate can cause lethal birth defects, it is usually inappropriate for pregnant women.

INSTRUCTIONS

Follow your doctor's instructions on dose and timing for methotrexate, which is taken **once a week** for psoriasis or rheumatoid arthritis. Do not drink alcohol or take salicylates such as aspirin or Pepto-Bismol while on this drug. Methotrexate can increase sensitivity to ultraviolet light, so protect your skin from exposure to sun or tanning lamps.

INTERACTION

People taking methotrexate for leukemia or other cancers may be more susceptible to infection than healthy people. Bactrim, Septra, and other brands of co-trimoxazole are useful for ear infections, urinary tract infections, and so forth. Reports indicate, however, that Bactrim or other sulfa antibiotics (including Gantanol and Gantrisin) can increase the toxicity of methotrexate to the blood system, resulting in bone marrow suppression, anemia, or changes in blood tests. *This interaction can be life threatening.* **Deaths have been reported.**

If both medications are prescribed, ask if another antibiotic would work as well. If both medicines are needed, the doctor should follow closely with frequent blood tests.
Symptoms of Methotrexate Toxicity
Nausea, vomiting, diarrhea, mouth sores, rash, itching, black sticky stools, stomach pain, sore throat, fever, chills, unusual bleeding or bruising, yellow skin or eyes, shortness of breath, cough, dark or bloody urine, and swelling of the legs or feet. Notify the physician immediately.

Never take or stop medication without your doctor's advice.

INTERACTION

LIFE THREATENING

Antibiotic
(CO-TRIMOXAZOLE)

Transplant Drug

BRAND NAME

Bactrim   Cotrim   Septra
SMZ-TMP   Sulfatrim   Uroplus
(All co-trimoxazole, formerly known as trimethoprim-sulfamethoxazole)

DESCRIPTION

Bactrim, Septra, and other brands of co-trimoxazole are often prescribed for urinary tract infections or ear infections. They may also be useful in treating traveler's diarrhea and certain types of bronchitis and pneumonia. Occasionally such antibiotics may result in superinfection that must be treated with a different drug. Some people become more sensitive to sunlight—and more susceptible to sunburn—when taking one of these drugs. Side effects may include gastrointestinal upset, headache, rash, and yellow skin and eyes.

INSTRUCTIONS

This drug is best absorbed when taken on an empty stomach, at least one hour before or two hours after a meal. It may be taken with food if it upsets the stomach. Drink at least eight cups of water a day to help keep the drug from crystallizing in the kidneys, and avoid large doses of vitamin C.

BRAND NAME

Sandimmune

GENERIC NAME

cyclosporine

DESCRIPTION

Sandimmune suppresses the immune system so that a person receiving a transplant does not reject this life-saving organ. Doctors have also tried using it in treating autoimmune diseases, in which the immune system attacks a person's own tissues. Multiple sclerosis is an example.

INSTRUCTIONS

Sandimmune comes as an oral solution with a taste reminiscent of castor oil. It should be mixed in a glass with milk, chocolate milk, or orange juice at room temperature and drunk at once. Then the glass (no plastic) should be rinsed and the rinsing fluid drunk to get the full dose. Do not take Sandimmune with grapefruit juice unless the physician is monitoring blood levels of the drug closely. (See page 43.) Due to a possible interaction between cyclosporine and oral contraceptives, barrier methods of contraception should be used while taking this drug.

Regular monitoring is important. Do not stop this medicine unless your doctor so directs.

INTERACTION

A transplant patient who comes down with an infection needs an antibiotic, and co-trimoxazole may be appropriate. This should be undertaken only with very careful follow-up and monitoring. Co-trimoxazole and other sulfa antibiotics may reduce the blood level of Sandimmune to a point so low that the drug becomes ineffective. Patients on this combination have experienced rejection episodes. *Although we are aware of no deaths, this interaction could be life threatening.*

In addition, kidney damage appears to occur more often with this combination of medications than with either drug alone. Frequent blood and urine tests may be required to detect a serious reaction.

Never take or stop medication without your doctor's advice.

INTERACTION

LIFE THREATENING

Antibiotic

(CO-TRIMOXAZOLE)

Diabetes Drugs

BRAND NAME

Bactrim   Cotrim   Septra
SMZ-TMP   Sulfatrim   Uroplus
(All co-trimoxazole, formerly known as trimethoprim-sulfamethoxazole)

DESCRIPTION

Bactrim, Septra, and other brands of co-trimoxazole are often prescribed for urinary tract infections or ear infections. They may also be useful in treating traveler's diarrhea and certain types of bronchitis and pneumonia. Occasionally such antibiotics may result in superinfection that must be treated with a different drug. Some people become more sensitive to sunlight—and more susceptible to sunburn—when taking one of these drugs. Side effects may include gastrointestinal upset, headache, rash, and yellow skin and eyes.

INSTRUCTIONS

This drug is best absorbed when taken on an empty stomach, at least one hour before or two hours after a meal. It may be taken with food if it upsets the stomach. Drink at least eight cups of water a day to help keep the drug from crystallizing in the kidneys, and avoid large doses of vitamin C.

BRAND NAME	GENERIC NAME
DiaBeta, Glynase, Micronase	glyburide
Diabinese	chlorpropamide
Dymelor	acetohexamide
Glucotrol	glipizide
Orinase	tolbutamide
Tolinase	tolazamide

DESCRIPTION

These pills are prescribed for non-insulin-dependent diabetics. They help control blood sugar by increasing the amount of insulin the pancreas makes and by making body tissues more sensitive to insulin. With diet, exercise, and blood sugar monitoring, they may reduce the risk of complications of diabetes. Low blood sugar (hypoglycemia) is the most common serious side effect. These medications interact with many others; check with a doctor or pharmacist before taking another drug.

INSTRUCTIONS

DiaBeta, Glucotrol, and Micronase should be taken 15 minutes to half an hour before meals. The others may be taken with food if they upset the stomach. Blood glucose monitoring is important. Notify the doctor immediately if you experience rash, fever, sore throat, or unusual bleeding or bruising.

INTERACTION

These oral diabetes drugs last longer in the body when a person also takes a sulfa antibiotic such as Bactrim or Septra. Some patients have experienced hypoglycemia as a consequence. Orinase and Diabinese have been implicated most frequently, but there is one case report of this interaction causing hypoglycemia in a patient on Glucotrol. *This interaction could be dangerous.* DiaBeta, Glynase, and Micronase do not appear to interact with co-trimoxazole to cause hypoglycemia. Still, if you are on any oral diabetes drug and need to take this antibiotic, monitor your blood sugar carefully and be alert for hypoglycemia.

Symptoms of Hypoglycemia (Low Blood Sugar)
Shaking, sweating, tiredness, low temperature, faintness, palpitations, hunger, headache, confusion, irritability, visual disturbances, coma. Close observation (preferably in the hospital) is recommended for two or three days after such a reaction.

INTERACTION

DANGEROUS

Antibiotic

(CO-TRIMOXAZOLE)

Amantadine

BRAND NAME

Bactrim   Cotrim   Septra
SMZ-TMP   Sulfatrim   Uroplus
(All co-trimoxazole, formerly known as trimethoprim-sulfamethoxazole)

DESCRIPTION

Bactrim, Septra, and other brands of co-trimoxazole are often prescribed for urinary tract infections or ear infections. They may also be useful in treating traveler's diarrhea and certain types of bronchitis and pneumonia. Occasionally such antibiotics may result in superinfection that must be treated with a different drug. Some people become more sensitive to sunlight—and more susceptible to sunburn—when taking one of these drugs. Side effects may include gastrointestinal upset, headache, rash, and yellow skin and eyes.

INSTRUCTIONS

This drug is best absorbed when taken on an empty stomach, at least one hour before or two hours after a meal. It may be taken with food if it upsets the stomach. Drink at least eight cups of water a day to help keep the drug from crystallizing in the kidneys, and avoid large doses of vitamin C.

BRAND NAME

Symadine   Symmetrel

DESCRIPTION

Amantadine is used for two completely different indications. It is frequently prescribed alone or with other drugs to control the symptoms of Parkinson's disease. Other people are prescribed amantadine either to prevent or to treat type-A influenza. In treating flu, it is most effective when begun as soon as possible after symptoms start. Older people may be more sensitive to side effects such as nausea, loss of appetite, dizziness, or insomnia, and may require lower doses than younger people. This drug is not generally appropriate for pregnant women, as it can cause birth defects in animals. Notify your doctor if you develop shortness of breath, swollen legs and feet, trouble urinating, or unexplained changes in mood.

INSTRUCTIONS

There is no information on whether amantadine should be taken with meals or on an empty stomach. It should not be discontinued suddenly, as that has triggered symptoms of Parkinson's disease in some patients.

INTERACTION

There is one case of an elderly man becoming very confused while taking this combination. When co-trimoxazole is taken in combination with amantadine, blood levels of both medications may be increased. *This interaction could be troublesome; stay alert for symptoms of confusion.*

Never take or stop medication without your doctor's advice.

INTERACTION

TROUBLESOME

Antibiotic

(CO-TRIMOXAZOLE)

Tuberculosis Drug

(RIFAMPIN)

BRAND NAME

Bactrim   Cotrim   Septra
SMZ-TMP   Sulfatrim   Uroplus
(All co-trimoxazole, formerly known as trimethoprim-sulfamethoxazole)

DESCRIPTION

Bactrim, Septra, and other brands of co-trimoxazole are often prescribed for urinary tract infections or ear infections. They may also be useful in treating traveler's diarrhea and certain types of bronchitis and pneumonia. Occasionally such antibiotics may result in superinfection that must be treated with a different drug. Some people become more sensitive to sunlight—and more susceptible to sunburn—when taking one of these drugs. Side effects may include gastrointestinal upset, headache, rash, and yellow skin and eyes.

INSTRUCTIONS

This drug is best absorbed when taken on an empty stomach, at least one hour before or two hours after a meal. It may be taken with food if it upsets the stomach. Drink at least eight cups of water a day to help keep the drug from crystallizing in the kidneys, and avoid large doses of vitamin C.

BRAND NAME	GENERIC NAME
Rifadin	rifampin
Rifamate	isoniazid/rifampin
Rimactane	rifampin

DESCRIPTION

Rifampin is used in combination with other medications to treat tuberculosis. To be effective, it needs to be taken faithfully for an extended period of time (at least six to nine months), as the doctor prescribes. Side effects may include digestive tract problems, menstrual irregularities, difficulty concentrating, fluid retention, and wheezing or shortness of breath. The orange discoloration of urine, saliva, and tears is not harmful, although it may stain contact lenses.

INSTRUCTIONS

Rifampin should be taken on an empty stomach, at least one hour before or two hours after meals. If you develop fever, chills, unusual tiredness, unusual bleeding or bruising, sore throat, muscle and bone pain, or yellow skin and eyes, contact your physician immediately.

INTERACTION

A urinary tract or other infection in a tuberculosis patient might require that these drugs be taken at the same time. Co-trimoxazole can raise blood levels of rifampin when these two medicines are taken together. *This interaction could be troublesome; notify your doctor of unusual symptoms.*

Symptoms of Rifampin Overdose
Nausea, lethargy, or even, rarely, abnormal liver function tests, liver tenderness, or yellow skin and eyes. Notify the physician promptly of any such symptoms.

Never take or stop medication without your doctor's advice.

INTERACTION

TROUBLESOME

Anticoagulant
(WARFARIN)
Coumadin

LIFE THREATENING

Antibiotic (co-trimoxazole)
Bactrim   Cotrim
Septra   SMZ-TMP
Sulfatrim   Uroplus

Antibiotic (metronidazole)
Flagyl   Protostat

Aspirin Arthritis Drugs (NSAIDs)

Barbiturates
Amytal   Butisol
Mebaral   Nembutal
phenobarbital   Seconal
Tuinal

Breast Cancer Drug
Nolvadex

Endometriosis Drug
Danocrine

Heart Drug
Cordarone

Ulcer Drug
Tagamet

DANGEROUS

Anabolic Steroids
Anadrol-50   Halotestin
Metandren   etc.

Antibiotics (macrolides)
Biaxin   E.E.S   E-Mycin
ERYC   EryPed   Ery-Tab
Erythrocin   Ilosone
PCE   Pediazole   etc.

Antibiotics (tetracyclines)
Achromycin V   doxycycline
Minocin   Vibramycin
etc.

Antidepressants (serotonin-based)
Paxil   Prozac   Zoloft

Antifungal Drugs
Diflucan   Monistat

Cholesterol Drug
Mevacor

Heart Drug (quinidine)
Cardioquin   Quinaglute
Quinidex   Quinora

TROUBLESOME

Anticonvulsant
Tegretol

Cholesterol Drugs
Colestid   Questran

Thyroid Hormone
Armour Thyroid   Cytomel
Levothroid   Synthroid
Thyroid Strong   etc.

Tuberculosis Drug (rifampin)
Rifadin   Rifamate
Rimactane

Vitamin E

Vitamin K

Interactions listed on this overview tree are the most important but not the only medicines with which warfarin interacts. See individual descriptions for details. Be sure to check with your physician and pharmacist if you must take any other drugs in combination with this anticoagulant.

LEVELS OF HAZARD: LIFE THREATENING   DANGEROUS   TROUBLESOME

Anticoagulant
(WARFARIN)

Antibiotic
(CO-TRIMOXAZOLE)

BRAND NAME   GENERIC NAME

Coumadin   warfarin

DESCRIPTION

Warfarin slows the liver's production of factors essential for the formation of blood clots. It is prescribed when there is a risk that a dangerous clot could form in a deep vein or a blood vessel leading to the lung, heart, or brain. The most serious complication of anticoagulant treatment is excessive bleeding. The dosage must be individually adjusted, requiring daily blood tests at first, then tests every four to six weeks. Other side effects may include nausea, loss of appetite, rash, fever, yellow eyes and skin, prolonged painful erection, and hair loss.

INSTRUCTIONS

Warfarin tablets can be swallowed with food or on an empty stomach. Try to avoid large variations in the quantity of vitamin-K–containing vegetables—such as broccoli, cabbage, or spinach—that you eat each day. Consuming much more or less than usual could change the action of the drug.

BRAND NAME

Bactrim   **Cotrim**   **Septra**
SMZ-TMP   **Sulfatrim**   **Uroplus**
(All co-trimoxazole, formerly known as trimethoprim-sulfamethoxazole)

DESCRIPTION

Bactrim, Septra, and other brands of co-trimoxazole are often prescribed for urinary tract infections or ear infections. They may also be useful in treating traveler's diarrhea and certain types of bronchitis or pneumonia. Occasionally such antibiotics may result in superinfection that must be treated with a different drug. Some peole become more sensitive to sunlight—and more susceptible to sunburn—when taking one of these drugs. Side effects may include gastrointestinal upset, headache, rash, and yellow skin and eyes.

INSTRUCTIONS

This drug is best absorbed when taken on an empty stomach, at least one hour before or two hours after a meal. It may be taken with food if it upsets the stomach. Drink at least eight cups of water a day to help keep the drug from crystallizing in the kidneys, and avoid large doses of vitamin C.

INTERACTION

Sulfa antibiotics such as Bactrim can substantially increase the effects of warfarin. *This interaction could trigger life-threatening bleeding.*

    Apparently, co-trimoxazole interferes with the metabolism of warfarin in the liver, leading to higher blood levels of the anticoagulant. When this combination of medications is required, the doctor will order frequent blood tests to check prothrombin (clotting) time.

Symptoms of Warfarin Overdose

There may be no early warning signs of danger. Blood tests are essential. Symptoms include any unusual bleeding, including rectal or urinary tract bleeding, excessive menstrual bleeding, nosebleeds, bleeding around gums, bruising, red or tar-black stools, vomiting blood, and red or dark-brown urine. Notify your doctor immediately if you suspect a problem.

INTERACTION

LIFE THREATENING

Anticoagulant
(WARFARIN)

Antibiotic
(METRONIDAZOLE)

BRAND NAME	GENERIC NAME
Coumadin	warfarin

DESCRIPTION

Warfarin slows the liver's production of factors essential for the formation of blood clots. It is prescribed when there is a risk that a dangerous clot could form in a deep vein or a blood vessel leading to the lung, heart, or brain. The most serious complication of anticoagulant treatment is excessive bleeding. The dosage must be individually adjusted, requiring daily blood tests at first, then tests every four to six weeks. Other side effects may include nausea, loss of appetite, rash, fever, yellow eyes and skin, prolonged painful erection, and hair loss.

INSTRUCTIONS

Warfarin tablets can be swallowed with food or on an empty stomach. Try to avoid large variations in the quantity of vitamin–K–containing vegetables—such as broccoli, cabbage, and spinach—that you eat each day. Consuming much more or less than usual could change the action of the drug.

BRAND NAME	GENERIC NAME
Flagyl	metronidazole
Protostat	metronidazole

DESCRIPTION

Metronidazole is most often prescribed to treat vaginal infections caused by *Trichomonas*. It is also useful in treating some serious abdominal, skin, and gynecologic infections, and certain cases of blood poisoning and meningitis. Side effects of this antibiotic may include digestive tract upset, seizures, confusion, depression, rash, and a metallic taste in the mouth. Darkened urine is common but not dangerous.

INSTRUCTIONS

Metronidazole may be taken with meals to reduce stomach upset. Avoid alcohol while on this drug and for a day after stopping it, because the combination could trigger flushing, headache, nausea, and vomiting.

INTERACTION

Metronidazole can interfere with the body's elimination of warfarin, leading to higher blood levels of the anticoagulant. *This interaction could trigger life-threatening bleeding.*

This interaction is expected in many or most patients taking both warfarin and metronidazole. The doctor will probably order frequent blood tests to see if the dose of warfarin should be adjusted. Contact your physician without delay if there are any signs of unusual bleeding.

Symptoms of Warfarin Overdose

There may be no early warning signs of danger. Blood tests are essential. Symptoms include any unusual bleeding, including rectal or urinary tract bleeding, excessive menstrual bleeding, nosebleeds, bleeding around gums, bruising, red or tar-black stools, vomiting blood, and red or dark-brown urine. Notify your doctor immediately if you suspect a problem.

Never take or stop medication without your doctor's advice.

INTERACTION

LIFE THREATENING

Anticoagulant
(WARFARIN)

Aspirin and Arthritis Drugs
(NSAIDS)

BRAND NAME	GENERIC NAME
Coumadin	warfarin

DESCRIPTION

Warfarin slows the liver's production of factors essential for the formation of blood clots. It is prescribed when there is a risk that a dangerous clot could form in a deep vein or a blood vessel leading to the lung, heart, or brain. The most serious complication of anticoagulant treatment is excessive bleeding. The dosage must be individually adjusted, requiring daily blood tests at first, then tests every four to six weeks. Other side effects may include nausea, loss of appetite, rash, fever, yellow eyes and skin, prolonged painful erection, and hair loss.

INSTRUCTIONS

Warfarin tablets can be swallowed with food or on an empty stomach. Try to avoid large variations in the quantity of vitamin-K–containing vegetables—such as broccoli, cabbage, or spinach—that you eat each day. Consuming much more or less than usual could change the action of the drug.

BRAND NAME	GENERIC NAME
Alka-Seltzer	acetylsalicylic acid
Anacin	acetylsalicylic acid
Ascriptin	acetylsalicylic acid
Bayer	acetylsalicylic acid
Ecotrin, etc.	acetylsalicylic acid

DESCRIPTION

Aspirin is a versatile and inexpensive medication used to alleviate pain such as headache, reduce inflammation, bring down fever, prevent heart attacks or strokes, and forestall blood clots. It may also lower the risk of gastrointestinal cancer, especially colon cancer. Aspirin may be irritating to the digestive tract, and chronic use can trigger the development of ulcers. Ringing in the ears and unusual bleeding are also potential side effects. For the interaction of anticoagulants with other arthritis drugs, see page 257.

INSTRUCTIONS

Aspirin may be taken with food or milk to reduce stomach upset, always with a full eight ounces of liquid. Pregnant women should take aspirin only under the doctor's supervision. Children with flu or chickenpox must avoid aspirin because it increases the risk of Reye's syndrome.

INTERACTION

Both aspirin and warfarin are effective anticlotting agents, although they work through different pathways. Large doses of aspirin can significantly increase bleeding in people taking warfarin. *This interaction could prove life threatening.*

Low doses of aspirin together with warfarin may only slightly increase the risk of bleeding. A study (CARS) currently underway will test this combination. Until the results are in, aspirin and warfarin should be combined only under close monitoring. Prothrombin time should be tested, but serious bleeding may occur even without major changes in this test.

Symptoms of Warfarin Overdose

There may be no early warning signs of danger. Blood tests are essential. Symptoms include any unusual bleeding, including rectal or urinary tract bleeding, excessive menstrual bleeding, nosebleeds, bleeding around gums, bruising, red or tar-black stools, vomiting blood, and red or dark-brown urine. Notify your doctor immediately if you suspect a problem.

Never take or stop medication without your doctor's advice.

INTERACTION

LIFE THREATENING

Anticoagulant
(WARFARIN)

Barbiturates

BRAND NAME	GENERIC NAME
Coumadin	warfarin

DESCRIPTION

Warfarin slows the liver's production of factors essential for the formation of blood clots. It is prescribed when there is a risk that a dangerous clot could form in a deep vein or a blood vessel leading to the lung, heart, or brain. The most serious complication of anticoagulant treatment is excessive bleeding. The dosage must be individually adjusted, requiring daily blood tests at first, then tests every four to six weeks. Other side effects may include nausea, loss of appetite, rash, fever, yellow eyes and skin, prolonged painful erection, and hair loss.

INSTRUCTIONS

Warfarin tablets can be swallowed with food or on an empty stomach. Try to avoid large variations in the quantity of vitamin-K–containing vegetables—such as broccoli, cabbage, or spinach—that you eat each day. Consuming much more or less than usual could change the action of the drug.

BRAND NAME	GENERIC NAME
Alurate	aprobarbital
Amytal	amobarbital
Butisol	butabarbital
Lotusate	talbutal
Mebaral	mephobarbital
Nembutal	pentobarbital
Seconal	secobarbital
Solfoton	phenobarbital
Tuinal	amobarbital/ secobarbital

DESCRIPTION

Barbiturates were once used as sleeping pills, but now they are prescribed to prevent seizures. These medications can cause dependence if used for an extended period of time. Stopping suddenly could trigger severe withdrawal symptoms. Barbiturates interact with many other drugs, so check with the pharmacist or physician before taking any other medications.

INSTRUCTIONS

Any of these medications can cause drowsiness and limit attention. Take them at a time when you will not need to drive or do other complicated tasks.

INTERACTION

Barbiturates can rev up the liver enzymes that process warfarin, thus lowering both the blood levels and the effectiveness of this anticoagulant. *In such a situation, there is a risk of dangerous blood clots. Even more serious is the risk of life-threatening bleeding when a person on warfarin stops taking a barbiturate.* People vary a great deal in their response to this interaction. It is essential, however, that prothrombin time be tested frequently during the two weeks a barbiturate is started and the two weeks after it is stopped. Dosage adjustments may be necessary.

Symptoms of Warfarin Overdose

There may be no early warning signs of danger. Blood tests are essential. Symptoms include any unusual bleeding, including rectal or urinary tract bleeding, excessive menstrual bleeding, nosebleeds, bleeding around gums, bruising, red or tar-black stools, vomiting blood, and red or dark-brown urine. Notify your doctor immediately if you suspect a problem.

Never take or stop medication without your doctor's advice.

INTERACTION

LIFE THREATENING

Anticoagulant
(WARFARIN)

Breast Cancer Drug
(TAMOXIFEN)

BRAND NAME **Coumadin** GENERIC NAME warfarin

BRAND NAME **Nolvadex** GENERIC NAME tamoxifen

DESCRIPTION

Warfarin slows the liver's production of factors essential for the formation of blood clots. It is prescribed when there is a risk that a dangerous clot could form in a deep vein or a blood vessel leading to the lung, heart, or brain. The most serious complication of anticoagulant treatment is excessive bleeding. The dosage must be individually adjusted, requiring daily blood tests at first, then tests every four to six weeks. Other side effects may include nausea, loss of appetite, rash, fever, yellow eyes and skin, prolonged painful erection, and hair loss.

DESCRIPTION

Doctors prescribe Nolvadex to help prevent recurrence in women who have had breast cancer. The drug has also been approved in the treatment of metastatic breast cancer. In rare circumstances, it might be prescribed for enlarged painful breasts and for cancer of the pancreas. Tamoxifen acts as an estrogen blocker in breast tissue, and discourages the growth of estrogen-sensitive tumors. Side effects include hot flashes, nausea and vomiting, and menstrual irregularities or vaginal bleeding. Changes in vision have been reported, so periodic eye exams are advisable.

INSTRUCTIONS

Warfarin tablets can be swallowed with food or on an empty stomach. Try to avoid large variations in the quantity of vitamin-K–containing vegetables—such as broccoli, cabbage, or spinach—that you eat each day. Consuming much more or less than usual could change the action of the drug.

INSTRUCTIONS

Nolvadex may be taken with or without food. If you experience exceptional weakness, sleepiness, confusion, shortness of breath, or swollen, painful areas in the legs, contact the doctor immediately.

INTERACTION

In one case, a 65-year-old woman nearly died of hemorrhage several weeks after she was put on tamoxifen to battle breast cancer. She had been on the same dose of warfarin for many years prior to starting tamoxifen. Apparently, tamoxifen increased her blood level of warfarin to a dangerous degree. The doctors were able to save her life in the hospital and she was sent home on both drugs, but with the warfarin dose much reduced. *This interaction may be rare, but it could be life threatening.*

Prudence suggests frequent blood tests to check on warfarin's effectiveness during the weeks after Nolvadex is started or stopped. Notify the doctor immediately of any signs of bleeding.

Symptoms of Warfarin Overdose

There may be no early warning signs of danger. Blood tests are essential. Symptoms include any unusual bleeding, including rectal or urinary tract bleeding, excessive menstrual bleeding, nosebleeds, bleeding around gums, bruising, red or tar-black stools, vomiting blood, and red or dark-brown urine. Notify your doctor immediately if you suspect a problem.

Never take or stop medication without your doctor's advice.

INTERACTION
LIFE THREATENING

Anticoagulant
(WARFARIN)

Endometriosis Drug
(DANAZOL)

BRAND NAME | GENERIC NAME
Coumadin | warfarin

DESCRIPTION

Warfarin slows the liver's production of factors essential for the formation of blood clots. It is prescribed when there is a risk that a dangerous clot could form in a deep vein or a blood vessel leading to the lung, heart, or brain. The most serious complication of anticoagulant treatment is excessive bleeding. The dosage must be individually adjusted, requiring daily blood tests at first, then tests every four to six weeks. Other side effects may include nausea, loss of appetite, rash, fever, yellow eyes and skin, prolonged painful erection, and hair loss.

INSTRUCTIONS

Warfarin tablets can be swallowed with food or on an empty stomach. Try to avoid large variations in the quantity of vitamin-K–containing vegetables—such as broccoli, cabbage, or spinach—that you eat each day. Consuming much more or less than usual could change the action of the drug.

BRAND NAME | GENERIC NAME
Danocrine | danazol

DESCRIPTION

Danocrine is prescribed to control the pain of endometriosis. It works by reducing the hormonal input to this tissue. It is also helpful in controlling the pain of fibrocystic breast disease, and is occasionally prescribed in cases of very heavy menstrual flow, or, in men, for breast enlargement. Because Danocrine interacts with insulin, diabetics must be monitored especially carefully when taking this drug. In some women Danocrine may cause acne, facial or body hair growth, a deeper voice, weight gain, or other symptoms of masculinization. Contact the physician if you notice any of these. Danocrine must never be taken during pregnancy.

INSTRUCTIONS

Danocrine may be taken either with food or on an empty stomach. During Danocrine therapy, sexually active women should use barrier contraceptives (such as a diaphragm or condoms).

INTERACTION

Danocrine seems to increase the body's sensitivity to warfarin and may increase bleeding dramatically. *This interaction could be life threatening.*

The physician will probably order frequent blood tests for a period of time if danazol is stopped or started in a patient taking warfarin, to see if the dose of warfarin should be adjusted. If you experience unusual bleeding, let the physician know at once.

Symptoms of Warfarin Overdose

There may be no early warning signs of danger. Blood tests are essential. Symptoms include any unusual bleeding, including rectal or urinary tract bleeding, excessive menstrual bleeding, nosebleeds, bleeding around gums, bruising, red or tar-black stools, vomiting blood, and red or dark-brown urine. Notify your doctor immediately if you suspect a problem.

Never take or stop medication without your doctor's advice.

INTERACTION

LIFE THREATENING

Anticoagulant
(WARFARIN)

Heart Drug
(AMIODARONE)

BRAND NAME **Coumadin**   GENERIC NAME warfarin

BRAND NAME **Cordarone**   GENERIC NAME amiodarone

DESCRIPTION

Warfarin slows the liver's production of factors essential for the formation of blood clots. It is prescribed when there is a risk that a dangerous clot could form in a deep vein or a blood vessel leading to the lung, heart, or brain. The most serious complication of anticoagulant treatment is excessive bleeding. The dosage must be individually adjusted, requiring daily blood tests at first, then tests every four to six weeks. Other side effects may include nausea, loss of appetite, rash, fever, yellow eyes and skin, prolonged painful erection, and hair loss.

INSTRUCTIONS

Warfarin tablets can be swallowed with food or on an empty stomach. Try to avoid large variations in the quantity of vitamin-K–containing vegetables—such as broccoli, cabbage, or spinach—that you eat each day. Consuming much more or less than usual could change the action of the drug.

DESCRIPTION

Cordarone is used to treat life-threatening heart rhythm problems affecting the ventricle, or lower part, of the heart. Some doctors prescribe a lower dose for other rhythm disturbances. This medication has potentially serious side effects, and occasionally may exacerbate heart rhythm problems. Hospitalization is recommended for the first doses, and the doctor should monitor your progress carefully.

INSTRUCTIONS

Follow the physician's directions carefully. Tell your doctor if you notice shortness of breath, or changes in vision, or if your skin turns blue.

INTERACTION

Complicated cardiovascular problems may call for both an anticoagulant and a powerful heart drug. Cordarone increases the effect of warfarin so much that severe bleeding may occur. The dose of warfarin may need to be cut 30 to 50 percent if Cordarone is added. *This interaction could be life threatening.* Frequent blood tests are needed during the first month of combined therapy to check the warfarin dose. Cordarone lingers in the body a long time. If it is discontinued, blood tests will be needed for several months so that the dose of warfarin can be adjusted to avoid the risk of serious clotting.

Symptoms of Warfarin Overdose

There may be no early warning signs of danger. Blood tests are essential. Symptoms include any unusual bleeding, including rectal or urinary tract bleeding, excessive menstrual bleeding, nosebleeds, bleeding around gums, bruising, red or tar-black stools, vomiting blood, and red or dark-brown urine. Notify your doctor immediately if you suspect a problem.

Never take or stop medication without your doctor's advice.

INTERACTION

LIFE THREATENING

Anticoagulant
(WARFARIN)

Ulcer Drug
(H₂ ANTAGONIST)

BRAND NAME	GENERIC NAME
Coumadin	warfarin

BRAND NAME	GENERIC NAME
Tagamet	cimetidine

DESCRIPTION

Warfarin slows the liver's production of factors essential for the formation of blood clots. It is prescribed when there is a risk that a dangerous clot could form in a deep vein or a blood vessel leading to the lung, heart, or brain. The most serious complication of anticoagulant treatment is excessive bleeding. The dosage must be individually adjusted, requiring daily blood tests at first, then tests every four to six weeks. Other side effects may include nausea, loss of appetite, rash, fever, yellow eyes and skin, prolonged painful erection, and hair loss.

INSTRUCTIONS

Warfarin tablets can be swallowed with food or on an empty stomach. Try to avoid large variations in the quantity of vitamin-K–containing vegetables—such as broccoli, cabbage, or spinach—that you eat each day. Consuming much more or less than usual could change the action of the drug.

DESCRIPTION

Tagamet has revolutionized the treatment of ulcers and serious heartburn (esophagitis) by blocking special receptors (the histamine H₂ receptors), thereby reducing the acid environment of the stomach. Cimetidine is usually well tolerated, and has few side effects, although headaches, dizziness, and mild diarrhea are potential reactions. Some men complain of antitestosterone effects. At higher doses, this may lead to enlarged breasts or sexual problems. Older people and those who are very ill may experience depression, mental confusion, or disorientation. The dose may need to be adjusted for them. Tagamet can affect the liver, modifying the metabolism and elimination of a number of medications. Higher blood levels of such drugs may lead to increased toxicity, so check with your doctor and pharmacist if you take cimetidine with another medicine.

INSTRUCTIONS

Tagamet is usually taken with meals and/or at bedtime. Antacids may reduce absorption of Tagamet; do not take one for at least two hours after taking Tagamet.

INTERACTION

Although warfarin may cause nausea, loss of appetite, stomach cramping, or diarrhea, taking Tagamet to treat these symptoms might trigger serious problems. Tagamet affects metabolism and increases Coumadin's blood-thinning potential. This prolongs prothrombin time (a measure of clotting) and could lead to serious hemorrhaging. *The interaction is potentially lethal.* Experts warn against this combination of drugs. If an ulcer medicine is needed with warfarin, the drugs Axid, Pepcid, or Zantac may be a safer alternative than Tagamet. Prothrombin time should be monitored when taking warfarin with an ulcer drug.

Symptoms of Warfarin Overdose

There may be no early warning signs of danger. Blood tests are essential. Symptoms include any unusual bleeding, including rectal or urinary tract bleeding, excessive menstrual bleeding, nosebleeds, bleeding around gums, bruising, red or tar-black stools, vomiting blood, and red or dark-brown urine. Notify your doctor immediately if you suspect a problem.

Never take or stop medication without your doctor's advice.

INTERACTION

LIFE THREATENING

Anticoagulant
(WARFARIN)

Anabolic Steroids

BRAND NAME | GENERIC NAME

Coumadin | warfarin

DESCRIPTION

Warfarin slows the liver's production of factors essential for the formation of blood clots. It is prescribed when there is a risk that a dangerous clot could form in a deep vein or a blood vessel leading to the lung, heart, or brain. The most serious complication of anticoagulant treatment is excessive bleeding. The dosage must be individually adjusted, requiring daily blood tests at first, then tests every four to six weeks. Other side effects may include nausea, loss of appetite, rash, fever, yellow eyes and skin, prolonged painful erection, and hair loss.

INSTRUCTIONS

Warfarin tablets can be swallowed with food or on an empty stomach. Try to avoid large variations in the quantity of vitamin-K–containing vegetables—such as broccoli, cabbage, or spinach—that you eat each day. Consuming much more or less than usual could change the action of the drug.

BRAND NAME | GENERIC NAME

Anadrol-50 | oxymetholone
Halotestin | fluoxymesterone
Metandren | methyltestosterone
Winstrol | stanozolol

DESCRIPTION

Anabolic steroids such as these promote the formation of body tissues and counteract breakdown. They may be prescribed to promote weight recovery after a severe prolonged illness, to offset the consequences of prolonged corticosteroid use, or to relieve the pain of bone breakdown due to osteoporosis. Such medicines are not appropriate during pregnancy. Possible side effects include detrimental changes in blood cholesterol and an increased risk of liver cysts and tumors. Acne, fluid retention, changes in sex drive, and the development of masculine characteristics in women may also occur.

INSTRUCTIONS

These drugs may cause nausea and vomiting. Tell the doctor if this becomes a problem, or if you develop swollen ankles or yellow skin. These medications may affect blood sugar control, so diabetics require close monitoring.

INTERACTION

Anabolic steroids increase the effects of warfarin against clotting. If one of these drugs is needed, prothrombin time should monitored closely to guide a possible adjustment in warfarin dose. Blood tests may also be required for several days after one of these medicines is discontinued. *This interaction could be dangerous.*

Symptoms of Warfarin Overdose

There may be no early warning signs of danger. Blood tests are essential. Symptoms include any unusual bleeding, including rectal or urinary tract bleeding, excessive menstrual bleeding, nosebleeds, bleeding around gums, bruising, red or tar-black stools, vomiting blood, and red or dark-brown urine. Notify your doctor immediately if you suspect a problem.

Never take or stop medication without your doctor's advice.

INTERACTION

DANGEROUS

Anticoagulant

(WARFARIN)

Antibiotics

(MACROLIDES)

BRAND NAME	GENERIC NAME
Coumadin	warfarin

DESCRIPTION

Warfarin slows the liver's production of factors essential for the formation of blood clots. It is prescribed when there is a risk that a dangerous clot could form in a deep vein or a blood vessel leading to the lung, heart, or brain. The most serious complication of anticoagulant treatment is excessive bleeding. The dosage must be individually adjusted, requiring daily blood tests at first, then tests every four to six weeks. Other side effects may include nausea, loss of appetite, rash, fever, yellow eyes and skin, prolonged painful erection, and hair loss.

INSTRUCTIONS

Warfarin tablets can be swallowed with food or on an empty stomach. Try to avoid large variations in the quantity of vitamin-K–containing vegetables—such as broccoli, cabbage, or spinach—that you eat each day. Consuming much more or less than usual could change the action of the drug.

BRAND NAME	GENERIC NAME
Biaxin	clarithromycin
E.E.S.	erythromycin
E-Mycin	erythromycin
ERYC	erythromycin
EryPed	erythromycin
Ery-Tab	erythromycin
Erythrocin	erythromycin
Ilosone	erythromycin
PCE	erythromycin
Pediazole	erythromycin
Tao	troleandomycin
Zithromax	azithromycin

DESCRIPTION

These broad-spectrum antibiotics are widely prescribed for respiratory tract, sinus, ear, and skin infections. They are also effective against *Chlamydia* and certain other infections of the reproductive tract.

INSTRUCTIONS

Some forms of erythromycin must be taken on an empty stomach; others may be taken with food. See the table of Food and Drug Compatibility on pages 59-73 for specifics. Biaxin can be taken without regard to meals. Zithromax is best taken on an empty stomach.

INTERACTION

Erythromycin increases the body's response to warfarin. In several cases, this has resulted in serious bleeding. Tests of prothrombin (clotting) time should be done frequently when erythromycin must be added to warfarin. Blood tests may also be required for several days after one of these medicines is discontinued. *This interaction could be dangerous.*

Biaxin and Zithromax may not interact with warfarin in the same way as the other macrolides. It would be wise, however, to consider the possibility of an interaction and to monitor prothrombin time closely if one of these antibiotics must be taken together with warfarin.

Symptoms of Warfarin Overdose

There may be no early warning signs of danger. Blood tests are essential. Symptoms include any unusual bleeding, including rectal or urinary tract bleeding, excessive menstrual bleeding, nosebleeds, bleeding around gums, bruising, red or tar-black stools, vomiting blood, and red or dark-brown urine. Notify your doctor immediately if you suspect a problem.

INTERACTION

DANGEROUS

Anticoagulant
(WARFARIN)

Antibiotics
(TETRACYCLINES)

BRAND NAME	GENERIC NAME
Coumadin	warfarin

DESCRIPTION

Warfarin slows the liver's production of factors essential for the formation of blood clots. It is prescribed when there is a risk that a dangerous clot could form in a deep vein or a blood vessel leading to the lung, heart, or brain. The most serious complication of anticoagulant treatment is excessive bleeding. The dosage must be individually adjusted, requiring daily blood tests at first, then tests every four to six weeks. Other side effects may include nausea, loss of appetite, rash, fever, yellow eyes and skin, prolonged painful erection, and hair loss.

INSTRUCTIONS

Warfarin tablets can be swallowed with food or on an empty stomach. Try to avoid large variations in the quantity of vitamin-K–containing vegetables—such as broccoli, cabbage, or spinach—that you eat each day. Consuming much more or less than usual could change the action of the drug.

BRAND NAME	GENERIC NAME
Achromycin V	tetracycline
Declomycin	demeclocycline
Doryx	doxycycline
Minocin	minocycline
Panmycin	tetracycline
Robitet	tetracycline
Rondomycin	methacycline
Sumycin	tetracycline
Terramycin	oxytetracycline
Uri-Tet	oxytetracycline
Vibramycin	doxycycline

DESCRIPTION

Tetracycline antibiotics are prescribed for a wide variety of infections, from Rocky Mountain spotted fever to common problems such as acne. Tetracycline is generally inappropriate for pregnant women and young children, because it may stain permanent teeth.

INSTRUCTIONS

Take most forms of tetracycline on an empty stomach. See the table of Food and Drug Compatibility on pages 59-73 for specifics. Do not take these drugs with antacids, calcium or iron supplements, or dairy products because they could interfere with absorption. Never take outdated tetracycline, which may be toxic to the kidneys.

INTERACTION

Tetracycline antibiotics appear capable of increasing warfarin's effects in some people. Prothrombin (clotting) time should be tested frequently when a tetracycline is started or stopped, and the dosage of warfarin adjusted accordingly; *otherwise, this interaction could lead to dangerous bleeding.*

Symptoms of Warfarin Overdose

There may be no early warning signs of danger. Blood tests are essential. Symptoms include any unusual bleeding, including rectal or urinary tract bleeding, excessive menstrual bleeding, nosebleeds, bleeding around gums, bruising, red or tar-black stools, vomiting blood, and red or dark-brown urine. Notify your doctor immediately if you suspect a problem.

INTERACTION

DANGEROUS

Anticoagulant
(WARFARIN)

Antidepressants
(SEROTONIN-BASED)

BRAND NAME	GENERIC NAME
Coumadin	warfarin

DESCRIPTION

Warfarin slows the liver's production of factors essential for the formation of blood clots. It is prescribed when there is a risk that a dangerous clot could form in a deep vein or a blood vessel leading to the lung, heart, or brain. The most serious complication of anticoagulant treatment is excessive bleeding. The dosage must be individually adjusted, requiring daily blood tests at first, then tests every four to six weeks. Other side effects may include nausea, loss of appetite, rash, fever, yellow eyes and skin, prolonged painful erection, and hair loss.

INSTRUCTIONS

Warfarin tablets can be swallowed with food or on an empty stomach. Try to avoid large variations in the quantity of vitamin-K–containing vegetables—such as broccoli, cabbage, or spinach—that you eat each day. Consuming much more or less than usual could change the action of the drug.

BRAND NAME	GENERIC NAME
Paxil	paroxetine
Prozac	fluoxetine
Zoloft	sertraline

DESCRIPTION

These antidepressants work by blocking the reuptake into brain cells of serotonin, a chemical messenger. Because they work differently from older antidepressants, they have different side effects and indications. Prozac, for instance, is also prescribed for obsessive-compulsive disorder and for bulimia. Older people and those with kidney or liver problems may need reduced doses. Prozac is cleared from the body very slowly and may linger weeks after discontinuation.

INSTRUCTIONS

Paxil and Zoloft are taken once a day, usually in the morning. Prozac is taken in the morning, or, if a higher dose has been prescribed, in the morning and at noon. It may be taken without regard to meals. Taking it with food may reduce stomach upset. A few patients experience serious weight loss on these medications. If this occurs, the doctor should be notified.

INTERACTION

Although there are only a few reports of interaction between any of these antidepressants and warfarin, it appears that in some cases these serotonin-based medications can increase the risk of bleeding associated with warfarin. *This interaction could be dangerous.*

It is possible that many patients will have no trouble with this combination, but the physician should monitor carefully for a potential interaction. Prothrombin time or international normalized ratio (INR) may be increased. Notify your physician immediately if you experience any symptoms of bleeding.

Symptoms of Warfarin Overdose

There may be no early warning signs of danger. Blood tests are essential. Symptoms include any unusual bleeding, including rectal or urinary tract bleeding, excessive menstrual bleeding, nosebleeds, bleeding around gums, bruising, red or tar-black stools, vomiting blood, and red or dark-brown urine. Notify your doctor immediately if you suspect a problem.

INTERACTION

DANGEROUS

Anticoagulant
(WARFARIN)

Antifungal Drugs

BRAND NAME	GENERIC NAME
Coumadin	warfarin

DESCRIPTION

Warfarin slows the liver's production of factors essential for the formation of blood clots. It is prescribed when there is a risk that a dangerous clot could form in a deep vein or a blood vessel leading to the lung, heart, or brain. The most serious complication of anticoagulant treatment is excessive bleeding. The dosage must be individually adjusted, requiring daily blood tests at first, then tests every four to six weeks. Other side effects may include nausea, loss of appetite, rash, fever, yellow eyes and skin, prolonged painful erection, and hair loss.

INSTRUCTIONS

Warfarin tablets can be swallowed with food or on an empty stomach. Try to avoid large variations in the quantity of vitamin-K–containing vegetables—such as broccoli, cabbage, or spinach—that you eat each day. Consuming much more or less than usual could change the action of the drug.

BRAND NAME	GENERIC NAME
Diflucan	fluconazole
Monistat	miconazole

DESCRIPTION

Diflucan is a strong antifungal drug used to treat serious yeast and yeastlike infections, including thrush and cryptococcal meningitis. While it can be lifesaving in such situations, in rare cases it also has potentially serious side effects. Diflucan may damage the liver, and liver enzymes should be monitored. Other side effects include nausea, vomiting, headache, skin rash, abdominal pain, and diarrhea. Notify your doctor if you experience any of these. The skin rash could become more serious.

Monistat is a vaginal cream used against vaginal yeast infections. It may cause hives or skin rash, but probably less circulates in the body than if it were taken as a pill or injection.

INSTRUCTIONS

Ask your doctor for precise instructions on how to take Diflucan. Doses are individualized, depending on the infection treated, and the first dose is often higher than the rest. Unprotected sexual intercourse should be avoided during Monistat treatment.

INTERACTION

Monistat is principally a vaginal preparation, but when given systemically (intravenously), it inhibits an important liver enzyme that processes warfarin. As a result, levels of the anticoagulant build up and prothrombin time may increase as much as four or five times. *This interaction could be dangerous, resulting in serious bleeding.* Even when Monistat is used as a vaginal cream, some is absorbed into the body. Precautions are appropriate. When either Diflucan or Monistat is taken together with warfarin, prothrombin time should be monitored frequently (at least every two days) and the dose of warfarin adjusted as necessary.

Symptoms of Warfarin Overdose

There may be no early warning signs of danger. Blood tests are essential. Symptoms include any unusual bleeding, including rectal or urinary tract bleeding, excessive menstrual bleeding, nosebleeds, bleeding around gums, bruising, red or tar-black stools, vomiting blood, and red or dark-brown urine. Notify your doctor immediately if you suspect a problem.

Never take or stop medication without your doctor's advice.

INTERACTION

DANGEROUS

Anticoagulant

(WARFARIN)

Cholesterol Drug

(LOVASTATIN)

BRAND NAME | GENERIC NAME

Coumadin   warfarin

DESCRIPTION

Warfarin slows the liver's production of factors essential for the formation of blood clots. It is prescribed when there is a risk that a dangerous clot could form in a deep vein or a blood vessel leading to the lung, heart, or brain. The most serious complication of anticoagulant treatment is excessive bleeding. The dosage must be individually adjusted, requiring daily blood tests at first, then tests every four to six weeks. Other side effects may include nausea, loss of appetite, rash, fever, yellow eyes and skin, prolonged painful erection, and hair loss.

INSTRUCTIONS

Warfarin tablets can be swallowed with food or on an empty stomach. Try to avoid large variations in the quantity of vitamin-K–containing vegetables—such as broccoli, cabbage, or spinach—that you eat each day. Consuming much more or less than usual could change the action of the drug.

BRAND NAME | GENERIC NAME

Mevacor   lovastatin

DESCRIPTION

Mevacor is a potent cholesterol-lowering agent that has become widely prescribed. Because of the association between high cholesterol and heart disease, Mevacor is given in the hope of preventing a heart attack. It reduces the body's production of cholesterol and speeds the removal of this fat from the bloodstream. Side effects of Mevacor include digestive distress, rash, and headache. Contact the physician if you experience muscle pain or weakness, because this could signal a serious reaction.

INSTRUCTIONS

Mevacor is best taken with the evening meal. It is most effective in combination with a prudent heart-healthy diet and a sensible exercise program.

INTERACTION

Mevacor appears to increase the effects of warfarin in some patients. Two middle-aged men requiring warfarin were later put on Mevacor for elevated cholesterol. Each of them developed unexpected bleeding and prolonged prothrombin times. *This interaction could be dangerous.* If Mevacor and warfarin are both needed, frequent blood tests will guide warfarin dose adjustment. There is no evidence that the other cholesterol-lowering drugs, Pravachol (generic: pravastatin) or Zocor (generic: simvastatin), interact with warfarin in the same fashion. Because they are similar to Mevacor, however, caution is probably advisable.

Symptoms of Warfarin Overdose

There may be no early warning signs of danger. Blood tests are essential. Symptoms include any unusual bleeding, including rectal or urinary tract bleeding, excessive menstrual bleeding, nosebleeds, bleeding around gums, bruising, red or tar-black stools, vomiting blood, and red or dark-brown urine. Notify your doctor immediately if you suspect a problem.

INTERACTION

DANGEROUS

Anticoagulant
(WARFARIN)

Heart Drug
(QUINIDINE)

BRAND NAME	GENERIC NAME
Coumadin	warfarin

DESCRIPTION

Warfarin slows the liver's production of factors essential for the formation of blood clots. It is prescribed when there is a risk that a dangerous clot could form in a deep vein or a blood vessel leading to the lung, heart, or brain. The most serious complication of anticoagulant treatment is excessive bleeding. The dosage must be individually adjusted, requiring daily blood tests at first, then tests every four to six weeks. Other side effects may include nausea, loss of appetite, rash, fever, yellow eyes and skin, prolonged painful erection, and hair loss.

INSTRUCTIONS

Warfarin tablets can be swallowed with food or on an empty stomach. Try to avoid large variations in the quantity of vitamin-K–containing vegetables—such as broccoli, cabbage, or spinach—that you eat each day. Consuming much more or less than usual could change the action of the drug.

BRAND NAME	GENERIC NAME
Cardioquin	quinidine
Quinaglute	quinidine
Quinidex	quinidine
Quinora	quinidine

DESCRIPTION

Quinidine is prescribed for a variety of heart rhythm disturbances. The first dose is considered a test to see if the patient will have a dangerous reaction. People with heart failure or with liver or kidney disease need close monitoring.

INSTRUCTIONS

Quinidine may upset the stomach and should be taken with food. Sustained-release tablets should not be chewed or crushed.

It may provoke visual disturbances, ringing in the ears, headache, dizziness, nausea, skin rash, or breathing difficulties. Notify your doctor if you develop any of these symptoms.

INTERACTION

Quinine derivatives, including the heart drug quinidine, may increase the effectiveness of warfarin. *This interaction could be dangerous, resulting in serious bleeding.*

Prothrombin time should be tested when any of these medicines must be started or stopped, because the dose of warfarin might need adjustment. Notify the doctor of any problems.

Symptoms of Warfarin Overdose

There may be no early warning signs of danger. Blood tests are essential. Symptoms include any unusual bleeding, including rectal or urinary tract bleeding, excessive menstrual bleeding, nosebleeds, bleeding around gums, bruising, red or tar-black stools, vomiting blood, and red or dark-brown urine. Notify your doctor immediately if you suspect a problem.

Never take or stop medication without your doctor's advice.

INTERACTION

DANGEROUS

Anticoagulant
(WARFARIN)

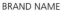

Anticonvulsant
(CARBAMAZEPINE)

BRAND NAME | GENERIC NAME
Coumadin | warfarin

DESCRIPTION

Warfarin slows the liver's production of factors essential for the formation of blood clots. It is prescribed when there is a risk that a dangerous clot could form in a deep vein or a blood vessel leading to the lung, heart, or brain. The most serious complication of anticoagulant treatment is excessive bleeding. The dosage must be individually adjusted, requiring daily blood tests at first, then tests every four to six weeks. Other side effects may include nausea, loss of appetite, rash, fever, yellow eyes and skin, prolonged painful erection, and hair loss.

INSTRUCTIONS

Warfarin tablets can be swallowed with food or on an empty stomach. Try to avoid large variations in the quantity of vitamin-K–containing vegetables—such as broccoli, cabbage, or spinach—that you eat each day. Consuming much more or less than usual could change the action of the drug.

BRAND NAME | GENERIC NAME
Tegretol | carbamazepine

DESCRIPTION

Carbamazepine is prescribed to prevent epileptic seizures, especially in people for whom other anticonvulsants have not worked well. It is also used to control severe facial pain related to the trigeminal nerve. Carbamazepine has the potential to trigger a lethal blood abnormality, so regular monitoring is critical, particularly during the first two months. This drug can cause drowsiness or dizziness; driving or other tasks requiring alertness may be impaired. Contact your doctor if you experience drowsiness, dizziness, confusion, mood or behavior changes, nausea, swollen legs and feet, pale stools, yellow skin and eyes, unusual bleeding or bruising, dark urine, sore throat, mouth sores, fever, or chills.

INSTRUCTIONS

Carbamazepine may upset the stomach; if so, take it with food or milk. Do not stop taking this drug suddenly; seizures could result. To maintain its strength, it must be stored away from humidity and heat in a tightly closed container.

INTERACTION

Carbamazepine apparently reduces circulating levels of warfarin. The result could be a greater risk of blood clots. *This interaction could be troublesome.*

When a person on warfarin needs to start or stop taking this anticonvulsant, close monitoring of prothrombin time is appropriate. A few case reports feature patients whose prothrombin time was five or six times greater upon discontinuing carbamazepine, a situation that could lead to dangerous bleeding. The physician may need to adjust the dose of warfarin when Tegretol is discontinued.

Symptoms of Warfarin Overdose

There may be no early warning signs of danger. Blood tests are essential. Symptoms include any unusual bleeding, including rectal or urinary tract bleeding, excessive menstrual bleeding, nosebleeds, bleeding around gums, bruising, red or tar-black stools, vomiting blood, and red or dark-brown urine. Notify your doctor immediately if you suspect a problem.

Never take or stop medication without your doctor's advice.

INTERACTION

TROUBLESOME

Anticoagulant
(WARFARIN)

Cholesterol Drugs

BRAND NAME | GENERIC NAME

Coumadin | warfarin

DESCRIPTION

Warfarin slows the liver's production of factors essential for the formation of blood clots. It is prescribed when there is a risk that a dangerous clot could form in a deep vein or a blood vessel leading to the lung, heart, or brain. The most serious complication of anticoagulant treatment is excessive bleeding. The dosage must be individually adjusted, requiring daily blood tests at first, then tests every four to six weeks. Other side effects may include nausea, loss of appetite, rash, fever, yellow eyes and skin, prolonged painful erection, and hair loss.

INSTRUCTIONS

Warfarin tablets can be swallowed with food or on an empty stomach. Try to avoid large variations in the quantity of vitamin-K–containing vegetables—such as broccoli, cabbage, or spinach—that you eat each day. Consuming much more or less than usual could change the action of the drug.

BRAND NAME | GENERIC NAME

Colestid | colestipol
Questran | cholestyramine

DESCRIPTION

Questran and Colestid are effective drugs for lowering total cholesterol and the particularly dangerous LDL (low-density lipoprotein) cholesterol, which is thought to contribute to coronary artery disease. They do this by binding to bile acids in the intestinal tract and removing them from circulation. Bile is made in the liver and used by the body to digest fats in food. When bile acids are reduced, the body has to work harder to convert cholesterol to make more bile. This is thought to reduce the amount of cholesterol circulating in the bloodstream.

INSTRUCTIONS

Questran and Colestid come in powder form and need to be mixed with a glassful of water. Questran should not be taken with carbonated beverages. These medications are usually taken before meals, but check with a physician or pharmacist for specific instructions.

INTERACTION

These cholesterol-lowering drugs appear to reduce the absorption of blood thinners such as Coumadin. This could lead to diminished effectiveness and increase the risk of blood clots. It would be better to avoid this interaction if at all possible. When that is not possible, at least six hours should separate the intake of Questran or Colestid and Coumadin. Maintain the same schedule each day to prevent variation in absorption. Blood should be monitored carefully to make sure proper anticoagulant action is obtained.

Never take or stop medication without your doctor's advice.

INTERACTION

TROUBLESOME

Anticoagulant

(WARFARIN)

Thyroid Hormone

BRAND NAME	GENERIC NAME
Coumadin	warfarin

DESCRIPTION

Warfarin slows the liver's production of factors essential for the formation of blood clots. It is prescribed when there is a risk that a dangerous clot could form in a deep vein or a blood vessel leading to the lung, heart, or brain. The most serious complication of anticoagulant treatment is excessive bleeding. The dosage must be individually adjusted, requiring daily blood tests at first, then tests every four to six weeks. Other side effects may include nausea, loss of appetite, rash, fever, yellow eyes and skin, prolonged painful erection, and hair loss.

INSTRUCTIONS

Warfarin tablets can be swallowed with food or on an empty stomach. Try to avoid large variations in the quantity of vitamin-K–containing vegetables—such as broccoli, cabbage, or spinach—that you eat each day. Consuming much more or less than usual could change the action of the drug.

BRAND NAME	GENERIC NAME
Armour Thyroid	dessicated thyroid
Cytomel	liothyronine
Levothroid	levothyroxine
Synthroid	levothyroxine
Thyroid Strong	dessicated thyroid
etc.	

DESCRIPTION

The thyroid gland controls the metabolic rate (oxygen use) of all the cells in the body and interacts in complex and important ways with virtually all the hormones the body produces. When the thyroid doesn't work properly, people often feel ill, but symptoms of thyroid dysfunction may be disconcertingly vague. When thyroid hormone is lacking, it is administered in pill form. When the dose is properly adjusted, a process that requires occasional blood tests, there should be few if any side effects.

INSTRUCTIONS

Thyroid hormone is best taken on an empty stomach at the same time each day. It should not be taken together with iron supplements, which reduce absorption.

INTERACTION

Thyroid hormone can have a major impact on bleeding associated with Coumadin, greatly increasing prothrombin time. People with underactive thyroids may need higher doses of warfarin than usual. If they are then started on thyroid hormone replacement, the anticoagulant may become significantly more effective (50 to 400 percent). *This reaction could result in troublesome bleeding.*

Symptoms of Warfarin Overdose

There may be no early warning signs of danger. Blood tests are essential. Symptoms include any unusual bleeding, including rectal or urinary tract bleeding, excessive menstrual bleeding, nosebleeds, bleeding around gums, bruising, red or tar-black stools, vomiting blood, and red or dark-brown urine. Notify your doctor immediately if you suspect a problem.

Never take or stop medication without your doctor's advice.

INTERACTION

TROUBLESOME

Anticoagulant
(WARFARIN)

Tuberculosis Drug
(RIFAMPIN)

BRAND NAME | GENERIC NAME
Coumadin | warfarin

DESCRIPTION

Warfarin slows the liver's production of factors essential for the formation of blood clots. It is prescribed when there is a risk that a dangerous clot could form in a deep vein or a blood vessel leading to the lung, heart, or brain. The most serious complication of anticoagulant treatment is excessive bleeding. The dosage must be individually adjusted, requiring daily blood tests at first, then tests every four to six weeks. Other side effects may include nausea, loss of appetite, rash, fever, yellow eyes and skin, prolonged painful erection, and hair loss.

INSTRUCTIONS

Warfarin tablets can be swallowed with food or on an empty stomach. Try to avoid large variations in the quantity of vitamin-K–containing vegetables—such as broccoli, cabbage, or spinach—that you eat each day. Consuming much more or less than usual could change the action of the drug.

BRAND NAME | GENERIC NAME
Rifadin | rifampin
Rifamate | isoniazid/rifampin
Rimactane | rifampin

DESCRIPTION

Rifampin is used in combination with other medications to treat tuberculosis. To be effective, it needs to be taken faithfully for an extended period of time (at least six to nine months), as the doctor prescribes. Side effects may include digestive tract problems, menstrual irregularities, difficulty concentrating, fluid retention, and wheezing or shortness of breath. The orange discoloration of urine, saliva, and tears is not harmful, although it may stain contact lenses.

INSTRUCTIONS

Rifampin should be taken on an empty stomach, at least one hour before or two hours after meals. If you develop fever, chills, unusual tiredness, unusual bleeding or bruising, sore throat, muscle and bone pain, or yellow skin and eyes, contact your physician immediately.

INTERACTION

Rifampin may speed the body's elimination of warfarin and thus decrease circulating levels of the anticoagulant. The result could be a greater risk of blood clots. *This interaction could be troublesome.*

When a person on warfarin needs to start or stop this tuberculosis treatment, close monitoring of prothrombin time is appropriate. Because rifampin increases the requirement for warfarin by as much as 50 percent, the dose must be adjusted downward carefully when rifampin is discontinued to avoid excess bleeding.

Symptoms of Warfarin Overdose

There may be no early warning signs of danger. Blood tests are essential. Symptoms include any unusual bleeding, including rectal or urinary tract bleeding, excessive menstrual bleeding, nosebleeds, bleeding around gums, bruising, red or tar-black stools, vomiting blood, and red or dark-brown urine. Notify your doctor immediately if you suspect a problem.

INTERACTION

TROUBLESOME

Anticoagulant
(WARFARIN)

Vitamin E

BRAND NAME	GENERIC NAME
Coumadin	warfarin

BRAND NAME	GENERIC NAME
Aquasol E	tocopherol
E-Complex	tocopherol
Vitamin E	tocopherol
Vita-Plus E	tocopherol

DESCRIPTION

Warfarin slows the liver's production of factors essential for the formation of blood clots. It is prescribed when there is a risk that a dangerous clot could form in a deep vein or a blood vessel leading to the lung, heart, or brain. The most serious complication of anticoagulant treatment is excessive bleeding. The dosage must be individually adjusted, requiring daily blood tests at first, then tests every four to six weeks. Other side effects may include nausea, loss of appetite, rash, fever, yellow eyes and skin, prolonged painful erection, and hair loss.

INSTRUCTIONS

Warfarin tablets can be swallowed with food or on an empty stomach. Try to avoid large variations in the quantity of vitamin-K–containing vegetables—such as broccoli, cabbage, or spinach—that you eat each day. Consuming much more or less than usual could change the action of the drug.

DESCRIPTION

Vitamin E is a fat-soluble vitamin derived from plant oils that acts as an antioxidant in the body and helps keep red blood cells from breaking down. While vitamin E deficiency is rare, supplements are prescribed for cystic fibrosis, and research is currently ongoing about the benefits of vitamin E in a wide range of situations, including heart attack prevention and protection from the effects of air pollution. Side effects are unusual at doses of 800 IU per day or less. People taking beta carotene supplements probably also need vitamin E supplements to maintain the proper balance between the two vitamins.

INSTRUCTIONS

Vitamin E may be taken with meals or on an empty stomach. A doctor's supervision is prudent for doses of 800 IU daily or more.

INTERACTION

Vitamin E alone helps prevent blood clotting by keeping platelets from sticking together. In combination with warfarin, theoretically it could have an additive effect and lead to unexpected bleeding. *This interaction could be troublesome.*

One patient got into trouble by taking up to 1,200 IU of vitamin E a day on his own, in addition to his prescribed warfarin. After two months, he experienced unusual bleeding and his prothrombin time was increased. Doses of vitamin E over 400 IU daily may be required to trigger this interaction, but it makes sense to be careful even at lower doses. If you plan to take vitamin E supplements, consult your doctor. More frequent blood tests may be appropriate.

Symptoms of Warfarin Overdose

There may be no early warning signs of danger. Blood tests are essential. Symptoms include any unusual bleeding, including rectal or urinary tract bleeding, excessive menstrual bleeding, nosebleeds, bleeding around gums, bruising, red or tar-black stools, vomiting blood, and red or dark-brown urine. Notify your doctor immediately if you suspect a problem.

Anticoagulant
(WARFARIN)

Vitamin K

BRAND NAME	GENERIC NAME
Coumadin	warfarin

DESCRIPTION

Warfarin slows the liver's production of factors essential for the formation of blood clots. It is prescribed when there is a risk that a dangerous clot could form in a deep vein or a blood vessel leading to the lung, heart, or brain. The most serious complication of anticoagulant treatment is excessive bleeding. The dosage must be individually adjusted, requiring daily blood tests at first, then tests every four to six weeks. Other side effects may include nausea, loss of appetite, rash, fever, yellow eyes and skin, prolonged painful erection, and hair loss.

INSTRUCTIONS

Warfarin tablets can be swallowed with food or on an empty stomach. Try to avoid large variations in the quantity of vitamin-K–containing vegetables—such as broccoli, cabbage, or spinach—that you eat each day. Consuming much more or less than usual could change the action of the drug.

DESCRIPTION

Vitamin K injections are sometimes administered to reverse the action of warfarin in the event of dangerous bleeding. In addition, this vitamin is found in liver, some legumes (such as soybeans, lentils, and chickpeas), dark leafy vegetables such as turnip or collard greens, and cabbage-family vegetables, including broccoli and brussels sprouts. Soybean oil, green tea, and seaweed are rich in vitamin K but not important sources in the usual diet.

INSTRUCTIONS

A healthy diet includes plenty of fruit, vegetables, legumes, and grains. The person on warfarin should try to maintain a relatively constant intake of such foods so that there will not be strong variations in the amount of dietary vitamin K.

INTERACTION

Vitamin K is essential for proper clotting of blood. Warfarin works by suppressing certain vitamin-K–dependent factors needed for the formation of blood clots, but giving enough extra vitamin K can overwhelm the system and diminish the effects of warfarin. *While this action is useful in the hospital when bleeding threatens, it could be troublesome if vitamin K intake were inadvertent.*

It is important not to vary intake of vitamin K sources greatly. If fluctuations are likely, prothrombin time should probably be monitored.

Symptoms of Warfarin Overdose
There may be no early warning signs of danger. Blood tests are essential. Symptoms include any unusual bleeding, including rectal or urinary tract bleeding, excessive menstrual bleeding, nosebleeds, bleeding around gums, bruising, red or tar-black stools, vomiting blood, and red or dark-brown urine. Notify your doctor immediately if you suspect a problem.

Never take or stop medication without your doctor's advice.

INTERACTION

TROUBLESOME

Anticonvulsant
(CARBAMAZEPINE)

Tegretol

LIFE THREATENING

Antibiotics (macrolides)
Biaxin   E.E.S.   E-Mycin
PCE   etc.

Pain Reliever (propoxyphene)
Darvocet-N   Darvon
Darvon-N   Wygesic

Ulcer Drug
Tagamet

Tuberculosis Drugs (isoniazid)
INH   Izonid   Laniazid
Nydrazid   Rifamate

Transplant Drug
Sandimmune

Oral Contraceptives

Lithium
Cibalith-S   Eskalith
Lithane   Lithobid
Lithonate   Lithotabs

Heart/Hypertension Drugs (calcium channel blockers)
Calan   Cardizem
Dilacor XR   Isoptin
Verelan

DANGEROUS

Anticonvulsant
Depakene   Depakote

Anticonvulsants (hydantoins)
Dilantin   Mesantoin
Peganone

Antidepressant (serotonin-based)
Prozac

Antidepressants (tricyclic)
Elavil   Norpramin
Pamelor   Tofranil
etc.

Asthma Drug (theophylline)
Elixophyllin   Quibron-T
Respbid   Slo-bid
Slo-Phyllin   Theobid
Theochron   Theoclear
Theo-Dur   Theolair
Theo-24   Theovent
etc.

Endometriosis Drug
Danocrine

TROUBLESOME

Antibiotic (doxycycline)
Doryx   Doxychel   Hyclate
Monodox   Vibramycin
Vibra-Tabs

Anticoagulant
Coumadin

Barbiturates
Amytal   Butisol
Mebaral   Nembutal
phenobarbital   Seconal
Tuinal

Drug for Schizophrenia
Haldol

Influenza Vaccine

Carbamazepine interacts with many other medications. Some of these interactions are potentially serious. We have included the most common, but be sure to check with your physician and pharmacist if you must take any other drugs in conjunction with this anticonvulsant.

LEVELS OF HAZARD: LIFE THREATENING   DANGEROUS   TROUBLESOME

Anticonvulsant

(CARBAMAZEPINE)

Antibiotics

(MACROLIDES)

BRAND NAME	GENERIC NAME
Tegretol	carbamazepine

DESCRIPTION

Carbamazepine is often prescribed to people for whom other anticonvulsants have not worked well. It is also used to control severe facial pain related to the trigeminal nerve. Carbamazepine may trigger a potentially lethal blood abnormality, so regular monitoring is critical, particularly during the first two months. This drug can cause drowsiness or dizziness; driving may be impaired. Contact your doctor if you experience drowsiness, dizziness, confusion, mood or behavior changes, nausea, swollen legs and feet, pale stools, yellow skin or eyes, unusual bleeding or bruising, dark urine, sore throat, mouth sores, fever, or chills.

INSTRUCTIONS

Carbamazepine may upset the stomach; if so, take it with food or milk. Do not stop this drug suddenly; seizures could result. To maintain its strength, it must be stored away from humidity and heat in a tightly closed container.

BRAND NAME	GENERIC NAME
Biaxin	clarithromycin
E.E.S.	erythromycin
E-Mycin	erythromycin
ERYC	erythromycin
EryPed	erythromycin
Ery-Tab	erythromycin
Erythrocin	erythromycin
Ilosone	erythromycin
PCE	erythromycin
Pediazole	erythromycin
Tao	troleandomycin
Zithromax	azithromycin

DESCRIPTION

These broad-spectrum antibiotics are widely prescribed for respiratory tract, sinus, ear, and skin infections. They are also effective against *Chlamydia* and certain other infections of the reproductive tract.

INSTRUCTIONS

Some forms of erythromycin must be taken on an empty stomach; others may be taken with food. See the table of Food and Drug Compatibility on pages 59-73 for specifics. Biaxin can be taken without regard to meals. Zithromax is best taken on an empty stomach.

INTERACTION

Erythromycin and other drugs in this category can interfere with the liver's processing of carbamazepine. The anticonvulsant can build up to toxic levels within a day or two. *This interaction can be life threatening, requiring hospitalization and resuscitation.*

If no other antibiotic is appropriate, carbamazepine levels must be monitored extremely closely. They may remain high for two or three days after the antibiotic is discontinued. The doctor may be able to adjust the dose of Tegretol to avoid a toxic reaction. Contact your physician without delay if there is any sign of problems.

Symptoms of Carbamazepine Toxicity

Nausea, vomiting, drowsiness, unsteadiness, incoordination, dizziness, muscle twitching or tremor, irregular breathing, rapid heartbeat, changes in blood pressure, changes in urination, and impaired consciousness. Notify your physician immediately of any such symptoms.

INTERACTION

LIFE THREATENING

Anticonvulsant

(CARBAMAZEPINE)

Pain Reliever

(PROPOXYPHENE)

BRAND NAME	GENERIC NAME
Tegretol	carbamazepine

DESCRIPTION

Carbamazepine is often prescribed to people for whom other anticonvulsants have not worked well. It is also used to control severe facial pain related to the trigeminal nerve. Carbamazepine may trigger a potentially lethal blood abnormality, so regular monitoring is critical, particularly during the first two months. This drug can cause drowsiness or dizziness; driving may be impaired. Contact your doctor if you experience drowsiness, dizziness, confusion, mood or behavior changes, nausea, swollen legs and feet, pale stools, yellow skin or eyes, unusual bleeding or bruising, dark urine, sore throat, mouth sores, fever, or chills.

INSTRUCTIONS

Carbamazepine may upset the stomach; if so, take it with food or milk. Do not stop this drug suddenly; seizures could result. To maintain its strength, it must be stored away from humidity and heat in a tightly closed container.

BRAND NAME	GENERIC NAME
Darvocet-N	propoxyphene/ acetaminophen
Darvon	propoxyphene
Darvon-N	propoxyphene
Wygesic	propoxyphene/ acetaminophen

DESCRIPTION

Darvon, Darvocet, and the generic forms of propoxyphene, alone or in combination with acetaminophen or aspirin (Darvon Compound), are popular prescription medicines for relieving moderate pain. Propoxyphene is a narcotic, about half as potent as codeine. It is more effective at preventing pain than at relieving pain that is already intense. This medicine may affect your ability to drive and do other complex tasks. Long-term use can lead to dependence. Side effects include nausea, vomiting, drowsiness, and dizziness. Tell your doctor if you become short of breath.

INSTRUCTIONS

Propoxyphene should be taken with food to reduce the risk of nausea. If it causes constipation, a stool softener or fiber bulk agent (such as Metamucil) may be used. Do not drink alcohol while taking propoxyphene.

INTERACTION

Propoxyphene interferes with liver metabolism of Tegretol and leads to high blood levels of carbamazepine. This will probably occur in most people taking both medications, with blood levels of the anticonvulsant ranging from 66 to 300 percent higher than normal. *This interaction can result in life-threatening carbamazepine toxicity, with possible coma.*

Generally, the doctor will be able to prescribe an alternate pain medication. If this is not possible, frequent monitoring of carbamazepine blood levels is necessary to prevent a dangerous interaction.

Symptoms of Carbamazepine Toxicity

Nausea, vomiting, drowsiness, unsteadiness, incoordination, dizziness, muscle twitching or tremor, irregular breathing, rapid heartbeat, changes in blood pressure, changes in urination, and impaired consciousness. Notify your physician immediately of any such symptoms.

Never take or stop medication without your doctor's advice.

INTERACTION

LIFE THREATENING

Anticonvulsant
(CARBAMAZEPINE)

Anticonvulsant
(VALPROIC ACID)

BRAND NAME	GENERIC NAME
Tegretol	carbamazepine

DESCRIPTION

Carbamazepine is often prescribed to people for whom other anticonvulsants have not worked well. It is also used to control severe facial pain related to the trigeminal nerve. Carbamazepine may trigger a potentially lethal blood abnormality, so regular monitoring is critical, particularly during the first two months. This drug can cause drowsiness or dizziness; driving may be impaired. Contact your doctor if you experience drowsiness, dizziness, confusion, mood or behavior changes, nausea, swollen legs and feet, pale stools, yellow skin or eyes, unusual bleeding or bruising, dark urine, sore throat, mouth sores, fever, or chills.

INSTRUCTIONS

Carbamazepine may upset the stomach; if so, take it with food or milk. Do not stop this drug suddenly; seizures could result. To maintain its strength, it must be stored away from humidity and heat in a tightly closed container.

BRAND NAME	GENERIC NAME
Depakene	valproic acid
Depakote	divalproex sodium

DESCRIPTION

Valproic acid is prescribed to prevent seizures, especially "petit mal" or absence seizures. It may be used in combination with other anticonvulsants, and is sometimes used to treat seizures associated with a sudden high fever in young children. Suddenly stopping this drug could trigger renewed seizure activity. This medication is not appropriate for patients with liver disease. Check with your doctor and pharmacist before taking any other drug.

INSTRUCTIONS

If this medicine upsets the stomach, it should be taken with food. Capsules should be swallowed whole, not chewed. Either of these medications can cause drowsiness and limit attention. Take them at a time when you will not need to drive or do other complicated tasks. Avoid alcohol, which may make drowsiness worse.

INTERACTION

Carbamazepine and valproic acid may both be prescribed for a complex seizure disorder. This combination may be complicated, because Tegretol can speed the elimination of Depakene and other valproates from the body. This may result in lower blood levels, and possibly a loss of effectiveness. *Because of the risk of seizures, this interaction is dangerous.*

Valproic acid can also affect carbamazepine levels. The action may vary from one person to another. Regular blood tests to monitor levels of both drugs are desirable for at least one month after starting or stopping this combination. Dosage adjustments may be necessary.

Symptoms of Carbamazepine Toxicity

Nausea, vomiting, drowsiness, unsteadiness, incoordination, dizziness, muscle twitching or tremor, irregular breathing, rapid heartbeat, changes in blood pressure, changes in urination, and impaired consciousness. Notify your physician immediately of any such symptoms.

INTERACTION

DANGEROUS

Anticonvulsant

(CARBAMAZEPINE)

Anticonvulsants

(HYDANTOINS)

BRAND NAME	GENERIC NAME
Tegretol	carbamazepine

DESCRIPTION

Carbamazepine is often prescribed to people for whom other anticonvulsants have not worked well. It is also used to control severe facial pain related to the trigeminal nerve. Carbamazepine may trigger a potentially lethal blood abnormality, so regular monitoring is critical, particularly during the first two months. This drug can cause drowsiness or dizziness; driving may be impaired. Contact your doctor if you experience drowsiness, dizziness, confusion, mood or behavior changes, nausea, swollen legs and feet, pale stools, yellow skin or eyes, unusual bleeding or bruising, dark urine, sore throat, mouth sores, fever, or chills.

INSTRUCTIONS

Carbamazepine may upset the stomach; if so, take it with food or milk. Do not stop this drug suddenly; seizures could result. To maintain its strength, it must be stored away from humidity and heat in a tightly closed container.

BRAND NAME	GENERIC NAME
Dilantin	phenytoin
Mesantoin	mephenytoin
Peganone	ethotoin

DESCRIPTION

These anticonvulsants are used to prevent epileptic seizures or seizures associated with brain surgery. Occasionally they may be prescribed to treat severe stabbing facial pain (trigeminal neuralgia). Tests may be needed to check blood cells, blood levels of the drug, liver function, and blood sugar. Special attention to oral hygiene is needed to prevent gum problems often associated with taking these anticonvulsants. Hydantoin anticonvulsants interact with many other drugs as well as alcohol, so check carefully with your physician and pharmacist before taking any other medication.

INSTRUCTIONS

Any of these medicines could upset the stomach. This is less likely if they are taken with food. All of them can cause drowsiness or blurred vision and could make driving dangerous.

INTERACTION

People who have had seizures often need more than one kind of medicine to prevent a recurrence. Carbamazepine and an anticonvulsant such as Dilantin may be prescribed together and can be helpful. They may interact in a complex and unpredictable way, however. Dilantin and similar drugs can lower blood levels of carbamazepine. No seizures have been reported as a result, but theoretically they are possible. In contrast, carbamazepine sometimes raises and sometimes lowers blood levels of Dilantin. Some cases of toxicity from excess phenytoin have been reported. *This interaction could well be dangerous.*

Frequent blood tests for both drugs are advised, especially when starting, stopping, or changing the dose of one of them. The dose of one or both may need to be adjusted.

Symptoms of Phenytoin Toxicity

Uncontrollable eye movements (nystagmus), unsteadiness, difficulty speaking clearly, dizziness, and stupor. Notify your physician immediately of any of these symptoms.

INTERACTION

DANGEROUS

Anticonvulsant
(CARBAMAZEPINE)

Antidepressant
(SEROTONIN-BASED)

BRAND NAME	GENERIC NAME
Tegretol	carbamazepine

DESCRIPTION

Carbamazepine is often prescribed to people for whom other anticonvulsants have not worked well. It is also used to control severe facial pain related to the trigeminal nerve. Carbamazepine may trigger a potentially lethal blood abnormality, so regular monitoring is critical, particularly during the first two months. This drug can cause drowsiness or dizziness; driving may be impaired. Contact your doctor if you experience drowsiness, dizziness, confusion, mood or behavior changes, nausea, swollen legs and feet, pale stools, yellow skin or eyes, unusual bleeding or bruising, dark urine, sore throat, mouth sores, fever, or chills.

INSTRUCTIONS

Carbamazepine may upset the stomach; if so, take it with food or milk. Do not stop this drug suddenly; seizures could result. To maintain its strength, it must be stored away from humidity and heat in a tightly closed container.

BRAND NAME	GENERIC NAME
Prozac	fluoxetine

DESCRIPTION

This antidepressant works by blocking the reuptake into brain cells of serotonin, a chemical messenger. Because it works differently from the older cyclic-type antidepressants, it has a different set of side effects and has become more popular. It may also work against a different array of problems, for instance, bulimia or obsessive-compulsive disorder. Older people and those with kidney or liver problems may need reduced doses. Prozac is cleared from the body very slowly and may linger weeks after discontinuation.

INSTRUCTIONS

Prozac is taken in the morning, or, if a higher dose has been prescribed, in the morning and at noon. It may be taken without regard to meals. Taking it with food may reduce stomach upset. A few patients experience serious weight loss on this medication. If this occurs, the doctor should be notified.

INTERACTION

A depressed person with epilepsy might need both Prozac and carbamazepine. This combination might also be prescribed to someone with bipolar depression who has not responded to the usual treatments. Prozac apparently interferes with carbamazepine metabolism and may increase blood levels of the anticonvulsant to the point of toxicity. *The interaction could be dangerous.*

Because Prozac can linger in the body, the problems may continue for some time even if the drug is discontinued. Notify your physician immediately if you experience symptoms. There are no documented problems with the related antidepressants Paxil and Zoloft, but be alert for such a possibility.

Symptoms of Carbamazepine Toxicity

Nausea, vomiting, drowsiness, unsteadiness, incoordination, dizziness, muscle twitching or tremor, irregular breathing, rapid heartbeat, changes in blood pressure, changes in urination, and impaired consciousness. Notify your physician immediately of any such symptoms.

Never take or stop medication without your doctor's advice.

INTERACTION

DANGEROUS

Anticonvulsant

(CARBAMAZEPINE)

Antidepressants

(TRICYCLIC)

BRAND NAME	GENERIC NAME
Tegretol	carbamazepine

DESCRIPTION

Carbamazepine is often prescribed to people for whom other anticonvulsants have not worked well. It is also used to control severe facial pain related to the trigeminal nerve. Carbamazepine may trigger a potentially lethal blood abnormality, so regular monitoring is critical, particularly during the first two months. This drug can cause drowsiness or dizziness; driving may be impaired. Contact your doctor if you experience drowsiness, dizziness, confusion, mood or behavior changes, nausea, swollen legs and feet, pale stools, yellow skin or eyes, unusual bleeding or bruising, dark urine, sore throat, mouth sores, fever, or chills.

INSTRUCTIONS

Carbamazepine may upset the stomach; if so, take it with food or milk. Do not stop this drug suddenly; seizures could result. To maintain its strength, it must be stored away from humidity and heat in a tightly closed container.

BRAND NAME	GENERIC NAME
Adapin, Sinequan	doxepin
Aventyl, Pamelor	nortriptyline
Elavil, Endep	amitriptyline
Norpramin,	
Pertofrane	desipramine
Tofranil	imipramine
etc.	

DESCRIPTION

Tricyclic antidepressants became popular during the 1970s and 1980s although they often caused unpleasant side effects (constipation, weight gain, sexual dysfunction, sluggishness, increased sun sensitivity, etc.). They are used to treat depression. Some of them may also be helpful in controlling chronic pain.

INSTRUCTIONS

Usually these medications are better taken with food, in the evening to avoid daytime drowsiness. A high-fiber diet may interfere with absorption, however. Sinequan Concentrate should be mixed with four ounces of milk, water, or juice just before taking, not ahead of time. Do not stop taking any of these drugs suddenly; if they must be discontinued, the doctor will supervise gradual phaseout.

INTERACTION

There are many reasons (including bipolar disorder) a patient might require both carbamazepine and a tricyclic antidepressant. There are indictions from the medical literature that people taking both types of drug may have lower blood levels of the tricyclic antidepressant. It is not clear how often this has an impact on effectiveness. Conversely, at least one patient developed carbamazepine toxicity when she started taking desipramine. Blood levels of the anticonvulsant were dangerously high. *No one knows how often this interaction may occur, but it could be dangerous.*

Blood levels of both carbamazepine and tricyclic antidepressants should be checked when a person starts or stops this combination. Report any unusual symptoms to your doctor.

Symptoms of Carbamazepine Toxicity

Nausea, vomiting, drowsiness, unsteadiness, incoordination, dizziness, muscle twitching or tremor, irregular breathing, rapid heartbeat, changes in blood pressure, changes in urination, and impaired consciousness. Notify the physician immediately of any such symptoms.

INTERACTION

DANGEROUS

Anticonvulsant

(CARBAMAZEPINE)

Asthma Drug

(THEOPHYLLINE)

BRAND NAME | GENERIC NAME

Tegretol   carbamazepine

DESCRIPTION

Carbamazepine is often prescribed to people for whom other anticonvulsants have not worked well. It is also used to control severe facial pain related to the trigeminal nerve. Carbamazepine may trigger a potentially lethal blood abnormality, so regular monitoring is critical, particularly during the first two months. This drug can cause drowsiness or dizziness; driving may be impaired. Contact your doctor if you experience drowsiness, dizziness, confusion, mood or behavior changes, nausea, swollen legs and feet, pale stools, yellow skin or eyes, unusual bleeding or bruising, dark urine, sore throat, mouth sores, fever, or chills.

INSTRUCTIONS

Carbamazepine may upset the stomach; if so, take it with food or milk. Do not stop this drug suddenly; seizures could result. To maintain its strength, it must be stored away from humidity and heat in a tightly closed container.

BRAND NAME

Aerolate	**Aquaphyllin**	**Asmalix**
Bronkodyl	**Elixomin**	**Elixophyllin**
Quibron-T	**Respbid**	**Slo-bid**
Slo-Phyllin	**Theobid**	**Theochron**
Theoclear	**Theo-Dur**	**Theolair**
Theo-24	**Theovent**	**Theo-X**
T-Phyl	**Uniphyl**	

DESCRIPTION

Theophylline helps to open airways, so it is generally used to treat and prevent asthma attacks. It may also be prescribed for people with emphysema or other chronic breathing problems. Babies and elderly men may need lower doses. The dose is monitored with regular blood tests to ensure that levels are less than 20 mcg/ml.

INSTRUCTIONS

Theophylline interacts with food in complex ways, so discuss this issue thoroughly with your doctor and pharmacist. Theophylline may upset the stomach. In some cases this problem can be alleviated by taking the drug with food. See the table of Food and Drug Interactions on pages 59-73 for more information.

INTERACTION

This interaction is complex and confusing, because carbamazepine may either increase or decrease blood levels of theophylline. Case reports confirm that both reactions occur.

Increased theophylline levels may lead to toxicity. Diminished levels may be associated with reduced efficacy. In addition, theophylline may reduce carbamazepine levels, leading to a seizure. *This interaction could be dangerous.*

It is important for your physician to check blood levels of both drugs. If you experience symptoms of toxicity, let your doctor know at once.

Symptoms of Theophylline Toxicity

Nausea, diarrhea, stomach pain, headache, insomnia, restlessness, and irritability. Severe toxicity (convulsions, heart rhythm changes, or death) may occur with no warning symptoms. Notify your doctor immediately if you suspect a problem.

INTERACTION

DANGEROUS

Anticonvulsant
(CARBAMAZEPINE)

Endometriosis Drug
(DANAZOL)

BRAND NAME	GENERIC NAME
Tegretol	carbamazepine

DESCRIPTION

Carbamazepine is often prescribed to people for whom other anticonvulsants have not worked well. It is also used to control severe facial pain related to the trigeminal nerve. Carbamazepine may trigger a potentially lethal blood abnormality, so regular monitoring is critical, particularly during the first two months. This drug can cause drowsiness or dizziness; driving may be impaired. Contact your doctor if you experience drowsiness, dizziness, confusion, mood or behavior changes, nausea, swollen legs and feet, pale stools, yellow skin or eyes, unusual bleeding or bruising, dark urine, sore throat, mouth sores, fever, or chills.

INSTRUCTIONS

Carbamazepine may upset the stomach; if so, take it with food or milk. Do not stop this drug suddenly; seizures could result. To maintain its strength, it must be stored away from humidity and heat in a tightly closed container.

BRAND NAME	GENERIC NAME
Danocrine	danazol

DESCRIPTION

Danocrine is prescribed to control the pain of endometriosis. It works by reducing the hormonal input to the affected tissue. It is also helpful in controlling the pain of fibrocystic breast disease, and is occasionally prescribed in cases of very heavy menstrual flow, or, in men, for breast enlargement. Because Danocrine interacts with insulin, diabetics must be monitored especially carefully when taking this drug. In some women Danocrine may cause acne, facial or body hair growth, a deeper voice, weight gain, or other symptoms of masculinization. Contact the physician if you notice any of these. Danocrine must never be taken during pregnancy.

INSTRUCTIONS

Danocrine may be taken either with food or on an empty stomach. During Danocrine therapy, sexually active women should use barrier contraceptives (such as a diaphragm or condoms).

INTERACTION

Danocrine may increase blood levels of carbamazepine to double the previous measurement. Several women on this combination of drugs experienced carbamazepine toxicity associated with high blood levels several days to a month after they added Danocrine to their regimen. *This interaction could be dangerous.*

A patient who requires both drugs should have carbamazepine blood levels monitored carefully when starting or stopping the Danocrine. She should also be aware that lethargy, dizziness, blurred vision, or unsteady gait may be signs of toxicity, and contact her doctor if she experiences any of them. The dose of carbamazepine may need adjustment.

Symptoms of Carbamazepine Toxicity

Nausea, vomiting, drowsiness, unsteadiness, incoordination, dizziness, muscle twitching or tremor, irregular breathing, rapid heartbeat, changes in blood pressure, changes in urination, and impaired consciousness. Notify your physician immediately of any such symptoms.

Never take or stop medication without your doctor's advice.

INTERACTION

DANGEROUS

Anticonvulsant
(CARBAMAZEPINE)

Heart/Blood Pressure Drugs
(CALCIUM CHANNEL BLOCKERS)

BRAND NAME	GENERIC NAME
Tegretol	carbamazepine

DESCRIPTION

Carbamazepine is often prescribed to people for whom other anticonvulsants have not worked well. It is also used to control severe facial pain related to the trigeminal nerve. Carbamazepine may trigger a potentially lethal blood abnormality, so regular monitoring is critical, particularly during the first two months. This drug can cause drowsiness or dizziness; driving may be impaired. Contact your doctor if you experience drowsiness, dizziness, confusion, mood or behavior changes, nausea, swollen legs and feet, pale stools, yellow skin or eyes, unusual bleeding or bruising, dark urine, sore throat, mouth sores, fever, or chills.

INSTRUCTIONS

Carbamazepine may upset the stomach; if so, take it with food or milk. Do not stop this drug suddenly; seizures could result. To maintain its strength, it must be stored away from humidity and heat in a tightly closed container.

BRAND NAME	GENERIC NAME
Calan, Isoptin	verapamil
Cardizem, Dilacor XR	diltiazem
Plendil	felodipine
Verelan	verapamil

DESCRIPTION

Calcium channel blockers such as Calan and Cardizem are popular drugs for lowering blood pressure, treating angina, and, in the case of verapamil, stabilizing irregular heart rhythms. Some of these drugs have been prescribed to prevent migraine or cluster headaches, ward off exercise-induced asthma, or treat congestive heart failure.

INSTRUCTIONS

These drugs come in a variety of doses; it is important to follow the doctor's directions to get the proper dose. Sustained-release forms, such as Calan SR or Dilacor XR, should not be chewed or crushed. Taking Plendil with grapefruit juice may lead to unexpectedly high blood levels. See the table of Food and Drug Interactions on pages 59-73 for specifics. If the drug must be discontinued, follow your doctor's instructions for gradual tapering.

INTERACTION

Both verapamil and diltiazem have been associated with elevated blood levels of carbamazepine, with the possibility of toxicity. *This interaction could be dangerous.*

Carbamazepine concentrations should be monitored closely if this drug is taken with a calcium channel blocker. Nifedipine may not interact, but the dose of carbamazepine may need to be reduced by as much as 50 percent when combined with verapamil. Monitoring is crucial if a patient on Tegretol stops taking a calcium channel blocker.

If a patient on Plendil takes carbamazepine, blood pressure may not be controlled with the normal dose of Plendil. One study found that patients on Tegretol had only about 6 percent the amount of Plendil in their bloodstreams as people taking the Plendil alone. In such a case, your doctor may want to adjust the dose of Plendil.

Symptoms of Carbamazepine Toxicity

Nausea, vomiting, drowsiness, unsteadiness, incoordination, dizziness, muscle twitching or tremor, irregular breathing, rapid heartbeat, changes in blood pressure, changes in urination, and impaired consciousness. Notify the physician immediately of any such symptoms.

Never take or stop medication without your doctor's advice.

INTERACTION

DANGEROUS

Anticonvulsant

(CARBAMAZEPINE)

Lithium

BRAND NAME
Tegretol

GENERIC NAME
carbamazepine

DESCRIPTION

Carbamazepine is often prescribed to people for whom other anticonvulsants have not worked well. It is also used to control severe facial pain related to the trigeminal nerve. Carbamazepine may trigger a potentially lethal blood abnormality, so regular monitoring is critical, particularly during the first two months. This drug can cause drowsiness or dizziness; driving may be impaired. Contact your doctor if you experience drowsiness, dizziness, confusion, mood or behavior changes, nausea, swollen legs and feet, pale stools, yellow skin or eyes, unusual bleeding or bruising, dark urine, sore throat, mouth sores, fever, or chills.

INSTRUCTIONS

Carbamazepine may upset the stomach; if so, take it with food or milk. Do not stop this drug suddenly; seizures could result. To maintain its strength, it must be stored away from humidity and heat in a tightly closed container.

BRAND NAME

Cibalith-S	**Eskalith**
Lithane	**Lithobid**
Lithonate	**Lithotabs**

DESCRIPTION

Lithium is most often used to treat bipolar depression, and seems to be especially helpful in easing the manic phases of this disorder. Regular blood tests are advisable for dose adjustment. The toxic dose is not a great deal higher than the effective dose, so your doctor should be notified of signs such as vomiting, diarrhea, unsteadiness in walking, weakness, or unusual drowsiness. This drug can affect the thyroid gland.

INSTRUCTIONS

Lithium should be taken immediately after meals or with food or milk to reduce stomach upset. It is essential to drink 8 to 12 glasses of water or other fluid each day while on lithium. This medication can affect alertness, so activities such as driving or operating machinery can be dangerous for people on lithium.

INTERACTION

Carbamazepine appears to make lithium more effective, without necessarily boosting blood levels noticeably. In some patients, this interaction has been of benefit, helping to control the manic phase better. In others, however, it has resulted in symptoms of lithium toxicity. *This interaction could be dangerous.*

Lithium may interact with carbamazepine to improve white blood cell counts that may be depressed by the anticonvulsant. Both drugs can affect thyroid function, however, and together may impact more heavily on the thyroid (lower circulating thyroid hormone) than either separately. Monitoring of clinical status is important when someone on lithium starts or stops carbamazepine. Blood tests for lithium levels may not tell the whole story. Patients on this combination should have thyroid function checked regularly.

Symptoms of Lithium Toxicity

Nausea, diarrhea, incoordination, muscle weakness, and difficulty walking may be signs of toxicity. Ringing in the ears, visual problems, dizziness, slurred speech, confusion, agitation, and incontinence are more serious. Notify the physician promptly of any such symptoms.

Never take or stop medication without your doctor's advice.

INTERACTION

DANGEROUS

Anticonvulsant

(CARBAMAZEPINE)

Oral Contraceptives

BRAND NAME

Tegretol

GENERIC NAME

carbamazepine

DESCRIPTION

Carbamazepine is often prescribed to people for whom other anticonvulsants have not worked well. It is also used to control severe facial pain related to the trigeminal nerve. Carbamazepine may trigger a potentially lethal blood abnormality, so regular monitoring is critical, particularly during the first two months. This drug can cause drowsiness or dizziness; driving may be impaired. Contact your doctor if you experience drowsiness, dizziness, confusion, mood or behavior changes, nausea, swollen legs and feet, pale stools, yellow skin or eyes, unusual bleeding or bruising, dark urine, sore throat, mouth sores, fever, or chills.

INSTRUCTIONS

Carbamazepine may upset the stomach; if so, take it with food or milk. Do not stop this drug suddenly; seizures could result. To maintain its strength, it must be stored away from humidity and heat in a tightly closed container.

BRAND NAME

Brevicon	**Demulen**	**Desogen**
Genora	**Levlen**	**Loestrin**
Lo/Ovral	**Modicon**	**N.E.E.**
Nelova	**Nordette**	**Norethin**
Norinyl	**Norlestrin**	**Ortho-**
Ortho-Novum	**Ovcon**	**Cyclen**
Ovral	**Triphasil**	

DESCRIPTION

Lower doses of estrogen and progestin make these drugs safer today than ever before. But women who smoke and take oral contraceptives still run an increased risk of strokes. These drugs are usually well tolerated, but side effects may include menstrual changes, nausea, migraine, depression, changes in vision, high blood pressure, liver tumors, gallbladder problems, blood clots, and heart attacks. Weigh the benefits and risks with your doctor when considering this form of contraception. Birth control pills interact with several other medications; check with your doctor or pharmacist before taking another drug in conjunction with oral contraceptives.

INSTRUCTIONS

For maximum effectiveness, oral contraceptives should be taken at the same time every day and precisely according to instructions. Missed doses can lead to an unwelcome pregnancy. Additional contraception is needed for at least the first week.

INTERACTION

A number of epileptic women (in one study, 3 out of 41) have become pregnant while taking oral contraceptives and carbamazepine. This seems to be the result of carbamazepine speeding clearance of both estrogen and progesterone from the body in less time than usual. *Because carbamazepine has also been associated with some birth defects, this interaction could be dangerous.*

A woman who must take carbamazepine should not rely on oral contraceptives alone.

Never take or stop medication without your doctor's advice.

INTERACTION

DANGEROUS

Anticonvulsant
(CARBAMAZEPINE)

Transplant Drug
(CYCLOSPORINE)

BRAND NAME	GENERIC NAME
Tegretol	carbamazepine

DESCRIPTION

Carbamazepine is often prescribed to people for whom other anticonvulsants have not worked well. It is also used to control severe facial pain related to the trigeminal nerve. Carbamazepine may trigger a potentially lethal blood abnormality, so regular monitoring is critical, particularly during the first two months. This drug can cause drowsiness or dizziness; driving may be impaired. Contact your doctor if you experience drowsiness, dizziness, confusion, mood or behavior changes, nausea, swollen legs and feet, pale stools, yellow skin or eyes, unusual bleeding or bruising, dark urine, sore throat, mouth sores, fever, or chills.

INSTRUCTIONS

Carbamazepine may upset the stomach; if so, take it with food or milk. Do not stop this drug suddenly; seizures could result. To maintain its strength, it must be stored away from humidity and heat in a tightly closed container.

BRAND NAME	GENERIC NAME
Sandimmune	cyclosporine

DESCRIPTION

Sandimmune suppresses the immune system so that a person receiving a transplant does not reject this life-saving organ. Doctors have also tried using it in treating autoimmune diseases, in which the immune system attacks a person's own tissues. Multiple sclerosis is an example.

INSTRUCTIONS

Sandimmune comes as an oral solution with a taste reminiscent of castor oil. It should be mixed in a glass with milk, chocolate milk, or orange juice at room temperature and drunk at once. Then the glass (no plastic) should be rinsed and the rinsing fluid drunk to get the full dose. Do not take Sandimmune with grapefruit juice unless the physician is monitoring blood levels of the drug closely. (See page 43.) Due to a possible interaction between cyclosporine and oral contraceptives, barrier methods of contraception should be used while taking this drug.

Regular monitoring is important. Do not stop this medicine unless your doctor so directs.

INTERACTION

Carbamazepine can increase the speed with which the body disposes of Sandimmune. In some cases, blood levels of Sandimmune drop below detectable limits after carbamazepine is added. *This interaction could be dangerous, with the possibility of a rejection episode resulting.*

Anticonvulsants containing valproic acid (Depakene, etc.) do not appear to affect Sandimmune concentrations in the same way and may offer an alternative. If both Sandimmune and carbamazepine are needed, blood tests for Sandimmune levels are recommended.

Never take or stop medication without your doctor's advice.

INTERACTION

DANGEROUS

Anticonvulsant
(CARBAMAZEPINE)

Tuberculosis Drug
(ISONIAZID)

BRAND NAME	GENERIC NAME
Tegretol	carbamazepine

DESCRIPTION

Carbamazepine is often prescribed to people for whom other anticonvulsants have not worked well. It is also used to control severe facial pain related to the trigeminal nerve. Carbamazepine may trigger a potentially lethal blood abnormality, so regular monitoring is critical, particularly during the first two months. This drug can cause drowsiness or dizziness; driving may be impaired. Contact your doctor if you experience drowsiness, dizziness, confusion, mood or behavior changes, nausea, swollen legs and feet, pale stools, yellow skin or eyes, unusual bleeding or bruising, dark urine, sore throat, mouth sores, fever, or chills.

INSTRUCTIONS

Carbamazepine may upset the stomach; if so, take it with food or milk. Do not stop this drug suddenly; seizures could result. To maintain its strength, it must be stored away from humidity and heat in a tightly closed container.

BRAND NAME	GENERIC NAME
INH	isoniazid
Izonid	isoniazid
Laniazid	isoniazid
Nydrazid	isoniazid
Rifamate	isoniazid/rifampin

DESCRIPTION

Isoniazid is used (in combination with other drugs) to treat tuberculosis and to prevent its progression. To be effective, it must be taken faithfully for an extended period of time as prescribed. Side effects may include numbness, tingling or pain in hands and feet, nausea, vomiting, stomachache, and elevated liver enzymes. If you develop fever, rash, weakness, or yellow eyes and skin, contact the doctor.

INSTRUCTIONS

Isoniazid is best taken on an empty stomach, at least one hour before meals or two hours after. It may be taken with food if it upsets the stomach. Alcohol increases the risk of a potentially fatal liver reaction, so don't drink. Foods high in tyramine interact with isoniazid to raise blood pressure dangerously; see the list on page 47. Fish such as skipjack and tuna may trigger an unpleasant histamine reaction. Symptoms of B_6 deficiency may develop; supplements may be required.

INTERACTION

Isoniazid can interfere with carbamazepine metabolism, leading to a buildup of the anticonvulsant in the body. Most patients on this combination will have higher blood levels of the anticonvulsant than they did before starting the tuberculosis drug. *This interaction can be dangerous, with carbamazepine toxicity developing rather quickly.*

There is some evidence that carbamazepine, in turn, can make isoniazid more toxic to the liver. If both drugs are required, blood levels of both carbamazepine and liver enzymes should be monitored closely. Contact your doctor at the first sign of trouble.

Symptoms of Carbamazepine Toxicity

Nausea, vomiting, drowsiness, unsteadiness, incoordination, dizziness, muscle twitching or tremor, irregular breathing, rapid heartbeat, changes in blood pressure, changes in urination, and impaired consciousness. Notify the physician immediately of any such symptoms.

INTERACTION

DANGEROUS

Anticonvulsant

(CARBAMAZEPINE)

Ulcer Drug

(H₂ ANTAGONIST)

BRAND NAME   GENERIC NAME

Tegretol   carbamazepine

DESCRIPTION

Carbamazepine is often prescribed to people for whom other anticonvulsants have not worked well. It is also used to control severe facial pain related to the trigeminal nerve. Carbamazepine may trigger a potentially lethal blood abnormality, so regular monitoring is critical, particularly during the first two months. This drug can cause drowsiness or dizziness; driving may be impaired. Contact your doctor if you experience drowsiness, dizziness, confusion, mood or behavior changes, nausea, swollen legs and feet, pale stools, yellow skin or eyes, unusual bleeding or bruising, dark urine, sore throat, mouth sores, fever, or chills.

INSTRUCTIONS

Carbamazepine may upset the stomach; if so, take it with food or milk. Do not stop this drug suddenly; seizures could result. To maintain its strength, it must be stored away from humidity and heat in a tightly closed container.

BRAND NAME   GENERIC NAME

Tagamet   cimetidine

DESCRIPTION

Tagamet has revolutionized the treatment of ulcers and serious heartburn (esophagitis) by blocking special receptors (the histamine H₂ receptors), thereby reducing the acid environment of the stomach. Cimetidine is usually well tolerated, and has few side effects, although headaches, dizziness, and mild diarrhea are potential reactions. Some men complain of anti-testosterone effects. At higher doses, this may lead to enlarged breasts or sexual problems. Older people and those who are very ill may experience depression, mental confusion, or disorientation. The dose may need to be adjusted for them. Tagamet can affect the liver, modifying the metabolism and elimination of a number of medications. Higher blood levels of such drugs may lead to increased toxicity, so check with your doctor and pharmacist if you take cimetidine with another medicine.

INSTRUCTIONS

Tagamet is usually taken with meals and/or at bedtime. Antacids may reduce absorption of Tagamet; do not take one for at least two hours after taking Tagamet.

INTERACTION

Tagamet appears to modify the metabolism of carbamazepine. The problem is that Tagamet affects liver enzymes and may make them less capable of processing these anticonvulsants. As a result, blood levels can rise. *This could lead to dangerous toxicity.*

    While Tagamet and Tegretol seem less likely to interact if Tegretol has been taken for longer than four weeks, physicians should be cautious when considering such a combination.

Symptoms of Carbamazepine Toxicity

Nausea, vomiting, drowsiness, unsteadiness, incoordination, dizziness, muscle twitching or tremor, irregular breathing, rapid heartbeat, changes in blood pressure, changes in urination, and impaired consciousness. Notify the physician immediately of any such symptoms.

INTERACTION

DANGEROUS

Anticonvulsant

(CARBAMAZEPINE)

Antibiotic

(DOXYCYCLINE)

BRAND NAME	GENERIC NAME
Tegretol	carbamazepine

DESCRIPTION

Carbamazepine is often prescribed to people for whom other anticonvulsants have not worked well. It is also used to control severe facial pain related to the trigeminal nerve. Carbamazepine may trigger a potentially lethal blood abnormality, so regular monitoring is critical, particularly during the first two months. This drug can cause drowsiness or dizziness; driving may be impaired. Contact your doctor if you experience drowsiness, dizziness, confusion, mood or behavior changes, nausea, swollen legs and feet, pale stools, yellow skin or eyes, unusual bleeding or bruising, dark urine, sore throat, mouth sores, fever, or chills.

INSTRUCTIONS

Carbamazepine may upset the stomach; if so, take it with food or milk. Do not stop this drug suddenly; seizures could result. To maintain its strength, it must be stored away from humidity and heat in a tightly closed container.

BRAND NAME	GENERIC NAME
Doryx	doxycycline
Doxi Film	doxycycline
Doxy-Caps	doxycycline
Doxychel Hyclate	doxycycline
Doxy-D	doxycycline
Monodox	doxycycline
Vibramycin	doxycycline
Vibra-Tabs	doxycycline

DESCRIPTION

Doxycycline is a form of tetracyline prescribed for a wide variety of infections, including serious ones such as Rocky Mountain spotted fever and Lyme disease, and common problems such as acne and traveler's diarrhea. Tetracycline is generally inappropriate for pregnant women and young children, as it may stain permanent teeth. This medicine makes many people more sensitive to ultraviolet light, so protect yourself from sunlight and tanning lamps.

INSTRUCTIONS

Doxycycline may be taken with food or milk to reduce stomach upset, always with a full eight ounces of liquid. Do not take this medicine with antacids, calcium supplements, or iron pills, as they could interfere with absorption of the drug. Never take outdated doxycycline, which may be toxic to the kidneys.

INTERACTION

Tegretol can speed the liver's processing of this antibiotic, potentially lowering blood levels and making it less effective. *This interaction could be troublesome, as the infection might not be eradicated.*

Other tetracyclines do not appear to interact with carbamazepine in this manner. If doxycycline is best, the doctor will want to keep a careful watch on the patient's progress, as a higher dose of doxycycline may be needed.

Never take or stop medication without your doctor's advice.

INTERACTION

TROUBLESOME

Anticonvulsant
(CARBAMAZEPINE)

Anticoagulant
(WARFARIN)

BRAND NAME	GENERIC NAME
Tegretol	carbamazepine

DESCRIPTION

Carbamazepine is often prescribed to people for whom other anticonvulsants have not worked well. It is also used to control severe facial pain related to the trigeminal nerve. Carbamazepine may trigger a potentially lethal blood abnormality, so regular monitoring is critical, particularly during the first two months. This drug can cause drowsiness or dizziness; driving may be impaired. Contact your doctor if you experience drowsiness, dizziness, confusion, mood or behavior changes, nausea, swollen legs and feet, pale stools, yellow skin or eyes, unusual bleeding or bruising, dark urine, sore throat, mouth sores, fever, or chills.

INSTRUCTIONS

Carbamazepine may upset the stomach; if so, take it with food or milk. Do not stop this drug suddenly; seizures could result. To maintain its strength, it must be stored away from humidity and heat in a tightly closed container.

BRAND NAME	GENERIC NAME
Coumadin	warfarin

DESCRIPTION

Warfarin slows the liver's production of factors essential for the formation of blood clots. It is prescribed when there is a risk that a dangerous clot could form in a deep vein or a blood vessel leading to the lung, heart, or brain. The most serious complication of anticoagulant treatment is excessive bleeding. The dosage must be individually adjusted, requiring daily blood tests at first, then tests every four to six weeks. Other side effects may include nausea, loss of appetite, rash, fever, yellow eyes and skin, prolonged painful erection, and hair loss.

INSTRUCTIONS

Warfarin tablets can be swallowed with food or on an empty stomach. Try to avoid large variations in the quantity of vitamin-K–containing vegetables—such as broccoli, cabbage, or spinach—that you eat each day. Consuming much more or less than usual could change the action of the drug.

INTERACTION

Carbamazepine apparently reduces circulating levels of warfarin. The result could be a greater risk of blood clots. *This interaction could be troublesome.*

When a person on warfarin needs to start or stop taking this anticonvulsant, close monitoring of prothrombin time is appropriate. A few case reports feature patients whose prothrombin time was five or six times greater upon discontinuing carbamazepine, a situation that could lead to dangerous bleeding. The physician may need to adjust the dose of warfarin when Tegretol is discontinued.

Symptoms of Warfarin Overdose

There may be no early warning signs of danger. Blood tests are essential. Symptoms include any unusual bleeding, including rectal or urinary tract bleeding, excessive menstrual bleeding, nosebleeds, bleeding around gums, bruising, red or tar-black stools, vomiting blood, and red or dark-brown urine. Notify your doctor immediately if you suspect a problem.

Never take or stop medication without your doctor's advice.

INTERACTION

TROUBLESOME

Anticonvulsant
(CARBAMAZEPINE)

Barbiturates

BRAND NAME	GENERIC NAME
Tegretol	carbamazepine

DESCRIPTION

Carbamazepine is often prescribed to people for whom other anticonvulsants have not worked well. It is also used to control severe facial pain related to the trigeminal nerve. Carbamazepine may trigger a potentially lethal blood abnormality, so regular monitoring is critical, particularly during the first two months. This drug can cause drowsiness or dizziness; driving may be impaired. Contact your doctor if you experience drowsiness, dizziness, confusion, mood or behavior changes, nausea, swollen legs and feet, pale stools, yellow skin or eyes, unusual bleeding or bruising, dark urine, sore throat, mouth sores, fever, or chills.

INSTRUCTIONS

Carbamazepine may upset the stomach; if so, take it with food or milk. Do not stop this drug suddenly; seizures could result. To maintain its strength, it must be stored away from humidity and heat in a tightly closed container.

BRAND NAME	GENERIC NAME
Alurate	aprobarbital
Amytal	amobarbital
Butisol	butabarbital
Lotusate	talbutal
Mebaral	mephobarbital
Mysoline	primidone
Nembutal	pentobarbital
Seconal	secobarbital
Solfoton	phenobarbital
Tuinal	amobarbital/ secobarbital

DESCRIPTION

Barbiturates were once used as sleeping pills, but now they are prescribed to prevent seizures. These medications can cause dependence if used for an extended period of time. Stopping suddenly could trigger severe withdrawal symptoms. Barbiturates interact with many other drugs, so check with the pharmacist or physician before taking any other medications.

INSTRUCTIONS

Any of these medications can cause drowsiness and limit attention. Take them at a time when you will not need to drive or do other complicated tasks. Never drink alcohol if you are taking a barbiturate.

INTERACTION

In complex seizure situations, a combination of carbamazepine and barbiturates may be appropriate for the control of epilepsy. Caution is required with this combination, however. Barbiturates can rev up the liver enzymes that process carbamazepine, speeding its elimination from the body. This generally leads to lower blood levels of the anticonvulsant than when it is taken alone. *This interaction might be troublesome if the anticonvulsant becomes less effective.*

Seizures are possible. They occurred in one case in which the barbiturate Mysoline evidently interfered with carbamazepine.

Never take or stop medication without your doctor's advice.

INTERACTION

TROUBLESOME

Anticonvulsant
(CARBAMAZEPINE)

Drug for Schizophrenia

BRAND NAME	GENERIC NAME
Tegretol	carbamazepine

DESCRIPTION

Carbamazepine is often prescribed to people for whom other anticonvulsants have not worked well. It is also used to control severe facial pain related to the trigeminal nerve. Carbamazepine may trigger a potentially lethal blood abnormality, so regular monitoring is critical, particularly during the first two months. This drug can cause drowsiness or dizziness; driving may be impaired. Contact your doctor if you experience drowsiness, dizziness, confusion, mood or behavior changes, nausea, swollen legs and feet, pale stools, yellow skin or eyes, unusual bleeding or bruising, dark urine, sore throat, mouth sores, fever, or chills.

INSTRUCTIONS

Carbamazepine may upset the stomach; if so, take it with food or milk. Do not stop this drug suddenly; seizures could result. To maintain its strength, it must be stored away from humidity and heat in a tightly closed container.

BRAND NAME	GENERIC NAME
Haldol	haloperidol

DESCRIPTION

Haldol is prescribed primarily for serious mental illness, agitation, and anxiety disorders. The drug can help control hallucinations and disorganized thinking. Haldol is also beneficial in treating the tics and verbalizations of Tourette's disorder.

This antipsychotic medication has a range of serious side effects and may affect the electrocardiogram. The QT interval (ECG readings that represent electrical heart activity) can be prolonged, and that could lead to serious heart rhythm disturbances.

INSTRUCTIONS

Haldol is best taken with food. The dose is highly variable depending on many factors and has to be individualized for each patient.

INTERACTION

This interaction is exceptionally confusing, because studies and clinical reports do not agree on its direction and impact. In some situations, patients do well on this combination of medications. Other reports show significantly (up to 60 percent) lower blood levels of Haldol when carbamazepine is added to the regimen. In some cases, this has resulted in lower efficacy, with a recurrence of hallucinations, delusions, and schizophrenic behavior. *This interaction could be troublesome.*

If a patient needs both medications, the doctor will need to monitor the clinical status carefully. The dosage of Haldol may require adjustment.

Never take or stop medication without your doctor's advice.

INTERACTION

TROUBLESOME

Anticonvulsant
(CARBAMAZEPINE)

Influenza Vaccine

BRAND NAME   GENERIC NAME

Tegretol   carbamazepine

DESCRIPTION

Carbamazepine is often prescribed to people for whom other anticonvulsants have not worked well. It is also used to control severe facial pain related to the trigeminal nerve. Carbamazepine may trigger a potentially lethal blood abnormality, so regular monitoring is critical, particularly during the first two months. This drug can cause drowsiness or dizziness; driving may be impaired. Contact your doctor if you experience drowsiness, dizziness, confusion, mood or behavior changes, nausea, swollen legs and feet, pale stools, yellow skin or eyes, unusual bleeding or bruising, dark urine, sore throat, mouth sores, fever, or chills.

INSTRUCTIONS

Carbamazepine may upset the stomach; if so, take it with food or milk. Do not stop this drug suddenly; seizures could result. To maintain its strength, it must be stored away from humidity and heat in a tightly closed container.

BRAND NAME

Fluogen
FluShield
Fluvirin
Fluzone
influenza virus vaccine trivalent

DESCRIPTION

Flu vaccine confers protection from influenza infection. It is reformulated every year to correspond to the strains of influenza virus current in the country. It takes approximately two weeks from the time of vaccination to develop immunity, which lasts for six months or so of the flu season.

INSTRUCTIONS

Vaccination is recommended for people over age 65, for those with chronic conditions, especially of the heart or lungs, and for the caregivers or household contacts of those at high risk. People who are allergic to chicken egg may also be allergic to the vaccine. Appropriate precautions are advised.

INTERACTION

Flu vaccine may interfere with the normal metabolism of carbamazepine, allowing blood levels of the anticonvulsant to rise. There is a possibility of carbamazepine toxicity for a few days following vaccination. Carbamazepine levels should be monitored. Notify your physician if you feel drowsy, lethargic, dizzy, or unsteady on your feet. *This interaction may be troublesome.*

Symptoms of Carbamazepine Toxicity

Nausea, vomiting, drowsiness, unsteadiness, incoordination, dizziness, muscle twitching or tremor, irregular breathing, rapid heartbeat, changes in blood pressure, changes in urination, and impaired consciousness. Notify your physician immediately of any such symptoms.

INTERACTION

TROUBLESOME

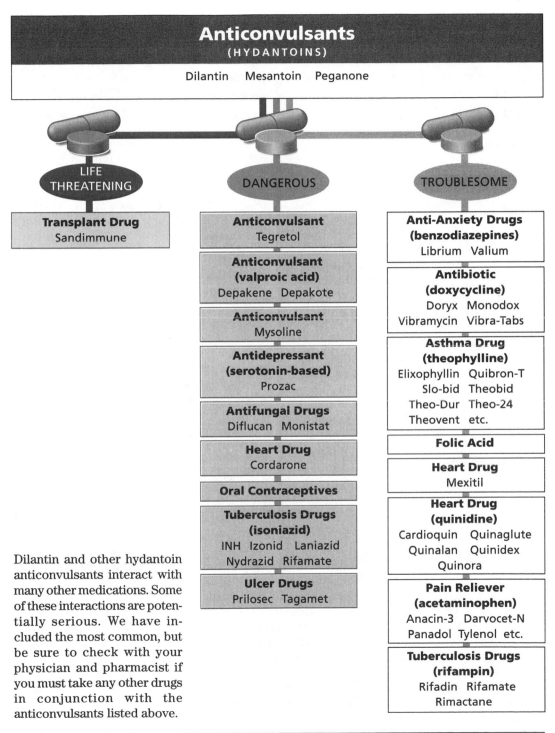

Anticonvulsants
(HYDANTOINS)

Dilantin   Mesantoin   Peganone

LIFE THREATENING

Transplant Drug
Sandimmune

DANGEROUS

Anticonvulsant
Tegretol

**Anticonvulsant
(valproic acid)**
Depakene   Depakote

Anticonvulsant
Mysoline

**Antidepressant
(serotonin-based)**
Prozac

Antifungal Drugs
Diflucan   Monistat

Heart Drug
Cordarone

Oral Contraceptives

**Tuberculosis Drugs
(isoniazid)**
INH   Izonid   Laniazid
Nydrazid   Rifamate

Ulcer Drugs
Prilosec   Tagamet

TROUBLESOME

**Anti-Anxiety Drugs
(benzodiazepines)**
Librium   Valium

**Antibiotic
(doxycycline)**
Doryx   Monodox
Vibramycin   Vibra-Tabs

**Asthma Drug
(theophylline)**
Elixophyllin   Quibron-T
Slo-bid   Theobid
Theo-Dur   Theo-24
Theovent   etc.

Folic Acid

Heart Drug
Mexitil

**Heart Drug
(quinidine)**
Cardioquin   Quinaglute
Quinalan   Quinidex
Quinora

**Pain Reliever
(acetaminophen)**
Anacin-3   Darvocet-N
Panadol   Tylenol   etc.

**Tuberculosis Drugs
(rifampin)**
Rifadin   Rifamate
Rimactane

Dilantin and other hydantoin anticonvulsants interact with many other medications. Some of these interactions are potentially serious. We have included the most common, but be sure to check with your physician and pharmacist if you must take any other drugs in conjunction with the anticonvulsants listed above.

LEVELS OF HAZARD: LIFE THREATENING   DANGEROUS   TROUBLESOME

Anticonvulsants

(HYDANTOINS)

Transplant Drug

(CYCLOSPORINE)

BRAND NAME	GENERIC NAME
Dilantin	phenytoin
Mesantoin	mephenytoin
Peganone	ethotoin

DESCRIPTION

These anticonvulsants are used to prevent epileptic seizures or seizures associated with brain surgery. Occasionally they may be prescribed to treat severe stabbing facial pain (trigeminal neuralgia). Tests may be needed to check blood cells, blood levels of the drug, liver function, and blood sugar. Special attention to oral hygiene is needed to prevent gum problems often associated with taking these anticonvulsants. Hydantoin anticonvulsants interact with many other drugs as well as alcohol, so check carefully with your physician and pharmacist before taking any other medication.

INSTRUCTIONS

Any of these medicines could upset the stomach. This is less likely if they are taken with food. All of them can cause drowsiness or blurred vision and could make driving dangerous.

BRAND NAME	GENERIC NAME
Sandimmune	cyclosporine

DESCRIPTION

Sandimmune suppresses the immune system so that a person receiving a transplant does not reject this lifesaving organ. Doctors have also tried using it in treating autoimmune diseases, in which the immune system attacks a person's own tissues. Multiple sclerosis is an example.

INSTRUCTIONS

Sandimmune comes as an oral solution with a taste reminiscent of castor oil. It should be mixed in a glass with milk, chocolate milk, or orange juice at room temperature and drunk at once. Then the glass (no plastic) should be rinsed and the rinsing fluid drunk to get the full dose. Do not take Sandimmune with grapefruit juice unless the physician is monitoring blood levels of the drug closely. (See page 43.)

Due to a possible interaction between cyclosporine and oral contraceptives, barrier methods of contraception should be used while taking this drug.

Regular monitoring is important. Do not stop this medicine unless your doctor so directs.

INTERACTION

Dilantin, and presumably the other drugs in its class, seems to interfere significantly with the absorption of Sandimmune. Patients on this combination have only half as much of the transplant drug circulating in their bodies as they had before starting Dilantin. The interaction sets in within two days of starting on Dilantin, and disappears within a week of stopping the anticonvulsant. Taking the medicines at different times does not seem to help. *Although we are aware of no deaths as a consequence of this interaction, such low levels of Sandimmune could lead to a life-threatening rejection episode.*

A person who needs both drugs should have Sandimmune levels monitored closely. The dose may need adjustment to maintain adequate blood levels. Contact your physician without delay if there is any sign of trouble.

Never take or stop medication without your doctor's advice.

INTERACTION

LIFE THREATENING

Anticonvulsants
(HYDANTOINS)

Anticonvulsant
(CARBAMAZEPINE)

BRAND NAME	GENERIC NAME
Dilantin	phenytoin
Mesantoin	mephenytoin
Peganone	ethotoin

DESCRIPTION

These anticonvulsants are used to prevent epileptic seizures or seizures associated with brain surgery. Occasionally they may be prescribed to treat severe stabbing facial pain (trigeminal neuralgia). Tests may be needed to check blood cells, blood levels of the drug, liver function, and blood sugar. Special attention to oral hygiene is needed to prevent gum problems often associated with taking these anticonvulsants. Hydantoin anticonvulsants interact with many other drugs as well as alcohol, so check carefully with your physician and pharmacist before taking any other medication.

INSTRUCTIONS

Any of these medicines could upset the stomach. This is less likely if they are taken with food. All of them can cause drowsiness or blurred vision and could make driving dangerous.

BRAND NAME	GENERIC NAME
Tegretol	carbamazepine

DESCRIPTION

Carbamazepine is often prescribed to people for whom other anticonvulsants have not worked well. It is also used to control severe facial pain related to the trigeminal nerve. Carbamazepine may trigger a potentially lethal blood abnormality, so regular monitoring is critical, particularly during the first two months. This drug can cause drowsiness or dizziness; driving may be impaired. Contact your doctor if you experience drowsiness, dizziness, confusion, mood or behavior changes, nausea, swollen legs and feet, pale stools, yellow skin or eyes, unusual bleeding or bruising, dark urine, sore throat, mouth sores, fever, or chills.

INSTRUCTIONS

Carbamazepine may upset the stomach; if so, take it with food or milk. Do not stop this drug suddenly; seizures could result. To maintain its strength, it must be stored away from humidity and heat in a tightly closed container.

INTERACTION

People who have had seizures often need more than one kind of medicine to prevent a recurrence. Carbamazepine and an anticonvulsant such as Dilantin may be prescribed together and can be helpful. They may interact in a complex and unpredictable way, however. Dilantin and similar drugs can lower blood levels of carbamazepine. No seizures have been reported as a result, but theoretically they are possible. In contrast, carbamazepine sometimes raises and sometimes lowers blood levels of Dilantin. Some cases of toxicity from excess phenytoin have been reported. *This interaction could well be dangerous.*

Frequent blood tests for both drugs are advised, especially when starting, stopping, or changing the dose of one of them. The dose of one or both may need to be adjusted.

Symptoms of Phenytoin Toxicity

Uncontrollable eye movements (nystagmus), unsteadiness, difficulty speaking clearly, dizziness, and stupor. Notify your physician immediately of any of these symptoms.

Never take or stop medication without your doctor's advice.

INTERACTION

DANGEROUS

Anticonvulsants
(HYDANTOINS)

Anticonvulsants
(VALPROIC ACID)

BRAND NAME	GENERIC NAME
Dilantin	phenytoin
Mesantoin	mephenytoin
Peganone	ethotoin

DESCRIPTION

These anticonvulsants are used to prevent epileptic seizures or seizures associated with brain surgery. Occasionally they may be prescribed to treat severe stabbing facial pain (trigeminal neuralgia). Tests may be needed to check blood cells, blood levels of the drug, liver function, and blood sugar. Special attention to oral hygiene is needed to prevent gum problems often associated with taking these anticonvulsants. Hydantoin anticonvulsants interact with many other drugs as well as alcohol, so check carefully with your physician and pharmacist before taking any other medication.

INSTRUCTIONS

Any of these medicines could upset the stomach. This is less likely if they are taken with food. All of them can cause drowsiness or blurred vision and could make driving dangerous.

BRAND NAME	GENERIC NAME
Depakene	valproic acid
Depakote	divalproex sodium

DESCRIPTION

Valproic acid is prescribed to prevent seizures, especially "petit mal" or absence seizures. It may be used in combination with other anticonvulsants, and is sometimes used to treat seizures associated with a sudden high fever in young children. Suddenly stopping this drug could trigger renewed seizure activity. This medication is not appropriate for patients with liver disease. Check with your doctor and pharmacist before taking any other drug.

INSTRUCTIONS

If this medicine upsets the stomach, it should be taken with food. Capsules should be swallowed whole, not chewed. Any of these medications can cause drowsiness and limit attention. Take them at a time when you will not need to drive or do other complicated tasks. Avoid alcohol, which may make drowsiness worse.

INTERACTION

Doctors may prescribe Dilantin and valproic acid together for a complex seizure disorder. Getting the dosage of the combination correct, however, may be complicated. Valproic acid competes with phenytoin for metabolic enzymes and carriers in the blood. The usual result is greater activity of Dilantin. Toxicity may occur even when blood levels are within the normal range.

Phenytoin may also reduce valproic acid levels, which might result in a loss of seizure control. Interpreting blood tests for these drugs is difficult because the interaction is extremely complex. Levels of both drugs should be monitored, however, so that doses can be adjusted if necessary. *The risk of toxicity or seizures makes this interaction dangerous.*

Symptoms of Phenytoin Toxicity

Uncontrollable eye movements (nystagmus), unsteadiness, difficulty speaking clearly, dizziness, and stupor. Notify your physician immediately of any of these symptoms.

INTERACTION

DANGEROUS

Anticonvulsants
(HYDANTOINS)

Anticonvulsant
(PRIMIDONE)

BRAND NAME	GENERIC NAME
Dilantin	phenytoin
Mesantoin	mephenytoin
Peganone	ethotoin

DESCRIPTION

These anticonvulsants are used to prevent epileptic seizures or seizures associated with brain surgery. Occasionally they may be prescribed to treat severe stabbing facial pain (trigeminal neuralgia). Tests may be needed to check blood cells, blood levels of the drug, liver function, and blood sugar. Special attention to oral hygiene is needed to prevent gum problems often associated with taking these anticonvulsants. Hydantoin anticonvulsants interact with many other drugs as well as alcohol, so check carefully with your physician and pharmacist before taking any other medication.

INSTRUCTIONS

Any of these medicines could upset the stomach. This is less likely if they are taken with food. All of them can cause drowsiness or blurred vision and could make driving dangerous.

BRAND NAME	GENERIC NAME
Mysoline	primidone

DESCRIPTION

This anticonvulsant is used alone or with other drugs to control "grand mal" or focal epileptic seizures. Tests may be needed every six months or so to check blood cells, blood levels of the drug, liver function, and blood sugar. Mysoline interacts with many other drugs as well as with alcohol, so check carefully before taking any other drugs in conjunction. The most common side effects—unsteadiness or clumsiness and vertigo—may become less troublesome after acclimating to the medicine. Do not stop this medicine suddenly, because seizures could result.

INSTRUCTIONS

This drug may upset the stomach. If so, it should be taken with food. It can cause drowsiness or blurred vision and could make driving or other complex tasks more dangerous.

INTERACTION

People who have had seizures may need more than one kind of medicine to prevent a recurrence. Dilantin and Mysoline may be prescribed together to good effect. Blood levels must be monitored when starting or stopping Dilantin, however, because this and similar drugs can alter the metabolism of primidone. Mysoline is broken down in the body into phenobarbital, among other chemicals, and blood levels of phenobarbital increase by up to 50 percent when primidone and Dilantin are taken together. There is a potential for primidone to reach toxic levels. *This interaction could be dangerous.*

Symptoms of Primidone Toxicity

Unsteadiness, nausea, vomiting, uncontrollable eye movements (nystagmus), dizziness, drowsiness, and impaired consciousness. Notify your physician immediately about any of these symptoms.

INTERACTION

DANGEROUS

Anticonvulsants

(HYDANTOINS)

Antidepressants

(SEROTONIN-BASED)

BRAND NAME	GENERIC NAME
Dilantin	phenytoin
Mesantoin	mephenytoin
Peganone	ethotoin

DESCRIPTION

These anticonvulsants are used to prevent epileptic seizures or seizures associated with brain surgery. Occasionally they may be prescribed to treat severe stabbing facial pain (trigeminal neuralgia). Tests may be needed to check blood cells, blood levels of the drug, liver function, and blood sugar. Special attention to oral hygiene is needed to prevent gum problems often associated with taking these anticonvulsants. Hydantoin anticonvulsants interact with many other drugs as well as alcohol, so check carefully with your physician and pharmacist before taking any other medication.

INSTRUCTIONS

Any of these medicines could upset the stomach. This is less likely if they are taken with food. All of them can cause drowsiness or blurred vision and could make driving dangerous.

BRAND NAME	GENERIC NAME
Prozac	fluoxetine

DESCRIPTION

This antidepressant works by blocking the reuptake into brain cells of serotonin, a chemical messenger. Because it works differently from the older cyclic-type antidepressants, it has a different set of side effects and has become more popular. It may also work against a different array of problems, for instance, bulimia or obsessive-compulsive disorder. Older people and those with kidney or liver problems may need reduced doses. Prozac is cleared from the body very slowly and may linger weeks after discontinuation.

INSTRUCTIONS

Prozac is taken in the morning, or, if a higher dose has been prescribed, in the morning and at noon. It may be taken without regard to meals. Taking it with food may reduce stomach upset. A few patients experience serious weight loss on this medication. If this occurs, the doctor should be notified.

INTERACTION

A depressed person with epilepsy might need both Prozac and an anticonvulsant medicine. Prozac apparently interferes with the metabolism of these compounds and may increase blood levels of Dilantin or similar anticonvulsants to the point of toxicity. *The interaction could be dangerous.*

 Because Prozac can linger in the body, interaction problems may continue for some time even if Prozac is discontinued. Notify your physician immediately if you experience symptoms such as unsteadiness, slurred speech, blurred vision, incoordination, dizziness, drowsiness, or confusion. Blood tests for a few weeks after starting or a few weeks after stopping Prozac are advisable.

Symptoms of Phenytoin Toxicity

Uncontrollable eye movements (nystagmus), unsteadiness, difficulty speaking clearly, dizziness, and stupor. Notify the physician immediately of any of these symptoms.

Never take or stop medication without your doctor's advice.

INTERACTION

DANGEROUS

Anticonvulsants

(HYDANTOINS)

Antifungal Drugs

BRAND NAME	GENERIC NAME
Dilantin	phenytoin
Mesantoin	mephenytoin
Peganone	ethotoin

DESCRIPTION

These anticonvulsants are used to prevent epileptic seizures or seizures associated with brain surgery. Occasionally they may be prescribed to treat severe stabbing facial pain (trigeminal neuralgia). Tests may be needed to check blood cells, blood levels of the drug, liver function, and blood sugar. Special attention to oral hygiene is needed to prevent gum problems often associated with taking these anticonvulsants. Hydantoin anticonvulsants interact with many other drugs as well as alcohol, so check carefully with your physician and pharmacist before taking any other medication.

INSTRUCTIONS

Any of these medicines could upset the stomach. This is less likely if they are taken with food. All of them can cause drowsiness or blurred vision and could make driving dangerous.

BRAND NAME	GENERIC NAME
Diflucan	fluconazole
Monistat	miconazole

DESCRIPTION

Diflucan is a strong antifungal drug used to treat serious yeast and yeastlike infections, including thrush and cryptococcal meningitis. While it can be lifesaving in such situations, in rare cases it also has potentially serious side effects. Diflucan may damage the liver, and liver enzymes should be monitored. Other side effects include nausea, vomiting, headache, skin rash, abdominal pain, and diarrhea. Notify your doctor if you experience any of these. The skin rash could become more serious.

Monistat is a vaginal cream used against vaginal yeast infections. It may cause hives or skin rash, but probably less circulates in the body than if it were taken as a pill or injection.

INSTRUCTIONS

Ask your doctor for precise instructions on how to take Diflucan. Doses are individualized, depending on the infection treated, and the first dose is often higher than the rest. Unprotected sexual intercourse should be avoided during Monistat treatment.

INTERACTION

Monistat is commonly used as a vaginal cream, which could result in blood levels too low to trigger this reaction. Clinical studies and case reports indicate that Diflucan can raise blood levels of Dilantin substantially and make it last longer. Toxicity is definitely a possibility. Toxicity associated with elevated phenytoin levels has also occurred when Monistat was given intravenously in conjunction with Dilantin. *This interaction could be dangerous.*

Blood levels of the anticonvulsant should be checked more frequently when someone must start or stop treatment with one of these antifungal drugs. Report any symptoms of toxicity to the doctor.

Symptoms of Phenytoin Toxicity

Uncontrollable eye movements (nystagmus), unsteadiness, difficulty speaking clearly, dizziness, and stupor. Notify the physician immediately of any of these symptoms.

Never take or stop medication without your doctor's advice.

INTERACTION

DANGEROUS

Anticonvulsants
(HYDANTOINS)

Heart Drug
(AMIODARONE)

BRAND NAME	GENERIC NAME
Dilantin	phenytoin
Mesantoin	mephenytoin
Peganone	ethotoin

DESCRIPTION

These anticonvulsants are used to prevent epileptic seizures or seizures associated with brain surgery. Occasionally they may be prescribed to treat severe stabbing facial pain (trigeminal neuralgia). Tests may be needed to check blood cells, blood levels of the drug, liver function, and blood sugar. Special attention to oral hygiene is needed to prevent gum problems often associated with taking these anticonvulsants. Hydantoin anticonvulsants interact with many other drugs as well as alcohol, so check carefully with your physician and pharmacist before taking any other medication.

INSTRUCTIONS

Any of these medicines could upset the stomach. This is less likely if they are taken with food. All of them can cause drowsiness or blurred vision and could make driving dangerous.

BRAND NAME	GENERIC NAME
Cordarone	amiodarone

DESCRIPTION

Cordarone is used to treat life-threatening heart rhythm problems affecting the ventricle, or lower part, of the heart. Some doctors prescribe a lower dose for other rhythm disturbances. This medication has potentially serious side effects, and occasionally may exacerbate heart rhythm problems. Hospitalization is recommended for the first doses, and the doctor should monitor your progress carefully.

INSTRUCTIONS

Follow the physician's directions carefully. Tell your doctor if you notice shortness of breath or changes in vision, or if your skin turns blue.

INTERACTION

Cordarone may interfere with the metabolism of Dilantin and similar drugs, leading to blood levels of the anticonvulsants that are twice as high as normal. In this case, a patient might experience symptoms of phenytoin toxicity. Cordarone is metabolized more rapidly in the presence of Dilantin. In theory, levels as much as 49 percent lower than normal could reduce its effectiveness against arrhythmias. *We are not aware of any cases, but the interaction could be quite dangerous.*

This interaction may show up slowly, so blood levels of phenytoin should be monitored. Be alert for signs of toxicity. Because Cordarone lasts a long time in the body, it may take weeks for blood levels to return to normal unless the doctor is able to adjust the dose.

Symptoms of Phenytoin Toxicity

Uncontrollable eye movements (nystagmus), unsteadiness, difficulty speaking clearly, dizziness, and stupor. Notify the physician immediately of any of these symptoms.

INTERACTION

DANGEROUS

Anticonvulsants

(HYDANTOINS)

Oral Contraceptives

BRAND NAME	GENERIC NAME
Dilantin	phenytoin
Mesantoin	mephenytoin
Peganone	ethotoin

BRAND NAME

Brevicon	**Demulen**	**Desogen**
Genora	**Levlen**	**Loestrin**
Lo/Ovral	**Modicon**	**N.E.E.**
Nelova	**Nordette**	**Norethin**
Norinyl	**Norlestrin**	**Ortho-**
Ortho-Novum	**Ovcon**	**Cyclen**
Ovral	**Triphasil**	

DESCRIPTION

These anticonvulsants are used to prevent epileptic seizures or seizures associated with brain surgery. Occasionally they may be prescribed to treat severe stabbing facial pain (trigeminal neuralgia). Tests may be needed to check blood cells, blood levels of the drug, liver function, and blood sugar. Special attention to oral hygiene is needed to prevent gum problems often associated with taking these anticonvulsants. Hydantoin anticonvulsants interact with many other drugs as well as alcohol, so check carefully with your physician and pharmacist before taking any other medication.

INSTRUCTIONS

Any of these medicines could upset the stomach. This is less likely if they are taken with food. All of them can cause drowsiness or blurred vision and could make driving dangerous.

DESCRIPTION

Lower doses of estrogen and progestin make these drugs safer today than ever before. But women who smoke and take oral contraceptives still run an increased risk of strokes. Side effects may include menstrual changes, nausea, migraine, depression, changes in vision, high blood pressure, liver tumors, gallbladder problems, blood clots, and heart attacks. Weigh the benefits and risks with your doctor when considering this form of contraception. Birth control pills interact with several other medications; check with your doctor or pharmacist before taking another drug in conjunction with oral contraceptives.

INSTRUCTIONS

Oral contraceptives should be taken at the same time every day and precisely according to instructions. Missed doses can lead to an unwelcome pregnancy. Additional contraception is needed for at least the first week.

INTERACTION

Epileptic women have become pregnant while taking oral contraceptives in conjunction with anticonvulsants. The risk is approximately 25 times higher than the normally very low risk of pregnancy using birth control pills. Hydantoins may speed clearance of both estrogen and progesterone from the body in less time than usual. *Because these anticonvulsants have been associated with some birth defects, this interaction could be dangerous.*

Oral contraceptives may also increase the blood levels of anticonvulsants such as Mesantoin, resulting in toxicity. Other contraceptive methods are advisable, if possible.

Symptoms of Phenytoin Toxicity

Uncontrollable eye movements (nystagmus), unsteadiness, difficulty speaking clearly, dizziness, and stupor. Notify the physician immediately of any of these symptoms.

Never take or stop medication without your doctor's advice.

INTERACTION

DANGEROUS

Anticonvulsants
(HYDANTOINS)

Tuberculosis Drug
(ISONIAZID)

BRAND NAME	GENERIC NAME
Dilantin	phenytoin
Mesantoin	mephenytoin
Peganone	ethotoin

DESCRIPTION

These anticonvulsants are used to prevent epileptic seizures or seizures associated with brain surgery. Occasionally they may be prescribed to treat severe stabbing facial pain (trigeminal neuralgia). Tests may be needed to check blood cells, blood levels of the drug, liver function, and blood sugar. Special attention to oral hygiene is needed to prevent gum problems often associated with taking these anticonvulsants. Hydantoin anticonvulsants interact with many other drugs as well as alcohol, so check carefully with your physician and pharmacist before taking any other medication.

INSTRUCTIONS

Any of these medicines could upset the stomach. This is less likely if they are taken with food. All of them can cause drowsiness or blurred vision and could make driving dangerous.

BRAND NAME	GENERIC NAME
INH	isoniazid
Izonid	isoniazid
Laniazid	isoniazid
Nydrazid	isoniazid
Rifamate	isoniazid/rifampin

DESCRIPTION

Isoniazid is used (in combination with other drugs) to treat tuberculosis and to prevent its progression. To be effective, it must be taken faithfully for an extended period of time as prescribed. Side effects may include numbness, tingling or pain in hands and feet, nausea, vomiting, stomachache, and elevated liver enzymes. If you develop fever, rash, weakness, or yellow eyes and skin, contact your doctor.

INSTRUCTIONS

Isoniazid is best taken on an empty stomach, at least one hour before meals or two hours after. It may be taken with food if it upsets the stomach. Alcohol increases the risk of a potentially fatal liver reaction, so don't drink. Foods high in tyramine interact with isoniazid to raise blood pressure dangerously; see the list on page 47. Fish such as skipjack and tuna may trigger an unpleasant histamine reaction. Symptoms of B_6 deficiency may develop; supplements may be required.

INTERACTION

One-tenth to almost a third of the people who must take both the tuberculosis medicine and one of these anticonvulsants will experience phenytoin toxicity. This is a far higher proportion than those who may have toxicity reactions while taking one of the hydantoins alone. *This interaction could be dangerous.*

It is important for your physician to check blood levels of Dilantin or a similar medication if you start or stop taking isoniazid. If you experience symptoms of toxicity, notify the doctor at once.

Symptoms of Phenytoin Toxicity

Uncontrollable eye movements (nystagmus), unsteadiness, difficulty speaking clearly, dizziness, and stupor. Notify your physician immediately of any of these symptoms.

INTERACTION

DANGEROUS

Anticonvulsants

(HYDANTOINS)

Ulcer Drugs

BRAND NAME	GENERIC NAME
Dilantin	phenytoin
Mesantoin	mephenytoin
Peganone	ethotoin

DESCRIPTION

These anticonvulsants are used to prevent epileptic seizures or seizures associated with brain surgery. Occasionally they may be prescribed to treat severe stabbing facial pain (trigeminal neuralgia). Tests may be needed to check blood cells, blood levels of the drug, liver function, and blood sugar. Special attention to oral hygiene is needed to prevent gum problems often associated with taking these anticonvulsants. Hydantoin anticonvulsants interact with many other drugs as well as alcohol, so check carefully with your physician and pharmacist before taking any other medication.

INSTRUCTIONS

Any of these medicines could upset the stomach. This is less likely if they are taken with food. All of them can cause drowsiness or blurred vision and could make driving dangerous.

BRAND NAME	GENERIC NAME
Prilosec	omeprazole
Tagamet	cimetidine

DESCRIPTION

Tagamet revolutionized the treatment of ulcers and serious heartburn by blocking special receptors, thereby reducing the acidity of the stomach. Cimetidine usually has few side effects, although headaches, dizziness, and mild diarrhea are potential reactions. Some men complain of antitestosterone effects. At higher doses, this may lead to enlarged breasts or sexual problems. Older people and those who are very ill may experience depression, mental confusion, or disorientation. The dose may need to be adjusted for them. Tagamet may modify the metabolism of a number of medications, so check with your doctor and pharmacist if you take cimetidine with another medicine.

Prilosec is a powerful acid suppressor that works through an entirely different mechanism. It too is effective for ulcers and severe heartburn.

INSTRUCTIONS

Tagamet is usually taken with meals and/or at bedtime. Antacids may reduce absorption of Tagamet; do not take one for at least two hours after taking Tagamet. Prilosec should be taken just before eating, preferably in the morning.

INTERACTION

Tagamet appears to modify the metabolism of Dilantin. Tagamet also seems likely to affect the metabolism of Mesantoin and Peganone, although this interaction has not yet been documented in the medical literature. The problem is that Tagamet affects liver enzymes so that they are less capable of processing these particular anticonvulsants. As a result, blood levels of the anticonvulsants can rise, leading to toxicity. A similar, but weaker, interaction has been noted in studies of Prilosec and Dilantin. *This interaction could be dangerous.*

Symptoms of Phenytoin Toxicity

Uncontrollable eye movements (nystagmus), unsteadiness, difficulty speaking clearly, dizziness, and stupor. Notify your physician immediately of any of these symptoms.

Never take or stop medication without your doctor's advice.

INTERACTION

DANGEROUS

Anticonvulsants
(HYDANTOINS)

Anti-Anxiety Drugs
(BENZODIAZEPINES)

BRAND NAME	GENERIC NAME
Dilantin	phenytoin
Mesantoin	mephenytoin
Peganone	ethotoin

DESCRIPTION

These anticonvulsants are used to prevent epileptic seizures or seizures associated with brain surgery. Occasionally they may be prescribed to treat severe stabbing facial pain (trigeminal neuralgia). Tests may be needed to check blood cells, blood levels of the drug, liver function, and blood sugar. Special attention to oral hygiene is needed to prevent gum problems often associated with taking these anticonvulsants. Hydantoin anticonvulsants interact with many other drugs as well as alcohol, so check carefully with your physician and pharmacist before taking any other medication.

INSTRUCTIONS

Any of these medicines could upset the stomach. This is less likely if they are taken with food. All of them can cause drowsiness or blurred vision and could make driving dangerous.

BRAND NAME	GENERIC NAME
Ativan	lorazepam
Dalmane	flurazepam
Doral	quazepam
Halcion	triazolam
Librium	chlordiazepoxide
Paxipam	halazepam
ProSom	estazolam
Restoril	temazepam
Serax	oxazepam
Tranxene	clorazepate
Valium	diazepam
Xanax	alprazolam

DESCRIPTION

Benzodiazepines are used primarily to treat anxiety disorders and insomnia. Some have also been employed to relieve panic attacks, seizures, muscle cramps, and contractions. Anesthesiologists often use such medications before certain surgical procedures.

Prolonged use may lead to dependence. Sudden withdrawal can produce unpleasant side effects and should always be supervised by a physician.

INSTRUCTIONS

These drugs may be taken with food, especially if they upset the digestive tract.

INTERACTION

This is a confusing interaction. The data are contradictory and no firm conclusions can be drawn. Nevertheless, there is some concern that Dilantin (phenytoin) levels may be increased by Valium or Librium. Some patients have apparently experienced symptoms of phenytoin toxicity as a result of this combination. Experts suggest that if patients need a benzodiazepine in addition to Dilantin, their blood phenytoin levels be monitored carefully, especially when starting or stopping the benzodiazepine. Although there is no information about anti-anxiety drugs other than Valium and Librium, the possibility exists that other benzodiazepines might interact with phenytoin as well.

Symptoms of Phenytoin Toxicity

Uncontrollable eye movements (nystagmus), unsteadiness, difficulty speaking clearly, dizziness, and stupor. Notify the physician immediately of any of these symptoms.

Never take or stop medication without your doctor's advice.

INTERACTION

TROUBLESOME

Anticonvulsants

(HYDANTOINS)

Antibiotic

(DOXYCYCLINE)

BRAND NAME	GENERIC NAME
Dilantin	phenytoin
Mesantoin	mephenytoin
Peganone	ethotoin

DESCRIPTION

These anticonvulsants are used to prevent epileptic seizures or seizures associated with brain surgery. Occasionally they may be prescribed to treat severe stabbing facial pain (trigeminal neuralgia). Tests may be needed to check blood cells, blood levels of the drug, liver function, and blood sugar. Special attention to oral hygiene is needed to prevent gum problems often associated with taking these anticonvulsants. Hydantoin anticonvulsants interact with many other drugs as well as alcohol, so check carefully with your physician and pharmacist before taking any other medication.

INSTRUCTIONS

Any of these medicines could upset the stomach. This is less likely if they are taken with food. All of them can cause drowsiness or blurred vision and could make driving dangerous.

BRAND NAME	GENERIC NAME
Doryx	doxycycline
Doxi Film	doxycycline
Doxy-Caps	doxycycline
Doxychel Hyclate	doxycycline
Doxy-D	doxycycline
Monodox	doxycycline
Vibramycin	doxycycline
Vibra-Tabs	doxycycline

DESCRIPTION

Doxycycline is a form of tetracyline prescribed for a wide variety of infections, including serious ones such as Rocky Mountain spotted fever and Lyme disease, and common problems such as acne and traveler's diarrhea. Tetracycline is generally inappropriate for pregnant women and young children, as it may stain permanent teeth. This medicine makes many people more sensitive to ultraviolet light, so protect yourself from sunlight and tanning lamps.

INSTRUCTIONS

Doxycycline may be taken with food or milk to reduce stomach upset, always with a full eight ounces of liquid. Do not take this medicine with antacids, calcium supplements, or iron pills, as they could interfere with absorption of the drug. Never take outdated doxycycline, which may be toxic to the kidneys.

INTERACTION

Dilantin, like Tegretol, can significantly reduce the amount of time it takes for the liver to process and eliminate doxycycline. As a consequence, blood levels of this antibiotic may be lower than expected when it is taken in conjunction with one of the hydantoins, and infections might not heal as quickly or as well as anticipated. *This interaction could certainly be troublesome.*

The doctor may decide to double the dose of doxycycline to ensure therapeutic success. In any event, progress on the antibiotic should be monitored closely in patients on hydantoin anticonvulsants.

INTERACTION

TROUBLESOME

Anticonvulsants
(HYDANTOINS)

Asthma Drug
(THEOPHYLLINE)

BRAND NAME	GENERIC NAME
Dilantin	phenytoin
Mesantoin	mephenytoin
Peganone	ethotoin

DESCRIPTION

These anticonvulsants are used to prevent epileptic seizures or seizures associated with brain surgery. Occasionally they may be prescribed to treat severe stabbing facial pain (trigeminal neuralgia). Tests may be needed to check blood cells, blood levels of the drug, liver function, and blood sugar. Special attention to oral hygiene is needed to prevent gum problems often associated with taking these anticonvulsants. Hydantoin anticonvulsants interact with many other drugs as well as alcohol, so check carefully with your physician and pharmacist before taking any other medication.

INSTRUCTIONS

Any of these medicines could upset the stomach. This is less likely if they are taken with food. All of them can cause drowsiness or blurred vision and could make driving dangerous.

BRAND NAME

Aerolate	**Aquaphyllin**	**Asmalix**
Bronkodyl	**Elixomin**	**Elixophyllin**
Quibron-T	**Respbid**	**Slo-bid**
Slo-Phyllin	**Theobid**	**Theochron**
Theoclear	**Theo-Dur**	**Theolair**
Theo-24	**Theovent**	**Theo-X**
T-Phyl	**Uniphyl**	

DESCRIPTION

Theophylline helps to open airways, so it is generally used to treat and prevent asthma attacks. It may also be prescribed for people with emphysema or other chronic breathing problems. Babies and elderly men may need lower doses. The dose is monitored with regular blood tests to ensure that levels are less than 20 mcg/ml.

INSTRUCTIONS

Theophylline interacts with food in complex ways, so discuss this issue thoroughly with your doctor and pharmacist. Theophylline may upset the stomach. In some cases this problem can be alleviated by taking the drug with food. See the table of Food and Drug Interactions on pages 59-73 for more information.

INTERACTION

This is a double interaction, because both theophylline and the anticonvulsants can lead to lower blood levels of the other drug. The effect of the anticonvulsants, especially Dilantin, is to speed up removal of theophylline from the system by as much as 65 percent. *This interaction could be troublesome, leading to asthma symptoms.*

The interaction may become noticeable within about five days of taking the two drugs together. If both are needed, blood levels of each should be monitored so that doses can be adjusted appropriately by your doctor.

Never take or stop medication without your doctor's advice.

INTERACTION

TROUBLESOME

Anticonvulsants

(HYDANTOINS)

Folic Acid

BRAND NAME	GENERIC NAME
Dilantin	phenytoin
Mesantoin	mephenytoin
Peganone	ethotoin

DESCRIPTION

These anticonvulsants are used to prevent epileptic seizures or seizures associated with brain surgery. Occasionally they may be prescribed to treat severe stabbing facial pain (trigeminal neuralgia). Tests may be needed to check blood cells, blood levels of the drug, liver function, and blood sugar. Special attention to oral hygiene is needed to prevent gum problems often associated with taking these anticonvulsants. Hydantoin anticonvulsants interact with many other drugs as well as alcohol, so check carefully with your physician and pharmacist before taking any other medication.

INSTRUCTIONS

Any of these medicines could upset the stomach. This is less likely if they are taken with food. All of them can cause drowsiness or blurred vision and could make driving dangerous.

BRAND NAME	GENERIC NAME
Folvite	folic acid

DESCRIPTION

Folic acid is a B vitamin essential for healthy red blood cells. Women who are planning to be become pregnant are now encouraged to take a moderate folic acid supplement, as this can reduce the risk of birth defects affecting the neural tube. Deficiency of this vitamin may produce megaloblastic anemia, but supplementing with folic acid alone could hide an underlying vitamin B_{12} deficiency (pernicious anemia).

INSTRUCTIONS

Fruits and vegetables, whole grains, and legumes are rich sources of this vitamin. Supplements of up to 800 micrograms (0.8 mg) are available without prescription, although most people maintain adequate stores of this vitamin on an intake of 100 to 200 micrograms daily.

INTERACTION

Dilantin can deplete folic acid levels, especially with long-term therapy. Relatively few patients develop frank megaloblastic anemia, but the clinician should be on the lookout for deficiency. Unfortunately, this interaction works both ways. Folic acid can reduce blood levels of phenytoin, so treatment should be supervised by an experienced physician. Occasionally folic acid supplementation (at levels greater than 2 mg/day) has reduced the efficacy of the anticonvulsant, with seizures occurring as a result. *This interaction could be troublesome.*

Dilantin has other potential nutritional impacts, and may lower levels of vitamin B_6, vitamin D, and vitamin K as well as folic acid. A person who expects to take this anticonvulsant for a long time might benefit from consultation with a knowledgeable dietitian.

INTERACTION

TROUBLESOME

Anticonvulsants
(HYDANTOINS)

Heart Drug
(MEXILETINE)

BRAND NAME   **GENERIC NAME**

Dilantin   phenytoin
Mesantoin   mephenytoin
Peganone   ethotoin

DESCRIPTION

These anticonvulsants are used to prevent epileptic seizures or seizures associated with brain surgery. Occasionally they may be prescribed to treat severe stabbing facial pain (trigeminal neuralgia). Tests may be needed to check blood cells, blood levels of the drug, liver function, and blood sugar. Special attention to oral hygiene is needed to prevent gum problems often associated with taking these anticonvulsants. Hydantoin anticonvulsants interact with many other drugs as well as alcohol, so check carefully with your physician and pharmacist before taking any other medication.

INSTRUCTIONS

Any of these medicines could upset the stomach. This is less likely if they are taken with food. All of them can cause drowsiness or blurred vision and could make driving dangerous.

BRAND NAME   **GENERIC NAME**

Mexitil   mexiletine

DESCRIPTION

Mexitil is used to treat severe, life-threatening heartbeat disturbances. Occasionally Mexitil aggravates heart rhythm irregularities, so careful monitoring is essential. Hospitalization is recommended for the first doses. This medicine interacts with many other drugs. Check with your physician and pharmacist before taking anything else.

INSTRUCTIONS

Mexitil may irritate the digestive tract, so it should be taken with food or an antacid. Dramatic changes in diet should be avoided. Notify the doctor immediately if fever, yellow skin and eyes, sore throat, or unusual tiredness develop.

INTERACTION

Dilantin and the other anticonvulsants in this class can affect the metabolism of Mexitil so that blood levels of this heart drug are reduced. This interaction was confirmed through a clinical study of healthy volunteers. There have been no reports to date, however, of lowered effectiveness resulting from the lower blood levels. *This interaction is potentially troublesome.*

Armed with knowledge of this interaction, the physician will wish to monitor blood levels of mexiletine when a patient starts or stops one of the hydantoin anticonvulsants. The doctor may need to adjust the dose of the heart medication.

INTERACTION

TROUBLESOME

Anticonvulsants

(HYDANTOINS)

Heart Drug

(QUINIDINE)

BRAND NAME	GENERIC NAME
Dilantin	phenytoin
Mesantoin	mephenytoin
Peganone	ethotoin

DESCRIPTION

These anticonvulsants are used to prevent epileptic seizures or seizures associated with brain surgery. Occasionally they may be prescribed to treat severe stabbing facial pain (trigeminal neuralgia). Tests may be needed to check blood cells, blood levels of the drug, liver function, and blood sugar. Special attention to oral hygiene is needed to prevent gum problems often associated with taking these anticonvulsants. Hydantoin anticonvulsants interact with many other drugs as well as alcohol, so check carefully with your physician and pharmacist before taking any other medication.

INSTRUCTIONS

Any of these medicines could upset the stomach. This is less likely if they are taken with food. All of them can cause drowsiness or blurred vision and could make driving dangerous.

BRAND NAME	GENERIC NAME
Cardioquin	quinidine
Quinaglute	quinidine
Quinalan	quinidine
Quinidex	quinidine
Quinora	quinidine

DESCRIPTION

Quinidine is prescribed for a variety of heart rhythm disturbances. The first dose is considered a test to see if the patient will have a dangerous reaction. People with heart failure, or with liver or kidney disease, need close monitoring.

INSTRUCTIONS

Quinidine may upset the stomach. Taking it with food may help alleviate this problem. Sustained-release tablets (Quinaglute Dura-Tabs, Quinalan, Quinidex Extentabs) should not be chewed or crushed.

Quinidine may provoke visual disturbances, ringing in the ears, headache, dizziness, nausea, skin rash, or breathing difficulties. Notify your doctor if you develop any of these symptoms. Do not stop this medicine unless your doctor so directs.

INTERACTION

Several case reports have demonstrated that Dilantin can speed elimination of quinidine from the system. It appears to do this through an effect on the liver enzymes responsible for metabolism. In some patients, quinidine levels are reduced by half, and the effectiveness of the medication is compromised. *This interaction could be troublesome.*

If phenytoin is to be added or deleted from a person's treatment regimen, blood levels of quinidine should be monitored carefully. The physician may need to adjust the dose.

Never take or stop medication without your doctor's advice.

INTERACTION

TROUBLESOME

Anticonvulsants
(HYDANTOINS)

BRAND NAME	GENERIC NAME
Dilantin	phenytoin
Mesantoin	mephenytoin
Peganone	ethotoin

DESCRIPTION

These anticonvulsants are used to prevent epileptic seizures or seizures associated with brain surgery. Occasionally they may be prescribed to treat severe stabbing facial pain (trigeminal neuralgia). Tests may be needed to check blood cells, blood levels of the drug, liver function, and blood sugar. Special attention to oral hygiene is needed to prevent gum problems often associated with taking these anticonvulsants. Hydantoin anticonvulsants interact with many other drugs as well as alcohol, so check carefully with your physician and pharmacist before taking any other medication.

INSTRUCTIONS

Any of these medicines could upset the stomach. This is less likely if they are taken with food. All of them can cause drowsiness or blurred vision and could make driving dangerous.

Pain Reliever
(ACETAMINOPHEN)

BRAND NAME	GENERIC NAME
Anacin-3	acetaminophen
Darvocet-N	acetaminophen/ propoxyphene
Panadol	acetaminophen
Tylenol	acetaminophen
Vicodin	acetaminophen/ hydrocodone

etc.

DESCRIPTION

Acetaminophen is widely available as an over-the-counter nonaspirin pain reliever, and is also found in a number of prescription pain medications, such as Darvocet and Percocet. In addition to relieving pain approximately as well as aspirin, acetaminophen is also good for bringing down fever. Regular alcohol consumption together with daily acetaminophen intake could increase the risk of liver problems.

INSTRUCTIONS

Acetaminophen may be taken with meals or on an empty stomach; pain relief is more rapid if it is taken without food. Fasting may make acetaminophen more dangerous to the liver. Never take large doses of acetaminophen if you are not able to eat regularly.

INTERACTION

Regular use of Dilantin or a similar anticonvulsant may make a person more susceptible to liver damage due to acetaminophen taken at high doses or for a long time. The more rapid metabolism of acetaminophen in the presence of hydantoins means it could be somewhat less effective. *This interaction could be troublesome.*

If acetaminophen does not appear to be offering the expected pain relief at normal doses, it would be more prudent to consider an alternate pain medication than to increase the dose of this drug. High doses could contribute to liver problems.

Never take or stop medication without your doctor's advice.

INTERACTION

TROUBLESOME

Anticonvulsants

(HYDANTOINS)

Tuberculosis Drug

(RIFAMPIN)

BRAND NAME	GENERIC NAME
Dilantin	phenytoin
Mesantoin	mephenytoin
Peganone	ethotoin

BRAND NAME	GENERIC NAME
Rifadin	rifampin
Rifamate	isoniazid/rifampin
Rimactane	rifampin

DESCRIPTION

These anticonvulsants are used to prevent epileptic seizures or seizures associated with brain surgery. Occasionally they may be prescribed to treat severe stabbing facial pain (trigeminal neuralgia). Tests may be needed to check blood cells, blood levels of the drug, liver function, and blood sugar. Special attention to oral hygiene is needed to prevent gum problems often associated with taking these anticonvulsants. Hydantoin anticonvulsants interact with many other drugs as well as alcohol, so check carefully with your physician and pharmacist before taking any other medication.

INSTRUCTIONS

Any of these medicines could upset the stomach. This is less likely if they are taken with food. All of them can cause drowsiness or blurred vision and could make driving dangerous.

DESCRIPTION

Rifampin is used in combination with other medications to treat tuberculosis. To be effective, it needs to be taken faithfully for an extended period of time (at least six to nine months), as the doctor prescribes. Side effects may include digestive tract problems, menstrual irregularities, difficulty concentrating, fluid retention, and wheezing or shortness of breath. The orange discoloration of urine, saliva, and tears is not harmful, although it may stain contact lenses.

INSTRUCTIONS

Rifampin should be taken on an empty stomach, at least one hour before or two hours after meals. If you develop fever, chills, unusual tiredness, unusual bleeding or bruising, sore throat, muscle and bone pain, or yellow skin and eyes, contact your physician immediately.

INTERACTION

A person who needs one of these tuberculosis medicines as well as Dilantin or a similar anticonvulsant may process the anticonvulsant more quickly. This could result in lower blood levels of the anticonvulsant than when it is taken alone. *This interaction might be troublesome, as the anticonvulsant could be less effective.*

Seizures are theoretically possible. Blood levels of Dilantin should be monitored when a person starts or stops rifampin therapy.

Never take or stop medication without your doctor's advice.

INTERACTION

TROUBLESOME

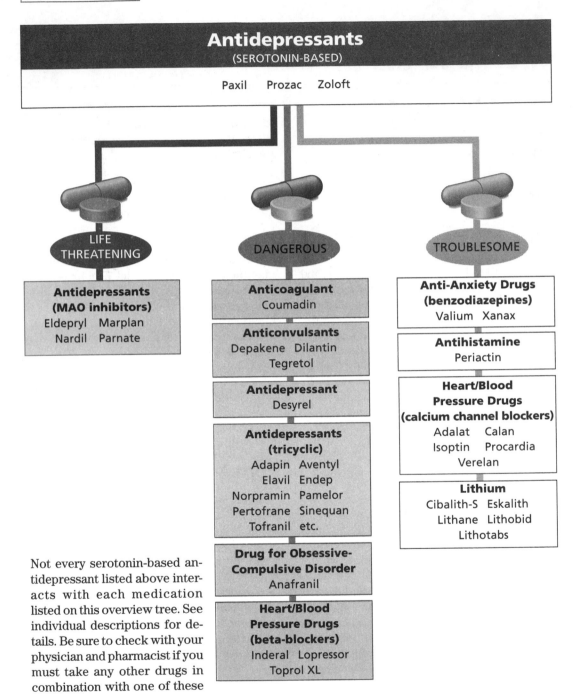

Antidepressants
(SEROTONIN-BASED)

Paxil   Prozac   Zoloft

LIFE THREATENING

DANGEROUS

TROUBLESOME

Antidepressants (MAO inhibitors)
Eldepryl   Marplan
Nardil   Parnate

Anticoagulant
Coumadin

Anticonvulsants
Depakene   Dilantin
Tegretol

Antidepressant
Desyrel

Antidepressants (tricyclic)
Adapin   Aventyl
Elavil   Endep
Norpramin   Pamelor
Pertofrane   Sinequan
Tofranil   etc.

Drug for Obsessive-Compulsive Disorder
Anafranil

Heart/Blood Pressure Drugs (beta-blockers)
Inderal   Lopressor
Toprol XL

Anti-Anxiety Drugs (benzodiazepines)
Valium   Xanax

Antihistamine
Periactin

Heart/Blood Pressure Drugs (calcium channel blockers)
Adalat   Calan
Isoptin   Procardia
Verelan

Lithium
Cibalith-S   Eskalith
Lithane   Lithobid
Lithotabs

Not every serotonin-based antidepressant listed above interacts with each medication listed on this overview tree. See individual descriptions for details. Be sure to check with your physician and pharmacist if you must take any other drugs in combination with one of these antidepressants.

LEVELS OF HAZARD: LIFE THREATENING   DANGEROUS   TROUBLESOME

Antidepressants
(SEROTONIN-BASED)

BRAND NAME	GENERIC NAME
Paxil	paroxetine
Prozac	fluoxetine
Zoloft	sertraline

DESCRIPTION

These antidepressants block the reuptake into brain cells of serotonin, a chemical messenger. Because they work differently from older antidepressants, they have different side effects and indications. Prozac is also prescribed for obsessive-compulsive disorder and for bulimia. Older people and those with kidney or liver problems may need reduced doses. Prozac is metabolized slowly and may linger weeks after discontinuation.

INSTRUCTIONS

Prozac, Paxil, and Zoloft are usually taken once a day, often in the morning. Prozac may be taken without regard to meals. Taking it with food may reduce stomach upset. A few patients experience serious weight loss on these medications. If this occurs, the doctor should be notified.

Antidepressants
(MAO INHIBITORS)

BRAND NAME	GENERIC NAME
Eldepryl	selegiline
Marplan	isocarboxazid
Nardil	phenelzine
Parnate	tranylcypromine

DESCRIPTION

These medications were among the earliest antidepressants to be developed and still work very well for some patients. Eldepryl, a drug used to treat Parkinson's disease, also has some monoamine oxidase (MAO) inhibitor activity and may interact with serotonin-based antidepressants. These drugs are slow to start acting, and may last in the body for a few weeks after medication is stopped.

INSTRUCTIONS

MAO inhibitors can interact in dangerous ways with tyramine-containing foods and beverages. See page 47. Consult your doctor before taking other prescription or over-the-counter drugs. Notify him or her if you notice a skin rash, severe headache, yellow eyes or skin, or dark urine. Do not stop this medicine unless your doctor so advises.

INTERACTION

When a patient does not get adequate relief of depression from one medication, the doctor may add a different antidepressant. The literature accompanying serotonin-based antidepressants warns against this combination. *Fatalities have resulted from this interaction.* Some people who have received this combination experience "serotonin syndrome," a very serious, potentially lethal reaction. Because these drugs last in the body for quite some time, at least two weeks should pass after discontinuing an MAO inhibitor before starting on Prozac, Zoloft, or Paxil. The manufacturer of Prozac recommends waiting five weeks after stopping Prozac before beginning an MAO inhibitor antidepressant. For Zoloft and Paxil, at least two weeks should elapse after stopping the serotonin-based antidepressant before beginning Marplan, Nardil, or Parnate. Eldepryl may also interact with the serotonin-based antidepressants.

Symptoms of Serotonin Syndrome

Severe shivering, agitation, confusion, restlessness, muscle twitches or rigidity, diarrhea, elevated temperature, sweating, changes in blood pressure, and coma. Notify your doctor at once if you experience any of these symptoms.

Never take or stop medication without your doctor's advice.

INTERACTION

LIFE THREATENING

Antidepressants
(SEROTONIN-BASED)

Anticoagulant
(WARFARIN)

BRAND NAME	GENERIC NAME
Paxil	paroxetine
Prozac	fluoxetine
Zoloft	sertraline

DESCRIPTION

These antidepressants work by blocking the reuptake into brain cells of serotonin, a chemical messenger. Because they work differently from older antidepressants, they have different side effects and indications. Prozac, for instance, is also prescribed for obsessive-compulsive disorder and for bulimia. Older people and those with kidney or liver problems may need reduced doses. Prozac is cleared from the body very slowly and may linger weeks after discontinuation.

INSTRUCTIONS

Paxil and Zoloft are taken once a day, usually in the morning. Prozac is taken in the morning, or, if a higher dose has been prescribed, in the morning and at noon. It may be taken without regard to meals. Taking it with food may reduce stomach upset. A few patients experience serious weight loss on these medications. If this occurs, the doctor should be notified.

BRAND NAME	GENERIC NAME
Coumadin	warfarin

DESCRIPTION

Warfarin slows the liver's production of factors essential for the formation of blood clots. It is prescribed when there is a risk that a dangerous clot could form in a deep vein or a blood vessel leading to the lung, heart, or brain. The most serious complication of anticoagulant treatment is excessive bleeding. The dosage must be individually adjusted, requiring daily blood tests at first, then tests every four to six weeks. Other side effects may include nausea, loss of appetite, rash, fever, yellow eyes and skin, prolonged painful erection, and hair loss.

INSTRUCTIONS

Warfarin tablets can be swallowed with food or on an empty stomach. Try to avoid large variations in the quantity of vitamin-K–containing vegetables—such as broccoli, cabbage, or spinach—that you eat each day. Consuming much more or less than usual could change the action of the drug.

INTERACTION

Although there are only a few reports of interaction between any of these antidepressants and warfarin, it appears that in some cases these serotonin-based medications can increase the risk of bleeding associated with warfarin. *This interaction could be dangerous.*

It is possible that many patients will have no trouble with this combination, but the physician should monitor carefully for a potential interaction. Prothrombin time or international normalized ratio (INR) may be increased. Notify your physician immediately if you experience any symptoms of bleeding.

Symptoms of Warfarin Overdose
There may be no early warning signs of danger. Blood tests are essential. Symptoms include any unusual bleeding, including rectal or urinary tract bleeding, excessive menstrual bleeding, nosebleeds, bleeding around gums, bruising, red or tar-black stools, vomiting blood, and red or dark-brown urine. Notify your doctor immediately if you suspect a problem.

Never take or stop medication without your doctor's advice.

INTERACTION

DANGEROUS

Antidepressant
(SEROTONIN-BASED)

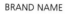

Anticonvulsants

BRAND NAME	GENERIC NAME
Prozac	fluoxetine

DESCRIPTION

This antidepressant works by blocking the reuptake into brain cells of serotonin, a chemical messenger. Because it works differently from the older cyclic-type antidepressants, it has a different set of side effects and has become more popular. It may also work against a different array of problems, for instance, bulimia or obsessive-compulsive disorder. Older people and those with kidney or liver problems may need reduced doses. Prozac is cleared from the body very slowly and may linger weeks after discontinuation.

INSTRUCTIONS

Prozac is taken in the morning, or, if a higher dose has been prescribed, in the morning and at noon. It may be taken without regard to meals. Taking it with food may reduce stomach upset. A few patients experience serious weight loss on this medication. If this occurs, the doctor should be notified.

BRAND NAME	GENERIC NAME
Depakene	valproic acid
Dilantin	phenytoin
Tegretol	carbamazepine

DESCRIPTION

These unrelated medicines are used to prevent seizures in patients with epilepsy. Dilantin or Tegretol may also be prescribed for a painful condition known as trigeminal neuralgia, while either Tegretol or Depakene may occasionally be used to treat bipolar ("manic") depression. Regular blood tests are needed for patients on Depakene or Tegretol to monitor for rare but serious adverse reactions.

INSTRUCTIONS

Do not discontinue any of these medicines unless your doctor supervises the process carefully. Suddenly stopping these drugs could trigger seizures. These pills should be taken with food to reduce the possibility of stomach upset. Notify the physician immediately of any unusual bruising, bleeding, or yellowing of the skin and eyes.

INTERACTION

A depressed person with epilepsy might need both Prozac and an anticonvulsant medicine. The combination might also be prescribed to someone with bipolar depression who has not responded to the usual treatments. Prozac apparently interferes with metabolism of these compounds and may increase blood levels of Tegretol, Dilantin, or Depakene to the point of toxicity. *The interaction could be dangerous.*

Because Prozac can linger in the body, interaction problems may continue for some time even if Prozac is discontinued. Contact your physician immediately if you experience symptoms such as unsteadiness, drowsiness, or confusion. Blood tests for a few weeks after starting or a few weeks after stopping Prozac are advisable.

Symptoms of Anticonvulsant Toxicity

Nausea, vomiting, digestive upset, slurred speech, blurred vision, incoordination, dizziness, confusion, yellow skin or eyes, unusual bleeding or bruising, headache, and fever. Notify your physician immediately of any of these symptoms.

INTERACTION

DANGEROUS

Antidepressants

(SEROTONIN-BASED)

Antidepressant

(TRAZODONE)

BRAND NAME	GENERIC NAME
Paxil	paroxetine
Prozac	fluoxetine

DESCRIPTION

These antidepressants work by blocking the reuptake into brain cells of serotonin, a chemical messenger. Because they work differently from the older cyclic-type antidepressants, they have a different set of side effects and have become more popular. They may also work against a different array of problems. Prozac, for instance, is also prescribed for obsessive-compulsive disorder. Older people and those with kidney or liver problems may need reduced doses. Prozac is cleared from the body very slowly and may linger weeks after discontinuation.

INSTRUCTIONS

Paxil is taken once a day, usually in the morning. Prozac is taken in the morning, or, if a higher dose has been prescribed, in the morning and at noon. Prozac may be taken without regard to meals. Taking it with food may reduce stomach upset. A few patients experience serious weight loss on these medications. If this occurs, the doctor should be notified.

BRAND NAME	GENERIC NAME
Desyrel	trazodone

DESCRIPTION

Desyrel is quite similar in action to the tricyclic antidepressants (see page 241). Side effects include palpitations, drowsiness, dizziness, dry mouth, lower sex drive, sluggishness, constipation, nasal congestion, and tremors. Weight gain may also be a problem for some people. Men occasionally develop prolonged and painful erections with this drug. If such an effect occurs it requires emergency treatment.

INSTRUCTIONS

Usually Desyrel is better taken with food, in the evening, to avoid daytime drowsiness. Activities that require mental attention such as driving or operating machinery can be dangerous for people on Desyrel. Never stop taking this drug suddenly. If Desyrel needs to be discontinued, this process should be monitored carefully by a physician.

INTERACTION

If a patient does not respond well to one antidepressant, the physician sometimes adds a different medication to try to reverse the depression. However, Prozac and Paxil slow down the liver enzyme that is essential to the metabolism of some older antidepressants such as Desyrel, and can cause blood levels of Desyrel to rise, potentially to toxic levels. *Although we are aware of no fatalities, this interaction could be quite serious.*

Because Prozac lasts a long time in the body, the problems may continue for a few weeks after it is discontinued. Generally, if both drugs are needed, the doctor should adjust the dose of each and monitor the effects closely.

Signs of Desyrel Overdose

Drowsiness, vomiting, dizziness, disorientation, difficulty speaking, difficulty walking, palpitations, prolonged penile erections, breathing difficulties, and seizures. Contact your physician immediately if any such signs of overdose appear.

INTERACTION

DANGEROUS

Antidepressants

(SEROTONIN-BASED)

Antidepressants

(TRICYCLIC)

BRAND NAME	GENERIC NAME
Paxil	paroxetine
Prozac	fluoxetine

DESCRIPTION

These antidepressants work by blocking the reuptake into brain cells of serotonin, a chemical messenger. Because they work differently from the older cyclic-type antidepressants, they have a different set of side effects and have become more popular. They may also work against a different array of problems. Prozac, for instance, is also prescribed for obsessive-compulsive disorder. Older people and those with kidney or liver problems may need reduced doses. Prozac is cleared from the body very slowly and may linger weeks after discontinuation.

INSTRUCTIONS

Paxil is taken once a day, usually in the morning. Prozac is taken in the morning, or, if a higher dose has been prescribed, in the morning and at noon. Prozac may be taken without regard to meals. Taking it with food may reduce stomach upset. A few patients experience serious weight loss on these medications. If this occurs, your doctor should be notified.

BRAND NAME	GENERIC NAME
Adapin, Sinequan	doxepin
Aventyl, Pamelor	nortriptyline
Elavil, Endep	amitriptyline
Norpramin, Pertofrane	desipramine
Tofranil	imipramine
etc.	

DESCRIPTION

Tricyclic antidepressants became popular during the 1970s and 1980s although they often caused unpleasant side effects (constipation, weight gain, sexual dysfunction, sluggishness, increased sun sensitivity, etc.). They are used to treat depression. Some of them may also be helpful in controlling chronic pain.

INSTRUCTIONS

Usually these medications are better taken with food, in the evening to avoid daytime drowsiness. A high-fiber diet may interfere with absorption, however. Sinequan Concentrate should be mixed with four ounces of milk, water, or juice just before taking, not ahead of time. Do not stop taking any of these drugs suddenly; if they must be discontinued, your doctor will supervise gradual phaseout.

INTERACTION

If a patient does not respond well to one antidepressant, the physician sometimes adds a different medication to try to reverse the depression. However, Prozac and Paxil slow down the liver enzyme that is essential to the metabolism of the older antidepressants listed above, and can cause blood levels of these medications to rise markedly, often 100 to 400 percent. This may result in toxic levels. *Although we are aware of no fatalities, this interaction is quite serious.*

Adverse effects may include, in extreme cases, delirium and seizures. Because Prozac lasts a long time in the body, the problems may continue for a few weeks after it is discontinued. Generally, if both drugs are needed, your doctor should adjust the dose of each and monitor the effects closely.

Symptoms of Tricyclic Antidepressant Overdose

Nausea, constipation, confusion, sleepiness, palpitations, dizziness, dry mouth, blurred vision, and fever. Contact the physician immediately if any such signs of overdose appear.

INTERACTION

DANGEROUS

Antidepressants
(SEROTONIN-BASED)

Drug for Obsessive-Compulsive Disorder
(CLOMIPRAMINE)

BRAND NAME	GENERIC NAME
Paxil	paroxetine
Prozac	fluoxetine

DESCRIPTION

These antidepressants work by blocking the reuptake into brain cells of serotonin, a chemical messenger. Because they work differently from the older cyclic-type antidepressants, they have a different set of side effects and have become more popular. They may also work against a different array of problems. Prozac, for instance, is also prescribed for obsessive-compulsive disorder. Older people and those with kidney or liver problems may need reduced doses. Prozac is cleared from the body very slowly and may linger weeks after discontinuation.

INSTRUCTIONS

Paxil is taken once a day, usually in the morning. Prozac is taken in the morning, or, if a higher dose has been prescribed, in the morning and at noon. Prozac may be taken without regard to meals. Taking it with food may reduce stomach upset. A few patients experience serious weight loss on these medications. If this occurs, your doctor should be notified.

BRAND NAME	GENERIC NAME
Anafranil	clomipramine

DESCRIPTION

Anafranil is prescribed to treat severe obsessive-compulsive disorder that interferes with a person's ability to function. It is related to the tricyclic antidepressants and may cause similar side effects. Sexual problems are a common side effect in men taking Anafranil.

INSTRUCTIONS

Anafranil is best taken with food, preferably in the evening to avoid daytime drowsiness. Do not stop taking Anafranil suddenly, because that could result in unpleasant withdrawal symptoms. If it must be discontinued, your doctor will supervise gradual phaseout.

INTERACTION

A doctor might prescribe both these medications for a patient with obsessive-compulsive disorder complicated by depression. In addition, Prozac may be prescribed for obsessions or compulsions and is often effective. If a patient does not respond well to one of these agents, however, the physician might try for a greater effect by adding the other. Both Prozac and Paxil slow down the liver enzyme critical for metabolizing Anafranil, and may cause blood levels of Anafranil to soar. *This interaction could be dangerous.*

Adverse effects may include, in extreme cases, delirium and seizures. Because Prozac lasts a long time in the body, the problems may continue for a few weeks after it is discontinued. Generally, if both drugs are needed, your doctor should adjust the dose of both and monitor the effects closely.

Symptoms of Anafranil Overdose

Nausea, constipation, confusion, sleepiness, palpitations, dizziness, dry mouth, blurred vision, and fever. Contact your physician immediately if any such signs of overdose appear.

INTERACTION

DANGEROUS

Antidepressant
(SEROTONIN-BASED)

Heart/Blood Pressure Drugs
(BETA-BLOCKERS)

BRAND NAME	GENERIC NAME
Prozac	fluoxetine

DESCRIPTION

This antidepressant works by blocking the reuptake into brain cells of serotonin, a chemical messenger. Because it works differently from the older cyclic-type antidepressants, it has a different set of side effects and has become more popular. It may also work against a different array of problems, for instance, bulimia or obsessive-compulsive disorder. Older people and those with kidney or liver problems may need reduced doses. Prozac is cleared from the body very slowly and may linger weeks after discontinuation.

INSTRUCTIONS

Prozac is taken in the morning, or, if a higher dose has been prescribed, in the morning and at noon. It may be taken without regard to meals. Taking it with food may reduce stomach upset. A few patients experience serious weight loss on this medication. If this occurs, your doctor should be notified.

BRAND NAME	GENERIC NAME
Inderal	propranolol
Lopressor	metoprolol
Toprol XL	metoprolol

DESCRIPTION

Beta-blockers such as these are often used to lower blood pressure, stabilize irregular heartbeats, relieve angina, or prevent migraines. Despite the great usefulness and versatility of these medicines, in general they are not appropriate for people with chronic breathing problems, because they can trigger airway tightening. Other side effects include changes in heart rate, cold hands and feet, and depression.

INSTRUCTIONS

Propranolol and metoprolol are best absorbed with meals, but consistency is the most important factor. These drugs should be taken at about the same time every day. Do not stop any of these medicines suddenly except on doctor's orders. Serious side effects could result.

INTERACTION

Because metoprolol and propranolol are both widely prescribed, it is likely that some people may take one of these drugs together with Prozac. There are a few case reports of increased toxicity of the beta-blocker attributed to this combination. One man developed a potentially life-threatening rhythm disturbance called heart block after adding Prozac to propranolol. A patient with angina experienced a dangerously slow pulse two days after Prozac was added to his heart medicine, metoprolol.

Anyone on a beta-blocker such as propranolol or metoprolol should be monitored very carefully if Prozac is added to the regimen. Dosage adjustments may be necessary. Because the effects of Prozac may persist in the body for up to two weeks after the drug is discontinued, caution must also be exercised if a beta-blocker is prescribed to someone who has recently stopped Prozac.

Symptoms of Beta-Blocker Toxicity

Slow heart rate, abnormal electrocardiogram, very low blood pressure, disorientation, lightheadedness, lethargy, or heart failure. Notify your physician immediately of any such symptoms.

INTERACTION

DANGEROUS

Antidepressant
(SEROTONIN-BASED)

Anti-Anxiety Drugs
(BENZODIAZEPINES)

BRAND NAME   GENERIC NAME

Prozac   fluoxetine

DESCRIPTION

This antidepressant works by blocking the reuptake into brain cells of serotonin, a chemical messenger. Because it works differently from the older cyclic-type antidepressants, it has a different set of side effects and has become more popular. It may also work against a different array of problems, for instance, bulimia or obsessive-compulsive disorder. Older people and those with kidney or liver problems may need reduced doses. Prozac is cleared from the body very slowly and may linger weeks after discontinuation.

INSTRUCTIONS

Prozac is taken in the morning, or, if a higher dose has been prescribed, in the morning and at noon. It may be taken without regard to meals. Taking it with food may reduce stomach upset. A few patients experience serious weight loss on this medication. If this occurs, your doctor should be notified.

BRAND NAME   GENERIC NAME

Valium   diazepam
Xanax   alprazolam

DESCRIPTION

The benzodiazepines have been used primarily to treat anxiety disorders and insomnia. Some have also been employed to relieve panic attacks, seizures, muscle cramps, and contractions. Anesthesiologists often give such medications prior to certain surgical procedures. Xanax has also been prescribed for agoraphobia (fear of crowds or open spaces), premenstrual tension, and psychological depression.

Prolonged use may lead to dependence. Sudden withdrawal can produce unpleasant side effects and should always be supervised by a physician.

INSTRUCTIONS

These drugs may be taken with food, especially if they upset the digestive tract.

INTERACTION

This is not a particularly worrisome interaction. In fact, physicians may often prescribe drugs such as Valium or Xanax to counteract the jittery feelings and insomnia that are sometimes associated with Prozac. If this combination is contemplated, however, there should be some consideration for the potential of these drugs to interact. Reports have surfaced linking Prozac to slightly higher blood levels of diazepam. Diazepam also lasted longer in the body when people were also taking Prozac. The clinical significance of this interaction is unclear. Data on Xanax and Prozac are contradictory. One study demonstrated a slight effect while another showed no impact. There may be no cause for concern, but until further research is done patients should be alert for increased effects from Valium or Xanax. Tasks that require coordination and attentiveness, like driving, could be affected.

Symptoms of Benzodiazepine Overdose

Disorientation, unsteadiness, confusion, slurred speech, drowsiness, dizziness, amnesia, or loss of motor coordination are tipoffs to overdose. Driving is hazardous! Contact your physician immediately if any such signs of overdose appear.

INTERACTION

TROUBLESOME

Antidepressant

(SEROTONIN-BASED)

Antihistamine

BRAND NAME	GENERIC NAME
Prozac	fluoxetine

DESCRIPTION

This antidepressant works by blocking the reuptake into brain cells of serotonin, a chemical messenger. Because it works differently from the older cyclic-type antidepressants, it has a different set of side effects and has become more popular. It may also work against a different array of problems, for instance, bulimia or obsessive-compulsive disorder. Older people and those with kidney or liver problems may need reduced doses. Prozac is cleared from the body very slowly and may linger weeks after discontinuation.

INSTRUCTIONS

Prozac is taken in the morning, or, if a higher dose has been prescribed, in the morning and at noon. It may be taken without regard to meals. Taking it with food may reduce stomach upset. A few patients experience serious weight loss on this medication. If this occurs, your doctor should be notified.

BRAND NAME	GENERIC NAME
Periactin	cyproheptadine

DESCRIPTION

Periactin is primarily prescribed for its antihistamine action to relieve allergy symptoms such as runny nose and red, itchy eyes, and hives. It has also been prescribed to stimulate appetite and increase weight. Side effects can include sleepiness, confusion, dizziness, nervousness, disorientation, dry mouth and nose, constipation, and difficult urination. Periactin also blocks the activity of the brain chemical serotonin. As a result it may interact with serotonin-based antidepressants such as Prozac.

INSTRUCTIONS

Periactin is best taken with food to reduce the risk of stomach upset or nausea. Because of the possibility of experiencing drowsiness, dizziness, confusion, and blurred vision people, should rarely, if ever, drive or operate machinery while taking Periactin.

INTERACTION

People who take Prozac may experience sexual side effects including lowered libido, difficulty ejaculating, and lack of orgasm. Because sexual dysfunction is thought to be caused by the serotonin-enhancing effect of Prozac, physicians have tried to reverse this unpleasant consequence by administering an antiserotonin drug such as Periactin. They were successful in restoring sexuality, but symptoms of depression also returned.

Two female patients taking Prozac for bulimia (binge eating and purging) also experienced a reemergence of their symptoms when Periactin was prescribed. It appears that the serotonin-blocking action of Periactin can reverse the benefits of Prozac. Although no reports have yet appeared regarding the interaction between Periactin and Paxil or Zoloft, there is every reason to believe it could be a problem. If depression returns, suicidal thoughts might occur. *This interaction could be troublesome.*

Never take or stop medication without your doctor's advice.

INTERACTION

TROUBLESOME

Antidepressant

(SEROTONIN-BASED)

Heart/Blood Pressure Drugs

(CALCIUM CHANNEL BLOCKERS)

BRAND NAME	GENERIC NAME
Prozac	fluoxetine

DESCRIPTION

This antidepressant works by blocking the reuptake into brain cells of serotonin, a chemical messenger. Because it works differently from the older cyclic-type antidepressants, it has a different set of side effects and has become more popular. It may also work against a different array of problems, for instance, bulimia or obsessive-compulsive disorder. Older people and those with kidney or liver problems may need reduced doses. Prozac is cleared from the body very slowly and may linger weeks after discontinuation.

INSTRUCTIONS

Prozac is taken in the morning, or, if a higher dose has been prescribed, in the morning and at noon. It may be taken without regard to meals. Taking it with food may reduce stomach upset. A few patients experience serious weight loss on this medication. If this occurs, your doctor should be notified.

BRAND NAME	GENERIC NAME
Adalat, Procardia	nifedipine
Calan, Isoptin,	
Verelan	verapamil

DESCRIPTION

These medications are prescribed primarily to treat angina or high blood pressure, or, in the case of verapamil, to stabilize irregular heart rhythms. They may also be prescribed to prevent migraine headaches or exercise-induced asthma, and to treat certain kinds of heart problems. They are usually well tolerated and are among the most popular cardiovascular drugs, but can cause gastrointestinal upset, dizziness, fluid retention, and other side effects. Elderly patients may require dosage adjustment.

INSTRUCTIONS

These drugs come in a variety of doses; follow the doctor's directions carefully to get the right dose. Sustained-release forms, such as Calan SR or Dilacor XR, should not be chewed or crushed and are best taken with food. Avoid taking Adalat or Procardia with grapefruit juice, as this could boost blood levels unexpectedly. See the table on pages 59-73 for specific instructions. Withdrawal symptoms, especially chest pain, may occur if these drugs are stopped suddenly. Follow the doctor's instructions for tapering slowly if the medicine must be discontinued.

INTERACTION

There are a few case reports of increased toxicity of calcium channel blockers such as Calan and Procardia due to this combination. *This interaction could be troublesome.*

Side Effects of Calcium Channel Blockers

Nausea, constipation, skin rash, dizziness, headache, drowsiness, insomnia, shortness of breath, fluid retention, and changes in heart rate or rhythm. Contact your physician promptly if any such adverse effects appear while you are on Prozac and one of the calcium channel blockers.

Never take or stop medication without your doctor's advice.

INTERACTION

TROUBLESOME

Antidepressant

(SEROTONIN-BASED)

Lithium

BRAND NAME | GENERIC NAME

Prozac | fluoxetine

DESCRIPTION

This antidepressant works by blocking the reuptake into brain cells of serotonin, a chemical messenger. Because it works differently from the older cyclic-type antidepressants, it has a different set of side effects and has become more popular. It may also work against a different array of problems, for instance, bulimia or obsessive-compulsive disorder. Older people and those with kidney or liver problems may need reduced doses. Prozac is cleared from the body very slowly and may linger weeks after discontinuation.

INSTRUCTIONS

Prozac is taken in the morning, or, if a higher dose has been prescribed, in the morning and at noon. It may be taken without regard to meals. Taking it with food may reduce stomach upset. A few patients experience serious weight loss on this medication. If this occurs, your doctor should be notified.

BRAND NAME

Cibalith-S
Eskalith
Lithane
Lithobid
Lithotabs

DESCRIPTION

Lithium is most often used to treat bipolar depression, and seems to be especially helpful in easing the manic phases of this disorder. Regular blood tests are advisable for dose adjustment. The toxic dose is not a great deal higher than the effective dose, so your doctor should be notified of signs such as vomiting, diarrhea, unsteadiness in walking, weakness, or unusual drowsiness. This drug can affect the thyroid gland.

INSTRUCTIONS

Lithium should be taken immediately after meals or with food or milk to reduce stomach upset. It is essential to drink 8 to 12 glasses of water or other fluid each day while on lithium. This medication can affect alertness, so activities such as driving or operating machinery can be dangerous for people on lithium.

INTERACTION

For someone with bipolar depression, the psychiatrist may prescribe both lithium, to prevent or treat the manic phase, and Prozac, to relieve the depressive stage. Paxil did not interact with lithium in a five-week study, and Zoloft resulted in an insignificant reduction in lithium levels. There is at least one report of a clinical interaction between lithium and Prozac, however. A 44-year-old woman who had been on lithium for 20 years with no problems developed dizziness, unsteadiness and difficulty walking, stiff arms and legs, and other signs of lithium toxicity shortly after starting Prozac. Her blood lithium levels were high and Prozac was stopped. She recovered fully. It is unclear how many others might also be susceptible to a similar reaction. *This interaction could be troublesome.*

Symptoms of Lithium Toxicity

Drowsiness, incoordination, dizziness, blurred vision, ringing in the ears, slurred speech, confusion, seizures, and coma. Notify your physician immediately of any of these symptoms.

Never take or stop medication without your doctor's advice.

INTERACTION

TROUBLESOME

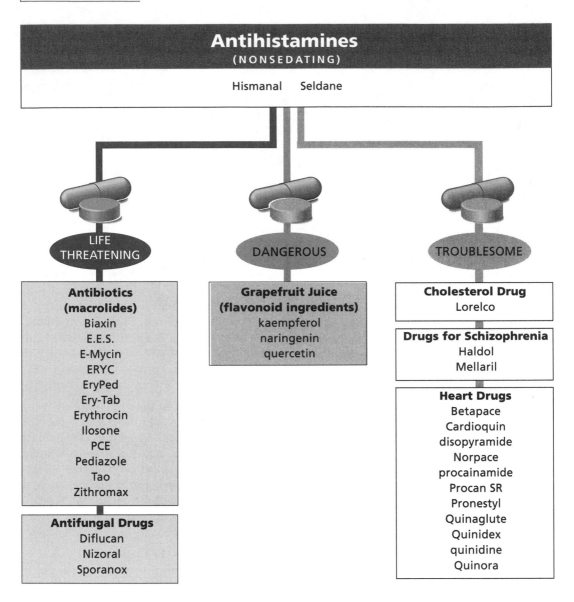

Antihistamines
(NONSEDATING)

Hismanal   Seldane

LIFE THREATENING

Antibiotics (macrolides)
Biaxin
E.E.S.
E-Mycin
ERYC
EryPed
Ery-Tab
Erythrocin
Ilosone
PCE
Pediazole
Tao
Zithromax

Antifungal Drugs
Diflucan
Nizoral
Sporanox

DANGEROUS

Grapefruit Juice (flavonoid ingredients)
kaempferol
naringenin
quercetin

TROUBLESOME

Cholesterol Drug
Lorelco

Drugs for Schizophrenia
Haldol
Mellaril

Heart Drugs
Betapace
Cardioquin
disopyramide
Norpace
procainamide
Procan SR
Pronestyl
Quinaglute
Quinidex
quinidine
Quinora

The most serious known interactions with these antihistamines are listed on this overview tree. See the individual summaries for details. Be sure to check with your pharmacist and physician before taking other drugs in combination with any nonsedating antihistamine.

LEVELS OF HAZARD: LIFE THREATENING   DANGEROUS   TROUBLESOME

Antihistamines
(NONSEDATING)

Antibiotics
(MACROLIDES)

BRAND NAME	GENERIC NAME
Hismanal	astemizole
Seldane	terfenadine

DESCRIPTION

Nonsedating antihistamines stifle sniffles and sneezes wihout making people feel like zombies. These drugs can also be effective for hives and other allergic skin conditions. Side effects are uncommon, but some people have reported dry mouth, jitteriness, nausea, fatigue, and headache. People on Seldane occasionally note hair loss, and some taking Hismanal may complain of increased appetite and weight gain. Drug toxicity can be very serious for individuals with liver problems. Older people may also be vulnerable to side effects, even on standard doses.

INSTRUCTIONS

Hismanal works best when taken on an empty stomach (either one hour before meals or two hours after eating). There are no special instructions for Seldane, although if it upsets the stomach this discomfort might be reduced by food.

BRAND NAME	GENERIC NAME
Biaxin	clarithromycin
E.E.S.	erythromycin
E-Mycin	erythromycin
ERYC	erythromycin
EryPed	erythromycin
Ery-Tab	erythromycin
Erythrocin	erythromycin
Ilosone	erythromycin
PCE	erythromycin
Pediazole	erythromycin
Tao	troleandomycin
Zithromax	azithromycin

DESCRIPTION

These broad-spectrum antibiotics are widely prescribed for respiratory tract, sinus, ear, and skin infections. They are also effective against *Chlamydia* and certain other infections of the reproductive tract.

INSTRUCTIONS

Some forms of erythromycin must be taken on an empty stomach; others may be taken with food. See the table of Food and Drug Compatibility on pages 59-73 for specifics. Biaxin can be taken without regard to meals. Zithromax is best taken on an empty stomach.

INTERACTION

People with allergies may be prone to ear, nose, throat, and respiratory tract infections that might call for one of the listed antibiotics. Unfortunately, these antibiotics affect the liver to slow metabolism of the antihistamines. Blood levels of Seldane and Hismanal may rise to dangerous levels. *The interaction is potentially lethal.* **Deaths have been reported.**

Abnormal electrocardiograms (prolongation of the QT interval), irregular heartbeats, and cardiac arrest are associated with elevated blood levels of Seldane or Hismanal. Erythromycin, Biaxin, and Tao have been reported to produce this effect. Although no case reports implicate Zithromax, it should be combined with these antihistamines only under careful medical supervision.

Symptoms of Seldane or Hismanal Toxicity

Except for subtle changes on an electrocardiogram, there may be no warning signs of danger. Heart palpitations, dizziness, fainting, chest discomfort, or shortness of breath require emergency treatment.

INTERACTION
LIFE THREATENING

Antihistamines
(NONSEDATING)

Antifungal Drugs

BRAND NAME	GENERIC NAME
Hismanal	astemizole
Seldane	terfenadine

DESCRIPTION

Nonsedating antihistamines stifle sniffles and sneezes wihout making people feel like zombies. These drugs can also be effective for hives and other allergic skin conditions. Side effects are uncommon, but some people have reported dry mouth, jitteriness, nausea, fatigue, and headache. People on Seldane occasionally note hair loss, and some taking Hismanal may complain of increased appetite and weight gain. Drug toxicity can be very serious for individuals with liver problems. Older people may also be vulnerable to side effects, even on standard doses.

INSTRUCTIONS

Hismanal works best when taken on an empty stomach (either one hour before meals or two hours after eating). There are no special instructions for Seldane, although if it upsets the stomach this discomfort might be reduced by food.

BRAND NAME	GENERIC NAME
Diflucan	fluconazole
Nizoral	ketoconazole
Sporanox	itraconazole

DESCRIPTION

Fungi can cause serious health problems, especially for those with weakened immune systems. Hard-to-treat infections of the mouth, throat, lungs, blood, brain, reproductive tract, skin, and nails have been fought with new and more powerful antifungal drugs such as Diflucan, Nizoral, and Sporanox. Although relatively rare, liver damage is a very serious adverse event associated with all three drugs. Liver enzymes should be monitored regularly and if symptoms develop (jaundice, fatigue, nausea, loss of appetite, pale stools, vomiting, dark urine), contact a physician immediately.

INSTRUCTIONS

Nizoral and Sporanox are best taken with food to reduce stomach upset. The dose of Diflucan must be individualized depending upon the type of infection being treated.

INTERACTION

Nizoral and Sporanox can affect the metabolism of the antihistamines Seldane and Hismanal. They do this by knocking out a crucial enzyme in the liver called cytochrome P-450-3A4. Without adequate amounts of this enzyme, blood levels of Seldane and Hismanal can rise, in some cases to dangerous levels. *The interaction is potentially lethal.* **Deaths have been reported.**

Abnormal electrocardiograms, irregular heartbeats, and cardiac arrest are associated with elevated blood levels of Seldane or Hismanal. At the time of this writing only Nizoral and Sporanox have been reported to interact with Hismanal and Seldane to produce this effect. It is not clear if Diflucan will also interact with nonsedating antihistamines. Caution is appropriate until more is known.

Symptoms of Seldane or Hismanal Toxicity

Except for subtle changes on an electrocardiogram, there may be no warning signs of danger. Heart palpitations, dizziness, fainting, chest discomfort, or shortness of breath require emergency treatment.

Never take or stop medication without your doctor's advice.

INTERACTION
LIFE THREATENING

Antihistamines
(NONSEDATING)

Grapefruit Juice

BRAND NAME	GENERIC NAME
Hismanal	astemizole
Seldane	terfenadine

FLAVONOID INGREDIENTS

kaempferol
naringenin
quercetin

DESCRIPTION

Nonsedating antihistamines stifle sniffles and sneezes wihout making people feel like zombies. These drugs can also be effective for hives and other allergic skin conditions. Side effects are uncommon, but some people have reported dry mouth, jitteriness, nausea, fatigue, and headache. People on Seldane occasionally note hair loss, and some taking Hismanal may complain of increased appetite and weight gain. Drug toxicity can be very serious for individuals with liver problems. Older people may also be vulnerable to side effects, even on standard doses.

INSTRUCTIONS

Hismanal works best when taken on an empty stomach (either one hour before meals or two hours after eating). There are no special instructions for Seldane, although if it upsets the stomach this discomfort might be reduced by food.

DESCRIPTION

Grapefruit juice contains ingredients called flavonoids that can have a profound effect on drug metabolism. Naringenin is present in highest concentrations and may impart the bitter aftertaste to grapefruit juice. It and other flavonoids can knock out an important enzyme in the liver (CYP-3A4) that is responsible for deactivating many medications. This can cause drug levels to climb and may lead to toxicity.

INSTRUCTIONS

Research on the effects of grapefruit juice on drug metabolism is still in its infancy. No one knows how many medications may be affected. To be on the safe side, do not take your medicines with grapefruit or grapefruit juice unless advised to do so by a physician. Preliminary data suggest that grapefruit is far less likely to affect blood levels if ingested four or more hours after taking medicine (Dr. David Flockhart, personal communication).

INTERACTION

The first warning that grapefruit juice could interact with drugs came during a study of the blood pressure medicine Plendil (felodipine). Blood levels of the drug jumped way beyond predicted levels when the medicine was swallowed with grapefruit juice. Other studies have confirmed that grapefruit juice magnifies the drug's effects and side effects.

A 1993 article in *The Journal of the American Medical Association* (Vol. 269, p. 1535-1536) suggested that grapefruit juice might also affect Seldane. This was later confirmed, and Hismanal too was found to be affected. When blood levels of these antihistamines rise there is a risk of dangerous, if not deadly, heart rhythm abnormalities. At the time of this writing there have been no cases reported, but the concern is great enough to discourage taking grapefruit juice with such pills.

Symptoms of Seldane or Hismanal Toxicity

Except for subtle changes on an electrocardiogram, there may be no warning signs of danger. Heart palpitations, dizziness, fainting, chest discomfort, or shortness of breath require emergency treatment.

Never take or stop medication without your doctor's advice.

INTERACTION

DANGEROUS

Antihistamines
(NONSEDATING)

Cholesterol Drug
(PROBUCOL)

BRAND NAME | GENERIC NAME
Hismanal | astemizole
Seldane | terfenadine

DESCRIPTION

Nonsedating antihistamines stifle sniffles and sneezes wihout making people feel like zombies. These drugs can also be effective for hives and other allergic skin conditions. Side effects are uncommon, but some people have reported dry mouth, jitteriness, nausea, fatigue, and headache. People on Seldane occasionally note hair loss, and some taking Hismanal may complain of increased appetite and weight gain. Drug toxicity can be very serious for individuals with liver problems. Older people may also be vulnerable to side effects, even on standard doses.

INSTRUCTIONS

Hismanal works best when taken on an empty stomach (either one hour before meals or two hours after eating). There are no special instructions for Seldane, although if it upsets the stomach this discomfort might be reduced by food.

BRAND NAME | GENERIC NAME
Lorelco | probucol

DESCRIPTION

Lorelco lowers cholesterol by roughly 10 to 15 percent. Unfortunately, it also diminishes good (HDL) cholesterol, which is thought to protect against heart disease. Lorelco has one unique benefit. It has strong antioxidant activity (like vitamin E and beta carotene) that may prevent bad (LDL) cholesterol from being deposited in the walls of arteries.

Lorelco can lead to digestive tract disturbances such as diarrhea. It may also affect the electrocardiogram. The QT interval (ECG readings that represent electrical heart activity) can be prolonged and that has led to serious heart rhythm disturbances.

INSTRUCTIONS

Lorelco is best taken with food to reduce stomach upset and improve absorption. The drug lingers in the body for a very long time (it is stored in fat) and can be measured in the bloodstream for up to six months after the drug has been stopped.

INTERACTION

This interaction is, at the time of this writing, purely theoretical. There have been, to our knowledge, no published reports of deaths or serious adverse reactions resulting from the combination of Lorelco and Seldane or Hismanal. Nevertheless, an article in *The Journal of the American Medical Association* (1993; Vol. 269, p. 1536) cautions physicians about "combining terfenadine [Seldane] therapy with other drugs that . . . prolong the QT interval."

Since both Lorelco and Hismanal may prolong the QT interval, the risk of a serious irregular heart rhythm must be weighed carefully by a physician before prescribing Lorelco together with either nonsedating antihistamine. *Such arrhythmias could be life threatening.*

Symptoms of Seldane or Hismanal Toxicity

Except for subtle changes on an electrocardiogram, there may be no warning signs of danger. Heart palpitations, dizziness, fainting, chest discomfort, or shortness of breath require emergency treatment.

Never take or stop medication without your doctor's advice.

INTERACTION

TROUBLESOME

Antihistamines

(NONSEDATING)

Drugs for Schizophrenia

BRAND NAME	GENERIC NAME
Hismanal	astemizole
Seldane	terfenadine

BRAND NAME	GENERIC NAME
Haldol	haloperidol
Mellaril	thioridazine

DESCRIPTION

Nonsedating antihistamines stifle sniffles and sneezes wihout making people feel like zombies. These drugs can also be effective for hives and other allergic skin conditions. Side effects are uncommon, but some people have reported dry mouth, jitteriness, nausea, fatigue, and headache. People on Seldane occasionally note hair loss, and some taking Hismanal may complain of increased appetite and weight gain. Drug toxicity can be very serious for individuals with liver problems. Older people may also be vulnerable to side effects, even on standard doses.

INSTRUCTIONS

Hismanal works best when taken on an empty stomach (either one hour before meals or two hours after eating). There are no special instructions for Seldane, although if it upsets the stomach this discomfort might be reduced by food.

DESCRIPTION

Haldol and Mellaril are prescribed primarily for serious mental illness, agitation, and anxiety disorders. The drugs can help control hallucinations and disorganized thinking. Haldol is also beneficial in treating the tics and verbalizations of Tourette's disorder.

These antipsychotic medications have a range of serious side effects and may affect the electrocardiogram. The QT interval on ECG readings, which represent electrical heart activity, can be prolonged, leading to serious heart rhythm disturbances.

INSTRUCTIONS

Haldol and Mellaril are best taken with food. The dose is highly variable, depending on many factors, and has to be individualized for each patient.

INTERACTION

This interaction is, at the time of this writing, purely theoretical. There have been, to our knowledge, no published reports of deaths or serious adverse reactions resulting from the combination of Haldol or Mellaril with Seldane or Hismanal. Nevertheless, an article in *The Journal of the American Medical Association* (1993; Vol. 269, p. 1536) cautions physicians about "combining terfenadine [Seldane] therapy with other drugs that . . . prolong the QT interval."

Seldane and Hismanal may prolong the QT interval, as can Haldol and Mellaril. Seldane is structurally similar to Haldol. The risk of a serious irregular heart rhythm must be weighed carefully by a physician before prescribing either Haldol or Mellaril with either of these nonsedating antihistamines. *Such arrhythmias could be life threatening.*

Symptoms of Seldane or Hismanal Toxicity

Except for subtle changes on an electrocardiogram, there may be no warning signs of danger. Heart palpitations, dizziness, fainting, chest discomfort, or shortness of breath require emergency treatment.

Never take or stop medication without your doctor's advice.

INTERACTION

TROUBLESOME

Antihistamines
(NONSEDATING)

Heart Drugs

BRAND NAME	GENERIC NAME
Hismanal	astemizole
Seldane	terfenadine

BRAND NAME	GENERIC NAME
Betapace	sotalol
Cardioquin	quinidine
Norpace	disopyramide
Procan SR	procainamide
Pronestyl	procainamide
Quinaglute	quinidine
Quinidex	quinidine
Quinora	quinidine

DESCRIPTION

Nonsedating antihistamines stifle sniffles and sneezes wihout making people feel like zombies. These drugs can also be effective for hives and other allergic skin conditions. Side effects are uncommon, but some people have reported dry mouth, jitteriness, nausea, fatigue, and headache. People on Seldane occasionally note hair loss, and some taking Hismanal may complain of increased appetite and weight gain. Drug toxicity can be very serious for individuals with liver problems. Older people may also be vulnerable to side effects, even on standard doses.

DESCRIPTION

Betapace, Norpace, procainamide, and quinidine are prescribed to control serious arrhythmias (irregular heart rhythms). These drugs may also promote arrhythmias and prolong the QT interval on ECG readings, which represent electrical heart activity. Cardiologists are often careful to reserve such medications for life threatening arrhythmias.

INSTRUCTIONS

Hismanal works best when taken on an empty stomach (either one hour before meals or two hours after eating). There are no special instructions for Seldane, although if it upsets the stomach this discomfort might be reduced by food.

INSTRUCTIONS

Quinidine is best taken with food to reduce stomach upset. Procainamide is absorbed better on an empty stomach but it causes GI problems and may be taken at mealtime. Check with a physician and pharmacist on proper dosing for all of these drugs because the dose must be individualized and timed carefully.

INTERACTION

This interaction is, at the time of this writing, purely theoretical. We know of no published reports of deaths or serious reactions resulting from the combination of antiarrhythmics and Seldane or Hismanal. Nevertheless, an article in *The Journal of the American Medical Association* (1993; Vol. 269, p. 1536) cautions physicians about combining Seldane with other drugs that prolong the QT interval or increase the risk of heart irregularities.

Mixing drugs that have the potential to cause heart rhythm disturbances could be dangerous. The risk of a serious arrhythmia must be weighed carefully by a physician before prescribing such heavy-duty heart pills with these nonsedating antihistamines. *Such arrhythmias could be life threatening.*

Symptoms of Seldane or Hismanal Toxicity

Except for subtle changes on an electrocardiogram, there may be no warning signs of danger. Heart palpitations, dizziness, fainting, chest discomfort, or shortness of breath require emergency treatment.

Never take or stop medication without your doctor's advice.

INTERACTION

TROUBLESOME

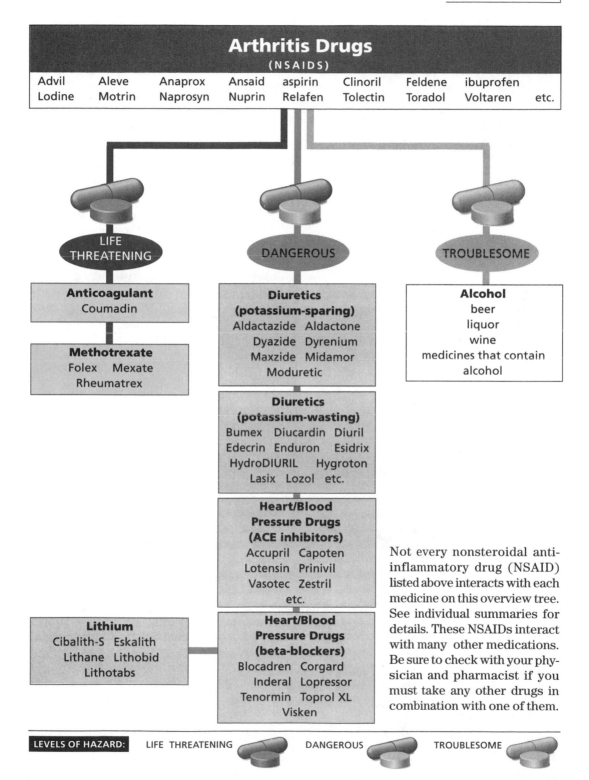

Arthritis Drugs
(NSAIDS)

Advil	Aleve	Anaprox	Ansaid	aspirin	Clinoril	Feldene	ibuprofen	
Lodine	Motrin	Naprosyn	Nuprin	Relafen	Tolectin	Toradol	Voltaren	etc.

LIFE THREATENING

Anticoagulant
Coumadin

Methotrexate
Folex   Mexate
Rheumatrex

Lithium
Cibalith-S   Eskalith
Lithane   Lithobid
Lithotabs

DANGEROUS

**Diuretics
(potassium-sparing)**
Aldactazide   Aldactone
Dyazide   Dyrenium
Maxzide   Midamor
Moduretic

**Diuretics
(potassium-wasting)**
Bumex   Diucardin   Diuril
Edecrin   Enduron   Esidrix
HydroDIURIL   Hygroton
Lasix   Lozol   etc.

**Heart/Blood
Pressure Drugs
(ACE inhibitors)**
Accupril   Capoten
Lotensin   Prinivil
Vasotec   Zestril
etc.

**Heart/Blood
Pressure Drugs
(beta-blockers)**
Blocadren   Corgard
Inderal   Lopressor
Tenormin   Toprol XL
Visken

TROUBLESOME

Alcohol
beer
liquor
wine
medicines that contain
alcohol

Not every nonsteroidal anti-inflammatory drug (NSAID) listed above interacts with each medicine on this overview tree. See individual summaries for details. These NSAIDs interact with many other medications. Be sure to check with your physician and pharmacist if you must take any other drugs in combination with one of them.

LEVELS OF HAZARD: LIFE THREATENING   DANGEROUS   TROUBLESOME

Arthritis Drugs
(NSAIDS)

Anticoagulant
(WARFARIN)

BRAND NAME	GENERIC NAME
Advil, Motrin, Nuprin	ibuprofen
Aleve, Naprosyn	naproxen
Ansaid	flurbiprofen
Aspirin	aspirin
Indocin	indomethacin
Lodine	etodolac
Relafen	nabumetone
Toradol	ketorolac
etc.	

DESCRIPTION

Nonsteroidal anti-inflammatory drugs (NSAIDs) can ease pain, lower a fever, and help control inflammation. They are frequently prescribed for arthritis, as well as for muscle strains, headaches, and other conditions. These medications can cause serious digestive tract upset, including heartburn, indigestion, and bleeding or perforated ulcers. Careful medical monitoring is essential.

INSTRUCTIONS

Take with food to reduce the risk of stomach irritation. (See table on pages 59-73.) Aspirin and OTC ibuprofen or naproxen should not be mixed with prescription NSAIDs or each other.

BRAND NAME	GENERIC NAME
Coumadin	warfarin

DESCRIPTION

Warfarin slows the liver's production of factors essential for the formation of blood clots. It is prescribed when there is a risk that a dangerous clot could form in a deep vein or a blood vessel leading to the lung, heart, or brain. The most serious complication of anticoagulant treatment is excessive bleeding. The dosage must be individually adjusted, requiring daily blood tests at first, then tests every four to six weeks. Other side effects may include nausea, loss of appetite, rash, fever, yellow eyes and skin, prolonged painful erection, and hair loss.

INSTRUCTIONS

Warfarin tablets can be swallowed with food or on an empty stomach. Try to avoid large variations in the quantity of vitamin-K–containing vegetables—such as broccoli, cabbage, or spinach—that you eat each day. Consuming much more or less than usual could change the action of the drug.

INTERACTION

Large doses of aspirin can significantly increase bleeding in people taking warfarin. *This interaction could prove life threatening.* See page 16 for recommendations on low-dose aspirin and Coumadin.

People who take NSAIDs for pain and inflammation and also warfarin may dramatically increase their risk of a bleeding ulcer. One study (*Arch. Intern. Med.*, Jul 26, 1993;153:1665-1670) reported that such combinations were associated with a 13-fold rise in GI hemorrhage. *Bleeding ulcers can be fatal.* If an arthritis medicine such as the ones listed here is prescribed with Coumadin, extreme caution must be exercised!

Symptoms of NSAID/Warfarin Adverse Interaction

Notify your doctor immediately if you detect any unusual bleeding, including rectal or urinary tract bleeding, excessive menstrual bleeding, bruising, red or tar-black stools, and red or dark brown urine. A silent or bleeding ulcer can occur with no symptoms. Indigestion, heartburn, anemia, fatigue, and weight loss may be early symptoms of trouble.

Never take or stop medication without your doctor's advice.

INTERACTION

LIFE THREATENING

Arthritis Drugs

(NSAIDS)

Methotrexate

BRAND NAME   GENERIC NAME

Advil, Motrin,
 Nuprin   ibuprofen
Aleve, Naprosyn naproxen
Ansaid   flurbiprofen
Aspirin   aspirin
Indocin   indomethacin
Lodine   etodolac
Relafen   nabumetone
Toradol   ketorolac
etc.

DESCRIPTION

Nonsteroidal anti-inflammatory drugs (NSAIDs) can ease pain, lower a fever, and help control inflammation. They are frequently prescribed for arthritis, as well as for muscle strains, headaches, and other conditions. These medications can cause serious digestive tract upset, including heartburn, indigestion, and bleeding or perforated ulcers. Careful medical monitoring is essential.

INSTRUCTIONS

Take with food to reduce the risk of stomach irritation. (See table on pages 59-73.) Aspirin and OTC ibuprofen or naproxen should not be mixed with prescription NSAIDs or each other.

BRAND NAME

Folex, Mexate, Rheumatrex

DESCRIPTION

Methotrexate interferes with folic acid metabolism in rapidly growing cells, making it useful for treating certain cancers and for severe psoriasis. It is also prescribed for rheumatoid arthritis. Methotrexate is a heavy-duty drug with potentially serious side effects, particularly for the liver. Frequent blood and urine tests will be needed to monitor lung, blood, liver, and kidney function. Let your doctor know if you have trouble with nausea, vomiting, loss of appetite, rash, hair loss, boils, or acne. Because methotrexate can cause lethal birth defects, it is usually inappropriate for pregnant women.

INSTRUCTIONS

Follow your doctor's instructions on dose and timing for methotrexate, which is taken **once a week** for psoriasis or rheumatoid arthritis. Do not drink alcohol or take salicylates such as aspirin or Pepto-Bismol while on this drug. Methotrexate can increase sensitivity to ultraviolet light, so protect your skin from exposure to sun or tanning lamps.

INTERACTION

Arthritis drugs (NSAIDs and aspirin) can make methotrexate far more toxic than when it is taken alone. Since methotrexate, by itself, has the potential for serious side effects, such an interaction can be extremely dangerous. Blood levels of methotrexate can climb unpredictably in the presence of NSAIDs and should be monitored closely. Kidney damage, digestive tract difficulties, bone marrow suppression, and immune system impairment are potential complications. *This interaction could be life threatening.* Lower doses of methotrexate used to treat rheumatoid arthritis or psoriasis may interact less severely, but careful medical supervision is crucial.

Symptoms of Methotrexate Toxicity

Nausea, vomiting, diarrhea, mouth sores, rash, itching, black sticky stools, stomach pain, sore throat, fever, chills, unusual bleeding or bruising, yellow skin or eyes, shortness of breath, cough, dark or bloody urine, or swelling of the legs or feet. Notify your physician immediately.

INTERACTION

LIFE THREATENING

Arthritis Drugs

(NSAIDS)

Diuretics

(POTASSIUM-SPARING)

BRAND NAME	GENERIC NAME
Advil, Motrin, Nuprin	ibuprofen
Aleve, Naprosyn	naproxen
Ansaid	flurbiprofen
Aspirin	aspirin
Indocin	indomethacin
Lodine	etodolac
Relafen	nabumetone
Voltaren	diclofenac
etc.	

DESCRIPTION

Nonsteroidal anti-inflammatory drugs (NSAIDs) can ease pain, lower a fever, and help control inflammation. They are frequently prescribed for arthritis, as well as for muscle strains, headaches, lower back discomfort, menstrual pain, and other conditions. These medications can cause serious digestive tract upset, including heartburn, indigestion, and bleeding or perforated ulcers. Careful medical monitoring is essential.

INSTRUCTIONS

Take with food to reduce the risk of stomach irritation. (See table on pages 59-73.) Aspirin and OTC ibuprofen or naproxen should not be mixed with prescription NSAIDs or each other.

BRAND NAME	GENERIC NAME
Aldactazide	spironolactone, HCTZ
Aldactone	spironolactone
Dyazide	triamterene, HCTZ
Dyrenium	triamterene
Maxzide	triamterene, HCTZ
Midamor	amiloride
Moduretic	amiloride, HCTZ

DESCRIPTION

Diuretics encourage the kidneys to eliminate excess fluid from the body. This can be useful in controlling high blood pressure, congestive heart failure, and certain other conditions. Spironolactone is also used to treat a hormonal condition called hyperaldosteronism. With other diuretics, important minerals (especially potassium and magnesium) are lost along with the fluid. With the above group of drugs, however, potassium is conserved.

INSTRUCTIONS

Midamor and Dyrenium may upset the stomach, so they are best taken right after meals. Maxzide can be taken without regard to meals. Midamor and Aldactone may interfere with the alertness and coordination necessary for driving. Periodic blood tests for magnesium and potassium are advisable.

INTERACTION

Some arthritis drugs may reduce the effectiveness of diuretics. Fluid may build up, posing a serious problem for patients with heart trouble. Thiazide diuretics such as hydrochlorothiazide (HCTZ) may be less effective in lowering blood pressure. If diuretics and arthritis drugs are taken simultaneously, blood pressure should be monitored carefully. Indocin may raise potassium levels to dangerous levels when combined with potassium-sparing diuretics like Moduretic. Measure potassium levels periodically. Potassium-sparing diuretics containing triamterene (Dyazide, Dyrenium, and Maxzide) may interact badly with ibuprofen, Indocin, or Voltaren (diclofenac). Kidney damage has been reported. Other arthritis drugs may also interact.

Symptoms of Heart and Kidney Problems

Notify your doctor of sudden weight gain, swollen legs and feet, change in the color of the urine, unusual back pain, fatigue, cough, or breathlessness. Elevated serum creatinine may mean kidney trouble. Monitor blood pressure frequently.

Never take or stop medication without your doctor's advice.

INTERACTION

DANGEROUS

Arthritis Drugs

(NSAIDS)

Diuretics

(POTASSIUM-WASTING)

BRAND NAME	GENERIC NAME
Advil, Motrin, Nuprin	ibuprofen
Aleve, Naprosyn	naproxen
Aspirin	aspirin
Clinoril	sulindac
Indocin	indomethacin
Lodine	etodolac
Relafen	nabumetone
Toradol	ketorolac
etc.	

BRAND NAME	GENERIC NAME
Bumex	bumetanide
Diachlor, Diuril	chlorothiazide
Diucardin, Saluron	hydroflumethiazide
Edecrin	ethacrynic acid
Enduron	methyclothiazide
Esidrix, HydroDIURIL	hydrochlorothiazide
Hygroton, Hylidone	chlorthalidone
Lasix	furosemide
Lozol	indapamide
etc.	

DESCRIPTION

Nonsteroidal anti-inflammatory drugs (NSAIDs) can ease pain, lower a fever, and help control inflammation. They are frequently prescribed for arthritis, as well as for muscle strains, headaches, lower back discomfort, menstrual pain, and other conditions. These medications can cause serious digestive tract upset, including heartburn, indigestion, and bleeding or perforated ulcers. Careful medical monitoring is essential.

INSTRUCTIONS

Take with food to reduce the risk of stomach irritation. (See table on pages 59-73.) Aspirin and OTC ibuprofen or naproxen should not be mixed with prescription NSAIDs or each other.

DESCRIPTION

Diuretics ("water pills") help the body eliminate excess fluid caused by congestive heart failure or kidney trouble, or as a side effect of other drugs. They are, however, most widely prescribed to lower blood pressure. While well tolerated, they may cause side effects, including stomach upset, sexual difficulties, and gout. Probably the most serious problem associated with these medications is a gradual depletion of potassium or magnesium, which could lead to irregular heart rhythms. Blood levels of these minerals should be monitored.

INSTRUCTIONS

If a diuretic is taken early in the day it may reduce nighttime urination. If it causes stomach upset the drug may be taken with food or milk. See the Food and Drug Interaction Table on pages 59-73 for specifics.

INTERACTION

NSAIDs such as ibuprofen and Indocin appear to reduce the effectiveness of diuretics such as Bumex and Lasix. (Clinoril may also affect Bumex.) Fluid may build up and symptoms of heart failure could become worse. This is a very serious situation for people with heart trouble. Thiazide diuretics such as chlorthalidone, chlorothiazide, and hydrochlorothiazide may be less effective in lowering blood pressure, but this interaction does not seem so serious. Blood pressure should be monitored to make sure adequate control is maintained.

Symptoms of Heart Problems
Fluid retention, fatigue, cough, and breathlessness are possible signs of congestive heart failure. Monitor blood pressure frequently. Notify the physician immediately of symptoms.

Never take or stop medication without your doctor's advice.

INTERACTION

DANGEROUS

Arthritis Drugs
(NSAIDS)

Heart/Blood Pressure Drugs
(ACE INHIBITORS)

BRAND NAME	GENERIC NAME
Advil, Motrin, Nuprin	ibuprofen
Aleve, Naprosyn	naproxen
Ansaid	flurbiprofen
Aspirin	aspirin
Indocin	indomethacin
Lodine	etodolac
Relafen	nabumetone
Toradol	ketorolac
etc.	

DESCRIPTION

Nonsteroidal anti-inflammatory drugs (NSAIDs) can ease pain, lower a fever, and help control inflammation. They are frequently prescribed for arthritis, as well as for muscle strains, headaches, lower back discomfort, menstrual pain, and other conditions. These medications can cause serious digestive tract upset, including heartburn, indigestion, and bleeding or perforated ulcers. Careful medical monitoring is essential.

INSTRUCTIONS

Take with food to reduce the risk of stomach irritation. (See table on pages 59-73.) Aspirin and OTC ibuprofen or naproxen should not be mixed with prescription NSAIDs or each other.

BRAND NAME	GENERIC NAME
Accupril	quinapril
Altace	ramipril
Capoten	captopril
Lotensin	benazepril
Monopril	fosinopril
Prinivil, Zestril	lisinopril
Vasotec	enalapril

DESCRIPTION

These medications are used to treat high blood pressure. They block angiotensin-converting enzyme, or ACE. Capoten and Vasotec can also be helpful in treating congestive heart failure. Capoten also helps conserve kidney function in diabetics. The ACE inhibitors are usually very well tolerated, but blood pressure may be lowered so much that a person starting on one of these medicines becomes dizzy or faints, especially upon standing up. Caution is advised. Some people on these medicines develop a nagging dry cough not helped by cough medicine.

INSTRUCTIONS

Capoten should be taken one hour before meals. High-fat meals may reduce absorption of Accupril. Food does not affect the other drugs in this class.

INTERACTION

Some of the arthritis drugs on this list can drastically diminish the effectiveness of blood pressure medicines such as Capoten and Vasotec. Indocin can wipe out the blood-pressure-lowering power of these drugs; ibuprofen can interact similarly with Capoten. Even aspirin given with or before Vasotec can reduce that drug's benefit for treating congestive heart failure. Although some people do not react badly to this combination, it makes sense to assume that any arthritis medicine could interfere with any ACE medication, and keep careful tabs on blood pressure and cardiac function if both drugs are needed. *This interaction could be dangerous.*

Kidney problems are a rare but serious reaction to both these classes of drugs. Taking them in combination may increase the risk of this problem. *Notify your doctor immediately of sudden weight gain, swollen legs and feet, change in the color of the urine, or unusual back pain.* A kidney function test may be in order. **Monitor blood pressure regularly.**

INTERACTION

DANGEROUS

Arthritis Drugs
(NSAIDS)

Heart/Blood Pressure Drugs
(BETA-BLOCKERS)

BRAND NAME	GENERIC NAME
Advil, Motrin,	
Nuprin	ibuprofen
Aleve, **Naprosyn**	naproxen
Ansaid	flurbiprofen
Aspirin	aspirin
Indocin	indomethacin
Lodine	etodolac
Relafen	nabumetone
Toradol	ketorolac
etc.	

DESCRIPTION

Nonsteroidal anti-inflammatory drugs (NSAIDs) can ease pain, lower a fever, and help control inflammation. They are prescribed for arthritis, muscle strains, headaches, and other conditions. These medications can cause serious digestive tract upset, including heartburn, indigestion, and bleeding or perforated ulcers. Careful medical monitoring is essential.

INSTRUCTIONS

Take with food to reduce the risk of stomach irritation. (See table on pages 59-73.) Aspirin and OTC ibuprofen or naproxen should not be mixed with prescription NSAIDs or each other.

BRAND NAME	GENERIC NAME
Blocadren	timolol
Corgard	nadolol
Inderal	propranolol
Lopressor, Toprol XL	metoprolol
Tenormin	atenolol
Visken	pindolol
(Other beta-blockers may also interact.)	

DESCRIPTION

Beta-blockers such as these are often used to lower blood pressure, stabilize irregular heartbeats, relieve angina, or prevent migraines. Despite the usefulness of these medicines, in general they are not appropriate for people with chronic breathing problems, because they can trigger airway tightening. Other side effects include changes in heart rate, cold hands and feet, and depression.

INSTRUCTIONS

Inderal and Lopressor are best absorbed with meals, but consistency is the most important factor. These drugs should be taken at about the same time every day. Do not stop any of these medicines suddenly except on doctor's orders. Serious side effects could result.

INTERACTION

This combination is of concern because so many people take beta-blockers for high blood pressure and heart problems. Millions rely on NSAIDs for pain relief. And people also consume huge quantities of over-the-counter aspirin, ibuprofen, and naproxen. Some interactions are likely to occur. NSAIDs may reduce the effectiveness of blood-pressure-lowering beta-blockers. Physicians and patients may not realize a beta-blocker is not working as efficiently as it should to control hypertension. Experts warn doctors to avoid this combination if possible. The arthritis drug Clinoril (sulindac) may be less likely to interact with beta-blockers, but no matter which arthritis drug is used, people taking an arthritis drug in combination with a beta-blocker will need to have blood pressure monitored frequently. If hypertension becomes a problem, the physician should adjust the dose of beta-blocker or reconsider treatment options.

Symptoms of Beta-Blocker Undertreatment

Blood pressure may climb and heart symptoms might appear. Be alert for chest pain or palpitations and notify your doctor immediately. Monitor blood pressure carefully.

Never take or stop medication without your doctor's advice.

INTERACTION

DANGEROUS

Arthritis Drugs

(NSAIDS)

Lithium

BRAND NAME | GENERIC NAME

Advil, Motrin,
Nuprin — ibuprofen
Aleve, Naprosyn — naproxen
Ansaid — flurbiprofen
Aspirin — aspirin
Indocin — indomethacin
Lodine — etodolac
Relafen — nabumetone
Toradol — ketorolac
etc.

DESCRIPTION

Nonsteroidal anti-inflammatory drugs (NSAIDs) can ease pain, lower a fever, and help control inflammation. They are frequently prescribed for arthritis, as well as for muscle strains, headaches, lower back discomfort, menstrual pain, and other conditions. These medications can cause serious digestive tract upset, including heartburn, indigestion, and bleeding or perforated ulcers. Careful medical monitoring is essential.

INSTRUCTIONS

Take with food to reduce the risk of stomach irritation. (See table on pages 59–73.) Aspirin and OTC ibuprofen or naproxen should not be mixed with prescription NSAIDs or each other.

BRAND NAME

Cibalith-S
Eskalith
Lithane
Lithobid
Lithotabs

DESCRIPTION

Lithium is most often used to treat bipolar depression, and seems to be especially helpful in easing the manic phases of this disorder. Regular blood tests are advisable for dose adjustment. The toxic dose is not a great deal higher than the effective dose, so the doctor should be notified of signs such as vomiting, diarrhea, unsteadiness in walking, weakness, or unusual drowsiness. This drug can affect the thyroid gland.

INSTRUCTIONS

Lithium should be taken immediately after meals or with food or milk to reduce stomach upset. It is essential to drink 8 to 12 glasses of water or other fluid each day while on lithium. This medication can affect alertness, so activities such as driving or operating machinery can be dangerous for people on lithium.

INTERACTION

Arthritis drugs can alter the way the body eliminates lithium, possibly through their effects on the kidney. The result is that lithium levels may climb, sometimes to toxic levels. It may take a week or two for this reaction to occur, so serum lithium levels should be measured several times during the first few weeks after starting or stopping one of these nonsteroidal anti-inflammatory drugs. People who are taking over-the-counter ibuprofen or Aleve (naproxen) should be sure to notify their doctors so that proper monitoring can be conducted.

Symptoms of Lithium Toxicity

Nausea, diarrhea, stomach pain, vomiting, incoordination, muscle weakness, and difficulty walking may be signs of early toxicity. Ringing in the ears, visual problems, dizziness, muscle twitching, difficulty speaking clearly, confusion, agitation, and incontinence are more serious signs of trouble. These symptoms require immediate medical attention.

Never take or stop medication without your doctor's advice.

INTERACTION

DANGEROUS

Arthritis Drugs
(NSAIDS)

Alcohol

BRAND NAME   GENERIC NAME

Advil, Motrin,
  Nuprin   ibuprofen
Aleve, Naprosyn   naproxen
Aspirin   aspirin
Indocin   indomethacin
Lodine   etodolac
Relafen   nabumetone
Toradol   ketorolac
etc.

DESCRIPTION

Nonsteroidal anti-inflammatory drugs (NSAIDs) can ease pain, lower a fever, and help control inflammation. They are frequently prescribed for arthritis, as well as for muscle strains, headaches, and other conditions. These medications can cause serious digestive tract upset, including heartburn, indigestion, and bleeding or perforated ulcers. Careful medical monitoring is essential.

INSTRUCTIONS

Take with food to reduce the risk of stomach irritation. (See table on pages 59-73.) Aspirin and OTC ibuprofen or naproxen should not be mixed with prescription NSAIDs or each other.

NAME

beer
liquor
wine
medicines that contain alcohol

DESCRIPTION

Alcohol comes in many guises. The obvious ones are liquor, beer, and wine. But you can also find substantial amounts of alcohol in certain medicines. Over-the-counter cough and cold products can contain up to 40 or 50 proof (20 to 25 percent by volume), which is a higher alcohol content than you would find in beer or wine. "Nighttime" remedies like NyQuil, Nytcold Medicine, and Pertussin PM Liquid are as much as 50 proof. This may not be a problem if all you take is a spoonful before bedtime, but some drugs may interact poorly with even modest amounts of alcohol.

INSTRUCTIONS

The absorption and effects of alcohol are magnified if you drink on an empty stomach. Fatty food can delay alcohol absorption. If you drink, do so in moderation, and never drive.

INTERACTION

Arthritis medicine (NSAIDs and aspirin) can be hard on the stomach. People often walk a tightrope between adequate pain relief and stomach upset or ulcers. Alcohol makes that balancing act far more difficult. Alcohol itself can be irritating to the digestive tract, and it also alters the natural protective lining of the stomach. Studies have shown that aspirin causes greater bleeding from the GI tract if people have been drinking. *This interaction could be troublesome.*

One study showed that normal doses of aspirin increase blood alcohol levels. The clinical significance of this research is controversial, but some people might have higher blood alcohol levels than expected if they take aspirin before a social drink. Don't combine aspirin or other NSAIDs and alcohol.

Symptoms of NSAID or Alcohol Toxicity

Nausea, stomach pain, indigestion, and heartburn are tipoffs to trouble. Bleeding from the stomach may occur with no symptoms. Ulcers and more serious digestive tract inflammation may not always be detectable without medical testing.

INTERACTION

TROUBLESOME

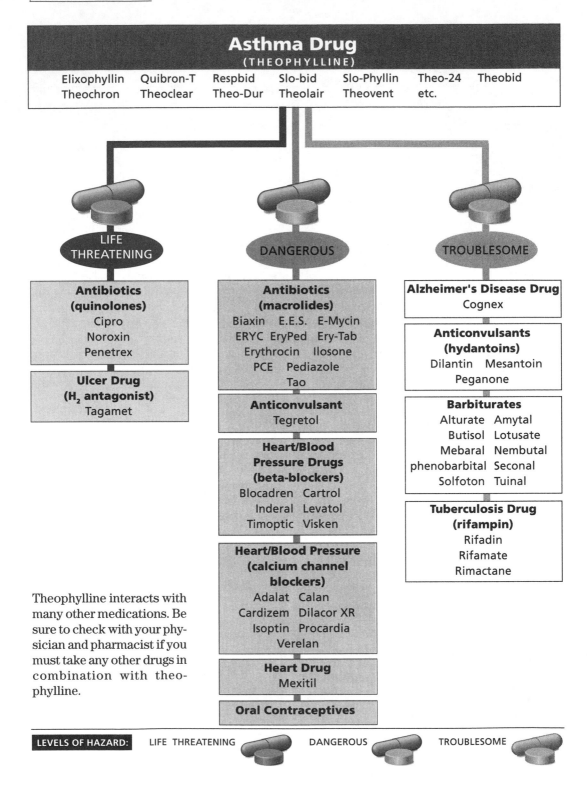

Asthma Drug
(THEOPHYLLINE)

Elixophyllin	Quibron-T	Respbid	Slo-bid	Slo-Phyllin	Theo-24	Theobid
Theochron	Theoclear	Theo-Dur	Theolair	Theovent	etc.	

LIFE THREATENING

Antibiotics (quinolones)
Cipro
Noroxin
Penetrex

Ulcer Drug (H₂ antagonist)
Tagamet

Theophylline interacts with many other medications. Be sure to check with your physician and pharmacist if you must take any other drugs in combination with theophylline.

DANGEROUS

Antibiotics (macrolides)
Biaxin   E.E.S.   E-Mycin
ERYC   EryPed   Ery-Tab
Erythrocin   Ilosone
PCE   Pediazole
Tao

Anticonvulsant
Tegretol

Heart/Blood Pressure Drugs (beta-blockers)
Blocadren   Cartrol
Inderal   Levatol
Timoptic   Visken

Heart/Blood Pressure (calcium channel blockers)
Adalat   Calan
Cardizem   Dilacor XR
Isoptin   Procardia
Verelan

Heart Drug
Mexitil

Oral Contraceptives

TROUBLESOME

Alzheimer's Disease Drug
Cognex

Anticonvulsants (hydantoins)
Dilantin   Mesantoin
Peganone

Barbiturates
Alturate   Amytal
Butisol   Lotusate
Mebaral   Nembutal
phenobarbital   Seconal
Solfoton   Tuinal

Tuberculosis Drug (rifampin)
Rifadin
Rifamate
Rimactane

LEVELS OF HAZARD: LIFE THREATENING   DANGEROUS   TROUBLESOME

Asthma Drug

(THEOPHYLLINE)

Antibiotics

(QUINOLONES)

BRAND NAME

Aerolate   **Aquaphyllin**   **Asmalix**
Bronkodyl   **Elixomin**   **Elixophyllin**
Quibron-T   **Respbid**   **Slo-bid**
Slo-Phyllin   **Theobid**   **Theochron**
Theoclear   **Theo-Dur**   **Theolair**
Theo-24   **Theovent**   **Theo-X**
T-Phyl   **Uniphyl**

DESCRIPTION

Theophylline helps to open airways, so it is generally used to treat and prevent asthma attacks. It may also be prescribed for people with emphysema or other chronic breathing problems. Babies and elderly men may need lower doses. The dose is monitored with regular blood tests to ensure that levels are less than 20 mcg/ml.

INSTRUCTIONS

Theophylline interacts with food in complex ways, so discuss this issue thoroughly with your doctor and pharmacist. Theophylline may upset the stomach. In some cases this problem can be alleviated by taking the drug with food. See the table of Food and Drug Compatibility on pages 59-73 for more information.

BRAND NAME	GENERIC NAME
Cipro	ciprofloxacin
Noroxin	norfloxacin
Penetrex	enoxacin

DESCRIPTION

These potent antibiotics are variously prescribed for infections of the respiratory tract (including ears and sinuses), skin, bones and joints, urinary tract, and reproductive organs. Occasionally bacteria not susceptible to these drugs may cause superinfection or serious diarrhea. Increased sensitivity to sunlight is also a potential problem. Side effects may include gastrointestinal upset, headache, rash, and restlessness.

INSTRUCTIONS

These drugs come in a variety of doses; it is important to follow the doctor's directions to get the proper dose. See the table of Food and Drug Compatibility on pages 59-73 for details on how to take each one. Antacids or other products containing aluminum, magnesium, iron, zinc, or bismuth should not be taken within two hours of the medicine. These medicines boost caffeine levels; it's best to drink less coffee, tea, or cola than usual.

INTERACTION

People with asthma are often susceptible to respiratory infections, for which these antibiotics are often prescribed. If both medications are needed, theophylline levels should be monitored carefully. Cipro, Noroxin, and Penetrex can raise blood levels of theophylline significantly, resulting in toxicity. *This interaction could be lethal.* **Deaths have been reported.**

Maxaquin and Floxin may not interact with theophylline in the same way. Still, the prudent doctor will monitor theophylline levels and the wise patient will report any symptoms of theophylline toxicity to the doctor.

Symptoms of Theophylline Toxicity

Nausea, diarrhea, stomach pain, headache, insomnia, restlessness, and irritability. Severe toxicity (convulsions, heart rhythm changes, or death) may occur with no warning symptoms. Notify your doctor immediately if you suspect a problem.

Never take or stop medication without your doctor's advice.

INTERACTION

LIFE THREATENING

Asthma Drug

(THEOPHYLLINE)

Ulcer Drug

(H₂ ANTAGONIST)

BRAND NAME

Aerolate	**Aquaphyllin**	**Asmalix**
Bronkodyl	**Elixomin**	**Elixophyllin**
Quibron-T	**Respbid**	**Slo-bid**
Slo-Phyllin	**Theobid**	**Theochron**
Theoclear	**Theo-Dur**	**Theolair**
Theo-24	**Theovent**	**Theo-X**
T-Phyl	**Uniphyl**	

DESCRIPTION

Theophylline helps to open airways, so it is generally used to treat and prevent asthma attacks. It may also be prescribed for people with emphysema or other chronic breathing problems. Babies and elderly men may need lower doses. The dose is monitored with regular blood tests to ensure that levels are less than 20 mcg/ml.

INSTRUCTIONS

Theophylline interacts with food in complex ways, so discuss this issue thoroughly with your doctor and pharmacist. Theophylline may upset the stomach. In some cases this problem can be alleviated by taking the drug with food. See the table of Food and Drug Compatibility on pages 59-73 for more information.

BRAND NAME | GENERIC NAME

Tagamet | cimetidine

DESCRIPTION

Tagamet has revolutionized the treatment of ulcers and serious heartburn (esophagitis) by blocking special receptors (the histamine H₂ receptors), thereby reducing the acid environment of the stomach. Cimetidine is usually well tolerated, and has few side effects, although headaches, dizziness, and mild diarrhea are potential reactions. Some men complain of antitestosterone effects. At higher doses, this may lead to enlarged breasts or sexual problems. Older people and those who are very ill may experience depression, mental confusion, or disorientation. The dose may need to be adjusted for them. Tagamet can affect the liver, modifying the metabolism and elimination of a number of medications. Higher blood levels of such drugs may lead to increased toxicity, so check with your doctor and pharmacist if you take cimetidine with another medicine.

INSTRUCTIONS

Tagamet is usually taken with meals and/or at bedtime. Antacids may reduce absorption of Tagamet; do not take one for at least two hours after taking Tagamet.

INTERACTION

One common side effect of theophylline is stomach upset, which may in some cases mimic the symptoms of an ulcer or chronic heartburn. If a patient taking theophylline is prescribed Tagamet for symptoms of stomach upset, blood levels of theophylline could reach toxic levels. *This interaction could be life threatening.*

Tagamet boosts blood levels of theophylline by a third to a half. Patients whose theophylline levels are already a bit high (over 15 mcg/ml) are at highest risk for trouble. Anyone who needs both of these medications should have blood levels of theophylline monitored closely. Notify the physician immediately of any symptoms of theophylline toxicity.

Symptoms of Theophylline Toxicity

Nausea, diarrhea, stomach pain, headache, insomnia, restlessness, and irritability. Severe toxicity (convulsions, heart rhythm changes, or death) may occur with no warning symptoms. Notify your doctor immediately if you suspect a problem.

Never take or stop medication without your doctor's advice.

INTERACTION

LIFE THREATENING

Asthma Drug

(THEOPHYLLINE)

Antibiotics

(MACROLIDES)

BRAND NAME

Aerolate	Aquaphyllin	Asmalix
Bronkodyl	Elixomin	Elixophyllin
Quibron-T	Respbid	Slo-bid
Slo-Phyllin	Theobid	Theochron
Theoclear	Theo-Dur	Theolair
Theo-24	Theovent	Theo-X
T-Phyl	Uniphyl	

DESCRIPTION

Theophylline helps to open airways, so it is generally used to treat and prevent asthma attacks. It may also be prescribed for people with emphysema or other chronic breathing problems. Babies and elderly men may need lower doses. The dose is monitored with regular blood tests to ensure that levels are less than 20 mcg/ml.

INSTRUCTIONS

Theophylline interacts with food in complex ways, so discuss this issue thoroughly with your doctor and pharmacist. Theophylline may upset the stomach. In some cases this problem can be alleviated by taking the drug with food. See the table of Food and Drug Compatibility on pages 59-73 for more information.

BRAND NAME	GENERIC NAME
Biaxin	clarithromycin
E.E.S.	erythromycin
E-Mycin	erythromycin
ERYC	erythromycin
EryPed	erythromycin
Ery-Tab	erythromycin
Erythrocin	erythromycin
Ilosone	erythromycin
PCE	erythromycin
Pediazole	erythromycin
Tao	troleandomycin

DESCRIPTION

These broad-spectrum antibiotics are widely prescribed for respiratory tract, sinus, ear, and skin infections. They are also effective against *Chlamydia* and certain other infections of the reproductive tract.

INSTRUCTIONS

Some forms of erythromycin must be taken on an empty stomach; others may be taken with food. See the table of Food and Drug Compatibility on pages 59-73 for specifics. Biaxin can be taken without regard to meals.

INTERACTION

People with asthma are often susceptible to respiratory infections, for which these antibiotics are often prescribed. If both medicines are needed, theophylline levels should be monitored carefully. Oral erythromycin and Tao are both capable of raising blood levels of theophylline. The result could be toxicity. *This interaction is dangerous.*

Because it is similar to erythromycin, Biaxin may also interact with theophylline. People vary greatly in their response to the interaction of theophylline and erythromycin. Those with high theophylline levels (over 15 mcg/ml) may be especially vulnerable. In addition, theophylline may reduce blood levels of erythromycin by as much as 30 percent. If you are on both drugs, stay in close touch with your doctor.

Symptoms of Theophylline Toxicity

Nausea, diarrhea, stomach pain, headache, insomnia, restlessness, and irritability. Severe toxicity (convulsions, heart rhythm changes, or death) may occur with no warning symptoms. Notify your doctor immediately if you suspect a problem.

Never take or stop medication without your doctor's advice.

INTERACTION

DANGEROUS

Asthma Drug

(THEOPHYLLINE)

Anticonvulsant

(CARBAMAZEPINE)

BRAND NAME

Aerolate	**Aquaphyllin**	**Asmalix**
Bronkodyl	**Elixomin**	**Elixophyllin**
Quibron-T	**Respbid**	**Slo-bid**
Slo-Phyllin	**Theobid**	**Theochron**
Theoclear	**Theo-Dur**	**Theolair**
Theo-24	**Theovent**	**Theo-X**
T-Phyl	**Uniphyl**	

BRAND NAME

Tegretol

GENERIC NAME

carbamazepine

DESCRIPTION

Theophylline helps to open airways, so it is generally used to treat and prevent asthma attacks. It may also be prescribed for people with emphysema or other chronic breathing problems. Babies and elderly men may need lower doses. The dose is monitored with regular blood tests to ensure that levels are less than 20 mcg/ml.

INSTRUCTIONS

Theophylline interacts with food in complex ways, so discuss this issue thoroughly with your doctor and pharmacist. Theophylline may upset the stomach. In some cases this problem can be alleviated by taking the drug with food. See the table of Food and Drug Compatibility on pages 59-73 for more information.

DESCRIPTION

Carbamazepine is often prescribed to people for whom other anticonvulsants have not worked well. It is also used to control severe facial pain related to the trigeminal nerve. Carbamazepine may trigger a potentially lethal blood abnormality, so regular monitoring is critical, particularly during the first two months. This drug can cause drowsiness or dizziness; driving may be impaired. Contact your doctor if you experience drowsiness, dizziness, confusion, mood or behavior changes, nausea, swollen legs and feet, pale stools, yellow skin or eyes, unusual bleeding or bruising, dark urine, sore throat, mouth sores, fever, or chills.

INSTRUCTIONS

Carbamazepine may upset the stomach; if so, take it with food or milk. Do not stop this drug suddenly; seizures could result. To maintain its strength, it must be stored away from humidity and heat in a tightly closed container.

INTERACTION

This interaction is complex and confusing, because carbamazepine may either increase or decrease blood levels of theophylline. Case reports confirm that both reactions occur.

Increased theophylline levels may lead to toxicity. Diminished levels may be associated with reduced efficacy. In addition, theophylline may reduce carbamazepine levels, leading to a seizure. *This interaction could be dangerous.*

It is important for your physician to check blood levels of both drugs. If you experience symptoms of toxicity, let your doctor know at once.

Symptoms of Theophylline Toxicity

Nausea, diarrhea, stomach pain, headache, insomnia, restlessness, and irritability. Severe toxicity (convulsions, heart rhythm changes, or death) may occur with no warning symptoms. Notify your doctor immediately if you suspect a problem.

INTERACTION

DANGEROUS

Asthma Drug
(THEOPHYLLINE)

Heart/Blood Pressure Drugs
(BETA-BLOCKERS)

BRAND NAME

Aerolate	Aquaphyllin	Asmalix
Bronkodyl	Elixomin	Elixophyllin
Quibron-T	Respbid	Slo-bid
Slo-Phyllin	Theobid	Theochron
Theoclear	Theo-Dur	Theolair
Theo-24	Theovent	Theo-X
T-Phyl	Uniphyl	

BRAND NAME	GENERIC NAME
Blocadren	timolol
Cartrol	carteolol
Inderal	propranolol
Levatol	penbutolol
Timoptic	timolol
Visken	pindolol

DESCRIPTION

Theophylline helps to open airways, so it is generally used to treat and prevent asthma attacks. It may also be prescribed for people with emphysema or other chronic breathing problems. Babies and elderly men may need lower doses. The dose is monitored with regular blood tests to ensure that levels are less than 20 mcg/ml.

DESCRIPTION

Beta-blockers are prescribed to lower blood pressure, stabilize irregular heartbeats, or prevent migraines. Timoptic eye drops help control glaucoma. Despite the usefulness and versatility of these medicines, in general they are not appropriate for people with chronic breathing problems, because they can trigger airway tightening. Other side effects include changes in heart rate, cold hands and feet, and depression.

INSTRUCTIONS

Theophylline interacts with food in complex ways, so discuss this issue thoroughly with your doctor and pharmacist. Theophylline may upset the stomach. In some cases this problem can be alleviated by taking the drug with food. See the table of Food and Drug Compatibility on pages 59-73 for more information.

INSTRUCTIONS

Cartrol, Levatol, and Visken are taken with or without food. Inderal is best absorbed with meals, but consistency is more important. It should be taken at roughly the same time every day. Ask your eye doctor to show you how to administer Timoptic drops so that their absorption is minimized. Do not stop any of these medicines suddenly except on doctor's orders. Serious side effects could result.

INTERACTION

Because beta-blockers can make breathing difficult, they are not often prescribed for people with asthma. The beta-blockers named above can reduce the body's ability to clear theophylline, resulting in increased blood levels of theophylline, with the potential for theophylline toxicity. *This interaction could be dangerous.*

Neither Corgard nor Tenormin interferes with theophylline clearance. It is uncommon but certainly not unknown for eye drops such as Timoptic to be absorbed into the body and produce systemic side effects. In that case, Timoptic could interact with theophylline.

Symptoms of Theophylline Toxicity

Nausea, diarrhea, stomach pain, headache, insomnia, restlessness, and irritability. Severe toxicity (convulsions, heart rhythm changes, or death) may occur with no warning symptoms. Notify your doctor immediately if you suspect a problem.

Never take or stop medication without your doctor's advice.

INTERACTION

DANGEROUS

Asthma Drug
(THEOPHYLLINE)

Heart/Blood Pressure Drugs
(CALCIUM CHANNEL BLOCKERS)

BRAND NAME

Aerolate	**Aquaphyllin**	**Asmalix**
Bronkodyl	**Elixomin**	**Elixophyllin**
Quibron-T	**Respbid**	**Slo-bid**
Slo-Phyllin	**Theobid**	**Theochron**
Theoclear	**Theo-Dur**	**Theolair**
Theo-24	**Theovent**	**Theo-X**
T-Phyl	**Uniphyl**	

DESCRIPTION

Theophylline helps to open airways, so it is generally used to treat and prevent asthma attacks. It may also be prescribed for people with emphysema or other chronic breathing problems. Babies and elderly men may need lower doses. The dose is monitored with regular blood tests to ensure that levels are less than 20 mcg/ml.

INSTRUCTIONS

Theophylline interacts with food in complex ways, so discuss this issue thoroughly with your doctor and pharmacist. Theophylline may upset the stomach. In some cases this problem can be alleviated by taking the drug with food. See the table of Food and Drug Compatibility on pages 59-73 for more information.

BRAND NAME / **GENERIC NAME**

Adalat, Procardia	nifedipine
Calan, Isoptin,	
Verelan	verapamil
Cardizem, Dilacor XR	diltiazem

DESCRIPTION

These medications are prescribed primarily to treat angina or high blood pressure, or, in the case of verapamil, to stabilize irregular heart rhythms. They are usually well tolerated and are among the most popular cardiovascular drugs, but can cause gastrointestinal upset, dizziness, fluid retention, and other side effects. Elderly patients may require dosage adjustment.

INSTRUCTIONS

These drugs come in a variety of doses; follow the doctor's directions carefully. Sustained-release forms, such as Calan SR or Dilacor XR, should not be chewed or crushed and are best taken with food. Avoid taking Adalat or Procardia with grapefruit juice, as this could boost blood levels unexpectedly. See the table on pages 59-73 for specific instructions. Withdrawal symptoms, especially chest pain, may occur if these drugs are stopped suddenly. Follow the doctor's instructions for tapering slowly if the medicine must be discontinued.

INTERACTION

Many medicines, including diltiazem and verapamil, are capable of elevating blood levels of theophylline by interfering with metabolism of the drug. People seem to vary in the degree to which they react to this interaction. *Although the documented increase in circulating theophylline is not large, it could be dangerous for someone whose blood levels were already high.*

Most studies indicate that Procardia has little effect on serum theophylline levels, but there are a few cases of patients who developed toxicity as a result of this interaction.

Symptoms of Theophylline Toxicity

Nausea, diarrhea, stomach pain, headache, insomnia, restlessness, and irritability. Severe toxicity (convulsions, heart rhythm changes, or death) may occur with no warning symptoms. Notify your doctor immediately if you suspect a problem.

Never take or stop medication without your doctor's advice.

INTERACTION

DANGEROUS

Asthma Drug
(THEOPHYLLINE)

Heart Drug
(MEXILETINE)

BRAND NAME

Aerolate	**Aquaphyllin**	**Asmalix**
Bronkodyl	**Elixomin**	**Elixophyllin**
Quibron-T	**Respbid**	**Slo-bid**
Slo-Phyllin	**Theobid**	**Theochron**
Theoclear	**Theo-Dur**	**Theolair**
Theo-24	**Theovent**	**Theox-X**
T-Phyl	**Uniphyl**	

DESCRIPTION

Theophylline helps to open airways, so it is generally used to treat and prevent asthma attacks. It may also be prescribed for people with emphysema or other chronic breathing problems. Babies and elderly men may need lower doses. The dose is monitored with regular blood tests to ensure that levels are less than 20 mcg/ml.

INSTRUCTIONS

Theophylline interacts with food in complex ways, so discuss this issue thoroughly with your doctor and pharmacist. Theophylline may upset the stomach. In some cases this problem can be alleviated by taking the drug with food. See the table of Food and Drug Compatibility on pages 59-73 for more information.

BRAND NAME   GENERIC NAME

Mexitil   mexiletine

DESCRIPTION

Mexitil is used to treat severe, life-threatening heartbeat disturbances. Occasionally Mexitil aggravates heart rhythm irregularities, so careful monitoring is essential. Hospitalization is recommended for the first doses. This medicine interacts with many other drugs. Check with your physician and pharmacist before taking anything else.

INSTRUCTIONS

Mexitil may irritate the digestive tract, so it should be taken with food or an antacid. Dramatic changes in diet should be avoided. Notify the doctor immediately if fever, yellow skin and eyes, sore throat, or unusual tiredness develop.

INTERACTION

Like many other medicines, Mexitil interferes with the metabolism of theophylline. Blood levels of theophylline can double, leading to symptoms of toxicity. Because Mexitil is given only to people vulnerable to heart rhythm changes, there is a possibility of serious heartbeat disturbances. *This interaction could be dangerous.*

Symptoms of Theophylline Toxicity

Nausea, diarrhea, stomach pain, headache, insomnia, restlessness, and irritability. Severe toxicity (convulsions, heart rhythm changes, or death) may occur with no warning symptoms. Notify your doctor immediately if you suspect a problem.

Never take or stop medication without your doctor's advice.

INTERACTION

DANGEROUS

Asthma Drug

(THEOPHYLLINE)

Oral Contraceptives

BRAND NAME

Aerolate **Aquaphyllin** **Asmalix**
Bronkodyl **Elixomin** **Elixophyllin**
Quibron-T **Respbid** **Slo-bid**
Slo-Phyllin **Theobid** **Theochron**
Theoclear **Theo-Dur** **Theolair**
Theo-24 **Theovent** **Theo-X**
T-Phyl **Uniphyl**

BRAND NAME

Brevicon **Demulen** **Desogen**
Genora **Levlen** **Loestrin**
Lo/Ovral **Modicon** **N.E.E.**
Nelova **Nordette** **Norethin**
Norinyl **Norlestrin** **Ortho-**
Ortho-Novum **Ovcon** **Cyclen**
Ovral **Triphasil**

DESCRIPTION

Theophylline helps to open airways, so it is generally used to treat and prevent asthma attacks. It may also be prescribed for people with emphysema or other chronic breathing problems. Babies and elderly men may need lower doses. The dose is monitored with regular blood tests to ensure that levels are less than 20 mcg/ml.

INSTRUCTIONS

Theophylline interacts with food in complex ways, so discuss this issue thoroughly with your doctor and pharmacist. Theophylline may upset the stomach. In some cases this problem can be alleviated by taking the drug with food. See the table of Food and Drug Compatibility on pages 59-73 for more information.

DESCRIPTION

Lower doses of estrogen and progestin make these drugs safer today than ever before. But women who smoke and take oral contraceptives still run an increased risk of strokes. Side effects may include menstrual changes, nausea, migraine, depression, changes in vision, high blood pressure, liver tumors, gallbladder problems, blood clots, and heart attacks. Weigh the benefits and risks with your doctor when considering this form of contraception. Birth control pills interact with several other medications; check with your doctor or pharmacist before taking another drug in conjunction with oral contraceptives.

INSTRUCTIONS

Oral contraceptives should be taken at the same time every day and precisely according to instructions. Missed doses can lead to an unwelcome pregnancy. Additional contraception is needed for at least the first week.

INTERACTION

In clinical studies, oral contraceptives appear to interfere with theophylline metabolism, and to raise blood levels of that drug. *This interaction could result in dangerous theophylline toxicity.*

Although we found no mention in the literature of postmenopausal estrogen therapy interacting with theophylline, theoretically such an interaction might be possible. Stay alert and notify your doctor of any symptoms of theophylline toxicity.

Symptoms of Theophylline Toxicity

Nausea, diarrhea, stomach pain, headache, insomnia, restlessness, and irritability. Severe toxicity (convulsions, heart rhythm changes, or death) may occur with no warning symptoms. Notify your doctor immediately if you suspect a problem.

Never take or stop medication without your doctor's advice.

INTERACTION

DANGEROUS

Asthma Drug

(THEOPHYLLINE)

Alzheimer's Disease Drug

BRAND NAME

Aerolate   **Aquaphyllin**   **Asmalix**
Bronkodyl   **Elixomin**   **Elixophyllin**
Quibron-T   **Respbid**   **Slo-bid**
Slo-Phyllin   **Theobid**   **Theochron**
Theoclear   **Theo-Dur**   **Theolair**
Theo-24   **Theovent**   **Theo-X**
T-Phyl   **Uniphyl**

DESCRIPTION

Theophylline helps to open airways, so it is generally used to treat and prevent asthma attacks. It may also be prescribed for people with emphysema or other chronic breathing problems. Babies and elderly men may need lower doses. The dose is monitored with regular blood tests to ensure that levels are less than 20 mcg/ml.

INSTRUCTIONS

Theophylline interacts with food in complex ways, so discuss this issue thoroughly with your doctor and pharmacist. Theophylline may upset the stomach. In some cases this problem can be alleviated by taking the drug with food. See the table of Food and Drug Compatibility on pages 59-73 for more information.

BRAND NAME   GENERIC NAME

Cognex   tacrine

DESCRIPTION

Cognex is used to treat Alzheimer's disease. While not a cure, it can slow mental deterioration in some patients. Some people experience substantial improvement, but such benefits are unpredictable. Side effects include elevated liver enzymes, nausea and digestive upset, headache, and fatigue.

INSTRUCTIONS

The dose must be individualized. Cognex should be taken between meals whenever possible. If it upsets the stomach, it may be taken with food. Liver enzymes should be monitored regularly.

INTERACTION

Cognex interferes with the normal metabolism of theophylline. This can lead to substantial elevations in theophylline levels (double the normal blood level). This might lead to theophylline toxicity. *This interaction could be troublesome.*

If theophylline must be prescribed in combination with Cognex, the doctor may need to adjust the dose of theophylline carefully. Frequent monitoring of blood levels is advisable.

Symptoms of Theophylline Toxicity

Nausea, diarrhea, stomach pain, headache, insomnia, restlessness, and irritability. Severe toxicity (convulsions, heart rhythm changes, or death) may occur with no warning symptoms. Notify your doctor immediately if you suspect a problem.

INTERACTION

TROUBLESOME

Asthma Drug
(THEOPHYLLINE)

Anticonvulsants
(HYDANTOINS)

BRAND NAME

Aerolate	**Aquaphyllin**	**Asmalix**
Bronkodyl	**Elixomin**	**Elixophyllin**
Quibron-T	**Respbid**	**Slo-bid**
Slo-Phyllin	**Theobid**	**Theochron**
Theoclear	**Theo-Dur**	**Theolair**
Theo-24	**Theovent**	**Theo-X**
T-Phyl	**Uniphyl**	

BRAND NAME | GENERIC NAME

Dilantin	phenytoin
Mesantoin	mephenytoin
Peganone	ethotoin

DESCRIPTION

Theophylline helps to open airways, so it is generally used to treat and prevent asthma attacks. It may also be prescribed for people with emphysema or other chronic breathing problems. Babies and elderly men may need lower doses. The dose is monitored with regular blood tests to ensure that levels are less than 20 mcg/ml.

INSTRUCTIONS

Theophylline interacts with food in complex ways, so discuss this issue thoroughly with your doctor and pharmacist. Theophylline may upset the stomach. In some cases this problem can be alleviated by taking the drug with food. See the table of Food and Drug Compatibility on pages 59-73 for more information.

DESCRIPTION

These anticonvulsants are used to prevent epileptic seizures or seizures associated with brain surgery. Occasionally they may be prescribed to treat severe stabbing facial pain (trigeminal neuralgia). Tests may be needed to check blood cells, blood levels of the drug, liver function, and blood sugar. Special attention to oral hygiene is needed to prevent gum problems often associated with taking these anticonvulsants. Hydantoin anticonvulsants interact with many other drugs as well as alcohol, so check carefully with your physician and pharmacist before taking any other medication.

INSTRUCTIONS

Any of these medicines could upset the stomach. This is less likely if they are taken with food. All of them can cause drowsiness or blurred vision and could make driving dangerous.

INTERACTION

This is a double interaction, because both theophylline and the anticonvulsants can lead to lower blood levels of the other drug. The effect of the anticonvulsants, especially Dilantin, is to speed up removal of theophylline from the system by as much as 65 percent. *This interaction could be troublesome, leading to asthma symptoms.*

The interaction may become noticeable within about five days of taking the two drugs together. If both are needed, blood levels of each should be monitored so that doses can be adjusted appropriately by the doctor.

Never take or stop medication without your doctor's advice.

INTERACTION

TROUBLESOME

Asthma Drug
(THEOPHYLLINE)

Barbiturates

BRAND NAME

Aerolate   **Aquaphyllin**   **Asmalix**
Bronkodyl   **Elixomin**   **Elixophyllin**
Quibron-T   **Respbid**   **Slo-bid**
Slo-Phyllin   **Theobid**   **Theochron**
Theoclear   **Theo-Dur**   **Theolair**
Theo-24   **Theovent**   **Theo-X**
T-Phyl   **Uniphyl**

BRAND NAME   GENERIC NAME

Alurate   aprobarbital
Amytal   amobarbital
Butisol   butabarbital
Lotusate   talbutal
Mebaral   mephobarbital
Nembutal   pentobarbital
Seconal   secobarbital
Solfoton   phenobarbital
Tuinal   amobarbital/
   secobarbital

DESCRIPTION

Theophylline helps to open airways, so it is generally used to treat and prevent asthma attacks. It may also be prescribed for people with emphysema or other chronic breathing problems. Babies and elderly men may need lower doses. The dose is monitored with regular blood tests to ensure that levels are less than 20 mcg/ml.

INSTRUCTIONS

Theophylline interacts with food in complex ways, so discuss this issue thoroughly with your doctor and pharmacist. Theophylline may upset the stomach. In some cases this problem can be alleviated by taking the drug with food. See the table of Food and Drug Compatibility on pages 59-73 for more information.

DESCRIPTION

Barbiturates were once used as sleeping pills, but now they are prescribed to prevent seizures. These medications can cause dependence if used for an extended period of time. Stopping suddenly could trigger severe withdrawal symptoms. Barbiturates interact with many other drugs, so check with the pharmacist or physician before taking any other medications.

INSTRUCTIONS

Any of these medications can cause drowsiness and limit attention. Take them at a time when you will not need to drive or do other complicated tasks.

INTERACTION

Barbiturates stimulate the body to get rid of theophylline more quickly than usual. Laboratory studies show that blood levels of theophylline could drop dramatically. In this event, the previous dose of theophylline might not be enough to allow easy breathing. Blood tests will tell if the dose of theophylline requires adjustment. *This interaction could be troublesome.*

INTERACTION

TROUBLESOME

Asthma Drug
(THEOPHYLLINE)

Tuberculosis Drug
(RIFAMPIN)

BRAND NAME

Aerolate	**Aquaphyllin**	**Asmalix**
Bronkodyl	**Elixomin**	**Elixophyllin**
Quibron-T	**Respbid**	**Slo-bid**
Slo-Phyllin	**Theobid**	**Theochron**
Theoclear	**Theo-Dur**	**Theolair**
Theo-24	**Theovent**	**Theo-X**
T-Phyl	**Uniphyl**	

DESCRIPTION

Theophylline helps to open airways, so it is generally used to treat and prevent asthma attacks. It may also be prescribed for people with emphysema or other chronic breathing problems. Babies and elderly men may need lower doses. The dose is monitored with regular blood tests to ensure that levels are less than 20 mcg/ml.

INSTRUCTIONS

Theophylline interacts with food in complex ways, so discuss this issue thoroughly with your doctor and pharmacist. Theophylline may upset the stomach. In some cases this problem can be alleviated by taking the drug with food. See the table of Food and Drug Compatibility on pages 59-73 for more information.

BRAND NAME	GENERIC NAME
Rifadin	rifampin
Rifamate	isoniazid/rifampin
Rimactane	rifampin

DESCRIPTION

Rifampin is used in combination with other medications to treat tuberculosis. To be effective, it needs to be taken faithfully for an extended period of time (at least six to nine months), as the doctor prescribes. Side effects may include digestive tract problems, menstrual irregularities, difficulty concentrating, fluid retention, and wheezing or shortness of breath. The orange discoloration of urine, saliva, and tears is not harmful, although it may stain contact lenses.

INSTRUCTIONS

Rifampin should be taken on an empty stomach, at least one hour before or two hours after meals. If you develop fever, chills, unusual tiredness, unusual bleeding or bruising, sore throat, muscle and bone pain, or yellow skin and eyes, contact your physician immediately.

INTERACTION

A person with tuberculosis might very well need both these medications, because the disease could contribute to wheezing and breathing difficulties. Alternatively, theophylline might be prescribed to treat shortness of breath developing as a side effect of rifampin. Rifampin speeds the metabolism of theophylline so that it disappears much more quickly from the body. This takes at least a week and often longer, but as it occurs, theophylline levels drop and asthma may become worse. *This interaction could be troublesome.*

It makes sense for the doctor to check blood levels of theophylline several times when rifampin is added or dropped. These tests will tell if a dosage adjustment is necessary.

Never take or stop medication without your doctor's advice.

INTERACTION

TROUBLESOME

Cholesterol Drugs

Mevacor Pravachol Zocor

LIFE THREATENING

Antibiotics (macrolides)
Biaxin   E.E.S.
E-Mycin   ERYC
EryPed   Ery-Tab
Erythrocin   Ilosone
PCE   Pediazole
Tao

Cholesterol Drugs
Lopid
niacin

Transplant Drug
Sandimmune

DANGEROUS

Anticoagulant
Coumadin

Not every cholesterol drug listed above interacts with each medicine on this overview tree. See individual summaries for details. Drugs shown here have the most serious known reactions with this type of cholesterol-lowering drug, but check with a health professional before taking any other medicine with one of these agents.

LEVELS OF HAZARD: LIFE THREATENING   DANGEROUS   TROUBLESOME

Cholesterol Drugs Antibiotics

(MACROLIDES)

BRAND NAME	GENERIC NAME
Mevacor	lovastatin
Pravachol	pravastatin
Zocor	simvastatin

DESCRIPTION

Mevacor and the newer related drugs, Pravachol and Zocor, are potent cholesterol-lowering agents that are widely prescribed. Because of the association between high cholesterol and heart disease, these drugs are given in the hope of preventing a heart attack. They reduce the body's production of cholesterol and speed the removal of this fat from the bloodstream. Side effects include digestive distress, rash, and headache. Contact the physician if you experience muscle pain or weakness, because this could signal a serious reaction.

INSTRUCTIONS

Mevacor is best taken with the evening meal. Zocor and Pravachol may be taken with or without food before bed. They are most effective in combination with a prudent heart-healthy diet and a sensible exercise program.

BRAND NAME	GENERIC NAME
Biaxin	clarithromycin
E.E.S.	erythromycin
E-Mycin	erythromycin
ERYC	erythromycin
EryPed	erythromycin
Ery-Tab	erythromycin
Erythrocin	erythromycin
Ilosone	erythromycin
PCE	erythromycin
Pediazole	erythromycin
Tao	troleandomycin

DESCRIPTION

These broad-spectrum antibiotics are widely prescribed for respiratory tract, sinus, ear, and skin infections. They are also effective against certain infections of the reproductive tract.

INSTRUCTIONS

Some erythromycins must be taken on an empty stomach; others may be taken with food. See the table of Food and Drug Interactions on pages 59-73 for specifics. Biaxin can be swallowed with food or on an empty stomach.

INTERACTION

There is a possibility that erythromycin antibiotics may interact with Mevacor to produce muscle destruction, possibly progressing to kidney failure. *This interaction, if confirmed by further research, could be life threatening, so we alert you to it now.*

Several cases of this reaction, called myopathy or rhabdomyolysis, have been reported when erythromycin was added to Mevacor. Because Mevacor can cause this reaction on its own (although this is rare), experts are uncertain that erythromycin is to blame. If you must take both drugs, however, be alert for signs of muscle weakness, tenderness, or pain, and contact your doctor immediately if they develop. Blood and urine tests will be required to determine if the reaction is serious. It is not known if Biaxin or Tao interacts with Mevacor; nor is it known if Pravachol or Zocor interacts with erythromycin in this way.

Symptoms of Myopathy to Watch For

Muscle weakness, change in gait, muscle pain, and muscles that are tender to the touch.

INTERACTION

LIFE THREATENING

Cholesterol Drugs Cholesterol Drugs

BRAND NAME	GENERIC NAME
Mevacor	lovastatin
Pravachol	pravastatin
Zocor	simvastatin

DESCRIPTION

Mevacor and the newer related drugs, Pravachol and Zocor, are potent cholesterol-lowering agents that are widely prescribed. Because of the association between high cholesterol and heart disease, these drugs are given in the hope of preventing a heart attack. They reduce the body's production of cholesterol and speed the removal of this fat from the bloodstream. Side effects include digestive distress, rash, and headache. Contact the physician if you experience muscle pain or weakness, because this could signal a serious reaction.

INSTRUCTIONS

Mevacor is best taken with the evening meal. Zocor and Pravachol may be taken with or without food before bed. They are most effective in combination with a prudent heart-healthy diet and a sensible exercise program.

BRAND NAME	GENERIC NAME
Lopid	gemfibrozil
Nicolar	niacin, nicotinic acid

DESCRIPTION

Lopid lowers triglycerides and raises beneficial HDL (high-density lipoprotein) levels. It is used to normalize blood cholesterol levels. Niacin, in the form of nicotinic acid, also lowers cholesterol without lowering HDL unduly. Lopid may cause digestive distress, headache, and rash. The most frequent adverse effects of niacin are bothersome rather than serious: flushing, tingling, or itching shortly after taking the medicine. Headache, stomachache, and rash are also possible.

INSTRUCTIONS

Lopid is to be taken one-half hour before morning and evening meals. Niacin is best taken with meals. A single aspirin tablet one-half hour before taking niacin may reduce flushing; check with your doctor. Both drugs work best in conjunction with a heart-healthy diet and sensible exercise.

INTERACTION

Some people with high cholesterol have a hard time getting it down with just one drug. Doctors may try a combination of cholesterol-lowering medications in such a case. Both niacin and Lopid have been used together with Mevacor, but there is a risk of serious interaction in both cases. In perhaps 3 or 4 percent of patients, Lopid can interact with Mevacor to produce muscle destruction, possibly progressing to kidney failure. Older women and people with preexisting kidney problems appear especially vulnerable. *Although we are aware of no deaths, this interaction could be life threatening.*

Several cases of this reaction, called myopathy or rhabdomyolysis, have also been reported with niacin and Mevacor. If you must take either drug with Mevacor, be alert for signs of muscle weakness, tenderness, or pain, and contact your doctor immediately if they develop. Blood and urine tests will be required to determine if the reaction is serious.

Zocor and Pravachol may also interact dangerously with Lopid.

Symptoms of Myopathy to Watch For

Muscle weakness, change in gait, muscle pain, and muscles that are tender to the touch.

Never take or stop medication without your doctor's advice.

INTERACTION

LIFE THREATENING

Cholesterol Drugs Transplant Drug

(CYCLOSPORINE)

BRAND NAME	GENERIC NAME
Mevacor	lovastatin
Pravachol	pravastatin
Zocor	simvastatin

DESCRIPTION

Mevacor and the newer related drugs, Pravachol and Zocor, are potent cholesterol-lowering agents that are widely prescribed. Because of the association between high cholesterol and heart disease, these drugs are given in the hope of preventing a heart attack. They reduce the body's production of cholesterol and speed the removal of this fat from the bloodstream. Side effects include digestive distress, rash, and headache. Contact the physician if you experience muscle pain or weakness, because this could signal a serious reaction.

INSTRUCTIONS

Mevacor is best taken with the evening meal. Zocor and Pravachol may be taken with or without food before bed.They are most effective in combination with a prudent heart-healthy diet and a sensible exercise program.

BRAND NAME	GENERIC NAME
Sandimmune	cyclosporine

DESCRIPTION

Sandimmune suppresses the immune system so that a person receiving a transplant does not reject this lifesaving organ. Doctors have also tried using it in treating autoimmune diseases, in which the immune system attacks a person's own tissues. Multiple sclerosis is an example.

INSTRUCTIONS

Sandimmune comes as an oral solution with a taste reminiscent of castor oil. It should be mixed in a glass with milk, chocolate milk, or orange juice at room temperature and drunk at once. Then the glass (no plastic) should be rinsed and the rinsing fluid drunk to get the full dose. Do not take Sandimmune with grapefruit juice unless the physician is monitoring blood levels of the drug closely. (See page 43.)

Due to a possible interaction between cyclosporine and oral contraceptives, barrier methods of contraception should be used while taking this drug.

Regular monitoring is important. Do not stop this medicine unless your doctor so directs.

INTERACTION

Although we are aware of no fatalities, the combination of Sandimmune and one of these cholesterol-lowering drugs could lead to a syndrome of muscle destruction (resulting in weakness and pain) and consequent kidney failure. This reaction, known as rhabdomyolysis, can occur with Mevacor alone, but adding Sandimmune increases the risk substantially. Some reports estimate that up to 30 percent of patients on this combination of drugs may experience muscle wasting. If you need both medications, stay alert and notify your doctor immediately of any symptoms of muscle problems. Blood and urine tests may be needed. *This interaction could be life threatening.*

Symptoms of Myopathy to Watch For

Muscle weakness, change in gait, muscle pain, and muscles that are tender to the touch.

Never take or stop medication without your doctor's advice.

INTERACTION

LIFE THREATENING

Cholesterol Drug

(LOVASTATIN)

Anticoagulant

(WARFARIN)

BRAND NAME | GENERIC NAME

Mevacor | lovastatin

DESCRIPTION

Mevacor is a potent cholesterol-lowering agent that has become widely prescribed. Because of the association between high cholesterol and heart disease, Mevacor is given in the hope of preventing a heart attack. It reduces the body's production of cholesterol and speeds the removal of this fat from the bloodstream. Side effects of Mevacor include digestive distress, rash, and headache. Contact the physician if you experience muscle pain or weakness, because this could signal a serious reaction.

INSTRUCTIONS

Mevacor is best taken with the evening meal. It is most effective in combination with a prudent heart-healthy diet and a sensible exercise program.

BRAND NAME | GENERIC NAME

Coumadin | warfarin

DESCRIPTION

Warfarin slows the liver's production of factors essential for the formation of blood clots. It is prescribed when there is a risk that a dangerous clot could form in a deep vein or a blood vessel leading to the lung, heart, or brain. The most serious complication of anticoagulant treatment is excessive bleeding. The dosage must be individually adjusted, requiring daily blood tests at first, then tests every four to six weeks. Other side effects may include nausea, loss of appetite, rash, fever, yellow eyes and skin, prolonged painful erection, and hair loss.

INSTRUCTIONS

Warfarin tablets can be swallowed with food or on an empty stomach. Try to avoid large variations in the quantity of vitamin-K–containing vegetables—such as broccoli, cabbage, or spinach—that you eat each day. Consuming much more or less than usual could change the action of the drug.

INTERACTION

Mevacor appears to increase the effects of warfarin in some patients. Two middle-aged men requiring warfarin were later put on Mevacor for elevated cholesterol. Each of them developed unexpected bleeding and prolonged prothrombin times. *This interaction could be dangerous.* If Mevacor and warfarin are both needed, frequent blood tests will guide warfarin dose adjustment. There is no evidence that the other cholesterol-lowering drugs, Pravachol (generic: pravastatin) or Zocor (generic: simvastatin), interact with warfarin in the same fashion. Because they are similar to Mevacor, however, caution is probably advisable.

Symptoms of Warfarin Overdose

There may be no early warning signs of danger. Blood tests are essential. Symptoms include any unusual bleeding, including rectal or urinary tract bleeding, excessive menstrual bleeding, nosebleeds, bleeding around gums, bruising, red or tar-black stools, vomiting blood, and red or dark-brown urine. Notify your doctor immediately if you suspect a problem.

Never take or stop medication without your doctor's advice.

INTERACTION

DANGEROUS

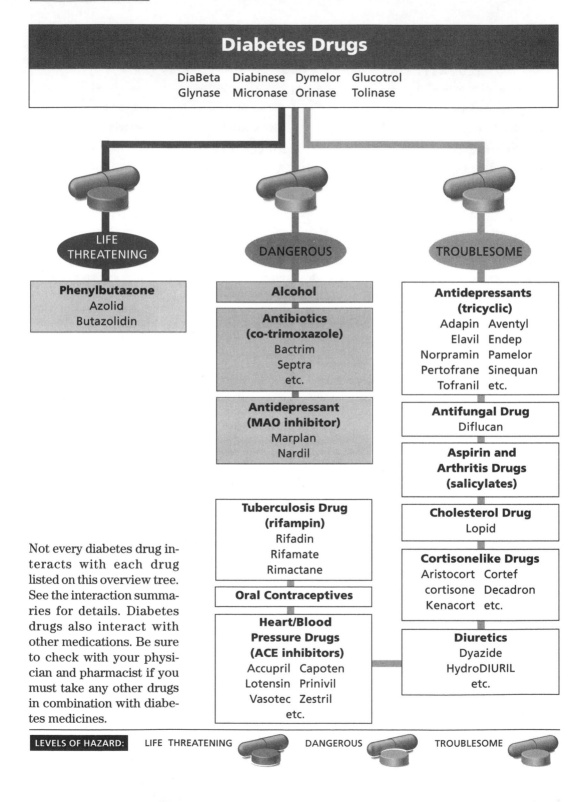

Diabetes Drugs

DiaBeta Diabinese Dymelor Glucotrol
Glynase Micronase Orinase Tolinase

LIFE THREATENING

Phenylbutazone
Azolid
Butazolidin

DANGEROUS

Alcohol

Antibiotics (co-trimoxazole)
Bactrim
Septra
etc.

Antidepressant (MAO inhibitor)
Marplan
Nardil

Tuberculosis Drug (rifampin)
Rifadin
Rifamate
Rimactane

Oral Contraceptives

Heart/Blood Pressure Drugs (ACE inhibitors)
Accupril Capoten
Lotensin Prinivil
Vasotec Zestril
etc.

TROUBLESOME

Antidepressants (tricyclic)
Adapin Aventyl
Elavil Endep
Norpramin Pamelor
Pertofrane Sinequan
Tofranil etc.

Antifungal Drug
Diflucan

Aspirin and Arthritis Drugs (salicylates)

Cholesterol Drug
Lopid

Cortisonelike Drugs
Aristocort Cortef
cortisone Decadron
Kenacort etc.

Diuretics
Dyazide
HydroDIURIL
etc.

Not every diabetes drug interacts with each drug listed on this overview tree. See the interaction summaries for details. Diabetes drugs also interact with other medications. Be sure to check with your physician and pharmacist if you must take any other drugs in combination with diabetes medicines.

LEVELS OF HAZARD: LIFE THREATENING DANGEROUS TROUBLESOME

Diabetes Drugs Phenylbutazone

BRAND NAME	GENERIC NAME
Diabinese	chlorpropamide
Dymelor	acetohexamide
Orinase	tolbutamide

DESCRIPTION

These pills are prescribed for non-insulin-dependent diabetics. They help control blood sugar by increasing the amount of insulin the pancreas makes and by making body tissues more sensitive to insulin. With diet, exercise, and blood sugar monitoring, they may reduce the risk of complications of diabetes. Low blood sugar (hypoglycemia) is the most common serious side effect. These medications interact with many others; check with your doctor or pharmacist before taking another drug.

INSTRUCTIONS

These diabetes drugs may be taken with food if they upset the stomach. Blood glucose monitoring is important. Notify the doctor immediately if you experience rash, fever, sore throat, or unusual bleeding or bruising.

BRAND NAME	GENERIC NAME
Azolid, Butazolidin	phenylbutazone

DESCRIPTION

This is a potent anti-inflammatory medicine used to treat painful joints caused by gout, rheumatoid arthritis, or degenerative arthritis. Older people (over 60) are more susceptible to adverse reactions and should take this medication for no longer than one week. Phenylbutazone interacts with many other medications and has a number of serious side effects. These may include abnormal blood counts, gastrointestinal upset, rash, and fluid retention. This medication may cause drowsiness and interfere with driving or other complex tasks.

INSTRUCTIONS

Phenylbutazone should be taken with food to minimize digestive upset. Notify the doctor immediately if you experience sore throat, mouth sores, unusual bleeding or bruising, swollen legs and feet, rash, blurred vision, fever, abdominal pain, black tarry stools, or sudden weight gain.

INTERACTION

Phenylbutazone can raise blood levels or lengthen the time that several of the oral diabetes drugs spend circulating in the body. The consequence of this can be unexpectedly low blood sugar, potentially leading to hypoglycemic coma. A person needing both medications should definitely monitor blood sugar more closely than usual. *This interaction could be lethal.* **At least one death has been reported.**

There have been no reports of interactions between phenylbutazone and the oral diabetes drugs DiaBeta and Glucotrol; nevertheless, it would be wise to monitor blood sugar closely if you take this combination of drugs.

Symptoms of Hypoglycemia (Low Blood Sugar)

Shaking, sweating, tiredness, low temperature, faintness, palpitations, hunger, headache, confusion, irritability, visual disturbances, and coma. Close observation (preferably in the hospital) is recommended for two or three days after such a reaction.

INTERACTION

LIFE THREATENING

Diabetes Drugs Alcohol

BRAND NAME	GENERIC NAME
Diabinese	chlorpropamide
Glucotrol	glipizide
Orinase	tolbutamide

NAME

beer
liquor
wine
medicines that contain alcohol

DESCRIPTION

These oral medications are prescribed for non-insulin-dependent diabetics. They help control blood sugar by increasing the amount of insulin the pancreas makes and by making body tissues more sensitive to insulin. When combined with a proper diet, exercise, and blood sugar monitoring, they may reduce the risk of complications of diabetes. Low blood sugar (hypoglycemia) is the most common serious side effect. These medications interact with many other drugs; check with a doctor or pharmacist before adding another medication.

INSTRUCTIONS

Glucotrol should be taken 15 minutes to half an hour before meals. The others may be taken with food, especially if they upset the stomach. Daily blood glucose monitoring is important. Notify the doctor immediately if you experience rash, fever, sore throat, or unusual bleeding or bruising.

DESCRIPTION

Alcohol comes in many guises. The obvious ones are liquor, beer, and wine. But you can also find substantial amounts of alcohol in certain medicines. Over-the-counter cough and cold products can contain up to 40 or 50 proof (20 to 25 percent by volume), which is a higher alcohol content than you would find in beer or wine. "Nighttime" remedies like NyQuil, Nytcold Medicine, and Pertussin PM Liquid are as much as 50 proof. This may not be a problem if all you take is a spoonful before bedtime, but some drugs may interact poorly with even modest amounts of alcohol.

INSTRUCTIONS

The absorption and effects of alcohol are magnified if you drink on an empty stomach. Fatty food can delay alcohol absorption. If you drink, do so in moderation, and never drive.

INTERACTION

The interaction between alcohol and oral diabetes drugs is complicated, and some aspects of this interaction are potentially dangerous. If patients taking Diabinese drink alcohol, they may experience an unpleasant reaction, with symptoms of nausea and vomiting, flushing, sweating, and throbbing headache. Alcohol may have other effects upon diabetes drugs. The person who drinks regularly may not be able to control blood sugar with the usual dose of Orinase (tolbutamide). On the other hand, if a person who doesn't often drink alcohol has several drinks, he or she may have a longer-than-expected effect from Glucotrol, with possible hypoglycemic symptoms. It is suggested that patients taking any of these oral diabetes drugs generally avoid alcohol. Remember that some liquid medicines contain alcohol (see page 154 for a list).

Symptoms of Hypoglycemia (Low Blood Sugar)

Shaking, sweating, tiredness, low temperature, faintness, palpitations, hunger, headache, confusion, irritability, visual disturbances, and coma. Close observation (preferably in the hospital) is recommended for two or three days after such a reaction.

Never take or stop medication without your doctor's advice.

INTERACTION

DANGEROUS

Diabetes Drugs

Antibiotics
(CO-TRIMOXAZOLE)

BRAND NAME	GENERIC NAME
DiaBeta, Glynase,	
Micronase	glyburide
Diabinese	chlorpropamide
Dymelor	acetohexamide
Glucotrol	glipizide
Orinase	tolbutamide
Tolinase	tolazamide

DESCRIPTION

These pills are prescribed for non-insulin-dependent diabetics. They help control blood sugar by increasing the amount of insulin the pancreas makes and by making body tissues more sensitive to insulin. With diet, exercise, and blood sugar monitoring, they may reduce the risk of complications of diabetes. Low blood sugar (hypoglycemia) is the most common serious side effect. These medications interact with many others; check with a doctor or pharmacist before taking another drug.

INSTRUCTIONS

DiaBeta, Glucotrol, and Micronase should be taken 15 minutes to half an hour before meals. The others may be taken with food if they upset the stomach. Blood glucose monitoring is important. Notify the doctor immediately if you experience rash, fever, sore throat, or unusual bleeding or bruising.

BRAND NAME

Bactrim, Cotrim, Septra, SMZ-TMP, Sulfatrim, Uroplus
(All co-trimoxazole, formerly known as trimethoprim-sulfamethoxazole)

DESCRIPTION

Bactrim, Septra, and other brands of co-trimoxazole are often prescribed for urinary tract infections or ear infections. They may also be useful in treating traveler's diarrhea and certain types of bronchitis or pneumonia. Occasionally use of such antibiotics may result in superinfection that must be treated with a different drug. Some people become more sensitive to sunlight—and more susceptible to sunburn—when taking one of these drugs. Side effects may include gastrointestinal upset, headache, rash, and yellow skin and eyes.

INSTRUCTIONS

This drug is best absorbed when taken on an empty stomach, at least one hour before or two hours after a meal. It may be taken with food if it upsets the stomach. Drink at least eight cups of water a day to help keep the drug from crystallizing in the kidney, and avoid large doses of vitamin C.

INTERACTION

These oral diabetes drugs last longer in the body when a person also takes a sulfa antibiotic such as Bactrim or Septra. Some patients have experienced hypoglycemia as a consequence. Orinase and Diabinese have been implicated most frequently, but there is one case report of this interaction causing hypoglycemia in a patient on Glucotrol. *This interaction could be dangerous.* DiaBeta, Glynase, and Micronase do not appear to interact with co-trimoxazole to cause hypoglycemia. Still, if you are on any oral diabetes drug and need to take this antibiotic, monitor your blood sugar carefully and be alert for hypoglycemia.

Symptoms of Hypoglycemia (Low Blood Sugar)

Shaking, sweating, tiredness, low temperature, faintness, palpitations, hunger, headache, confusion, irritability, visual disturbances, and coma. Close observation (preferably in the hospital) is recommended for two or three days after such a reaction.

Never take or stop medication without your doctor's advice.

INTERACTION

DANGEROUS

Diabetes Drugs Antidepressant

(MAO INHIBITOR)

BRAND NAME	GENERIC NAME
DiaBeta, Glynase, Micronase	glyburide
Diabinese	chlorpropamide
Glucotrol	glipizide
Orinase	tolbutamide
Tolinase	tolazamide

DESCRIPTION

These pills are prescribed for non-insulin-dependent diabetics. They help control blood sugar by increasing the amount of insulin the pancreas makes and by making body tissues more sensitive to insulin. With diet, exercise, and blood sugar monitoring, they may reduce the risk of complications of diabetes. Low blood sugar (hypoglycemia) is the most common serious side effect. These medications interact with many others; check with a doctor or pharmacist before taking another drug.

INSTRUCTIONS

DiaBeta, Glucotrol, and Micronase should be taken 15 minutes to half an hour before meals. The others may be taken with food if they upset the stomach. Blood glucose monitoring is important. Notify the doctor immediately if you experience rash, fever, sore throat, or unusual bleeding or bruising.

BRAND NAME	GENERIC NAME
Nardil	phenelzine

DESCRIPTION

This medication was among the earliest antidepressants to be developed and still works very well for some patients. These drugs are slow to start acting, and may last in the body for a few weeks after medication is stopped.

INSTRUCTIONS

MAO inhibitors can interact in dangerous ways with tyramine-containing foods and beverages. See page 47. Consult your doctor before taking other prescription or over-the-counter drugs. Notify him or her if you notice a skin rash, severe headache, yellow eyes or skin, or dark urine. Do not stop this medicine unless your doctor so advises.

INTERACTION

Nardil, an MAO inhibitor, can increase the glucose-lowering effects of the oral diabetes drugs and also of insulin. *Since severe hypoglycemia could result, this interaction may be dangerous.*

   If you need both medications, monitor blood sugar more carefully so that the doctor can help you adjust the dose of medication if necessary. This is not a do-it-yourself project. Notify your doctor if you develop hypoglycemia. The MAO inhibitor Parnate does not appear to lower blood sugar in the same way.

Symptoms of Hypoglycemia (Low Blood Sugar)

Shaking, sweating, tiredness, low temperature, faintness, palpitations, hunger, headache, confusion, irritability, visual disturbances, and coma. Close observation (preferably in the hospital) is recommended for two or three days after such a reaction.

Diabetes Drugs Antidepressants
(TRICYCLIC)

BRAND NAME	GENERIC NAME
DiaBeta, Glynase, Micronase	glyburide
Diabinese	chlorpropamide
Glucotrol	glipizide
Orinase	tolbutamide
Tolinase	tolazamide

BRAND NAME	GENERIC NAME
Adapin, Sinequan	doxepin
Aventyl, Pamelor	nortriptyline
Elavil, Endep	amitriptyline
Norpramin, Pertofrane	desipramine
Tofranil	imipramine
etc.	

DESCRIPTION

These pills are prescribed for non-insulin-dependent diabetics. They help control blood sugar by increasing the amount of insulin the pancreas makes and by making body tissues more sensitive to insulin. With diet, exercise, and blood sugar monitoring, they may reduce the risk of complications of diabetes. Low blood sugar (hypoglycemia) is the most common serious side effect. These medications interact with many others; check with your doctor or pharmacist before taking another drug.

INSTRUCTIONS

DiaBeta, Glucotrol, and Micronase should be taken 15 minutes to half an hour before meals. The others may be taken with food if they upset the stomach. Blood glucose monitoring is important. Notify the doctor immediately if you experience rash, fever, sore throat, or unusual bleeding or bruising.

DESCRIPTION

Tricyclic antidepressants became popular during the 1970s and 1980s though they often caused unpleasant side effects (constipation, weight gain, sexual dysfunction, sluggishness, increased sun sensitivity, etc.). They are used to treat depression. Some of them may also be helpful in controlling chronic pain.

INSTRUCTIONS

Usually these medications are better taken with food, in the evening to avoid daytime drowsiness. A high-fiber diet may interfere with absorption, however. Sinequan Concentrate should be mixed with four ounces of milk, water, or juice just before taking, not ahead of time. Do not stop taking any of these drugs suddenly; if they must be discontinued, your doctor will supervise gradual phaseout.

INTERACTION

This interaction has been deduced from case reports and needs confirmation from clinical studies. Tricyclic antidepressants are apparently capable of increasing the effects of oral diabetes drugs, so that a person might experience severe hypoglycemia. *This interaction could be troublesome.*

If you must take an antidepressant together with your oral diabetes drug, measure your blood sugar more frequently. Let your doctor know if you have an episode of low blood sugar.

Symptoms of Hypoglycemia (Low Blood Sugar)

Shaking, sweating, tiredness, low temperature, faintness, palpitations, hunger, headache, confusion, irritability, visual disturbances, and coma. Close observation (preferably in the hospital) is recommended for two or three days after such a reaction.

Never take or stop medication without your doctor's advice.

INTERACTION

TROUBLESOME

Diabetes Drug   Antifungal Drug

BRAND NAME	GENERIC NAME	BRAND NAME	GENERIC NAME
Orinase	tolbutamide	**Diflucan**	fluconazole

DESCRIPTION

This oral medication is prescribed for non-insulin-dependent diabetics. It helps control blood sugar by increasing the amount of insulin the pancreas makes and by making body tissues more sensitive to insulin. When combined with a proper diet, exercise, and blood sugar monitoring, it may reduce the risk of complications of diabetes. Low blood sugar (hypoglycemia) is the most common serious side effect. This medication interacts with many other drugs; check with your doctor or pharmacist before adding another medication.

INSTRUCTIONS

Tolbutamide may be taken with food, especially if it upsets the stomach. Daily blood glucose monitoring is important. Notify the doctor immediately if you experience rash, fever, sore throat, or unusual bleeding or bruising.

DESCRIPTION

Diflucan is a strong antifungal drug used to treat serious yeast and yeastlike infections, including thrush and cryptococcal meningitis. While it can be lifesaving in such situations, in rare cases it also has potentially serious side effects. Diflucan may damage the liver, and liver enzymes should be monitored. Other side effects include nausea, vomiting, headache, skin rash, abdominal pain, and diarrhea. Notify your doctor if you experience any of these. The skin rash could become more serious.

INSTRUCTIONS

Ask your doctor for precise instructions on how to take Diflucan. Doses are individualized, depending on the infection treated, and the first dose is often higher than the rest.

INTERACTION

Diflucan can boost blood levels of Orinase or generic tolbutamide. In the study that established this interaction, none of the healthy young men experienced dangerous changes in blood sugar level. However, diabetics might discover that this antifungal could make their Orinase more effective than expected. Hypoglycemia is theoretically possible. *This interaction could be troublesome.*

There is no indication that Diflucan interacts with other diabetes drugs, but it was not tested to rule out such an interaction. If you must take both medications, monitor your blood sugar carefully and notify your doctor if it is low.

Symptoms of Hypoglycemia (Low Blood Sugar)

Shaking, sweating, tiredness, low temperature, faintness, palpitations, hunger, headache, confusion, irritability, visual disturbances, and coma. Close observation (preferably in the hospital) is recommended for two or three days after such a reaction.

INTERACTION
TROUBLESOME

Diabetes Drugs

Aspirin and Arthritis Drugs

(SALICYLATES)

BRAND NAME	GENERIC NAME
DiaBeta, Glynase, Micronase	glyburide
Diabinese	chlorpropamide
Glucotrol	glipizide
Orinase	tolbutamide
Tolinase	tolazamide

DESCRIPTION

These pills are prescribed for non-insulin-dependent diabetics. They help control blood sugar by increasing the amount of insulin the pancreas makes and by making body tissues more sensitive to insulin. With diet, exercise, and blood sugar monitoring, they may reduce the risk of complications of diabetes. Low blood sugar (hypoglycemia) is the most common serious side effect. These medications interact with many others; check with your doctor or pharmacist before taking another drug.

INSTRUCTIONS

DiaBeta, Glucotrol, and Micronase should be taken 15 minutes to half an hour before meals. The others may be taken with food if they upset the stomach. Blood glucose monitoring is important. Notify the doctor immediately if you experience rash, fever, sore throat, or unusual bleeding or bruising.

BRAND NAME	GENERIC NAME
Alka-Seltzer	acetylsalicylic acid
Anacin	acetylsalicylic acid
Arthropan	choline salicylate
Ascriptin	acetylsalicylic acid
aspirin	acetylsalicylic acid
Bayer	acetylsalicylic acid
Bufferin	acetylsalicylic acid
Disalcid	salsalate
Ecotrin	acetylsalicylic acid
Uracel 5	sodium salicylate

DESCRIPTION

Aspirin is a versatile and inexpensive medication used to alleviate pain such as headache, reduce inflammation, bring down fever, prevent heart attacks or strokes, and forestall blood clots. It may also lower the risk of gastrointestinal cancer, especially colon cancer. Aspirin may be irritating to the digestive tract, and chronic use can trigger the development of ulcers. Ringing in the ears and unusual bleeding are also potential side effects.

INSTRUCTIONS

Aspirin may be taken with food or milk to reduce stomach upset, always with a full eight ounces of liquid. Pregnant women should take aspirin only under the doctor's supervision. Children with flu or chicken pox must avoid aspirin as it increases the risk of Reye's Syndrome.

INTERACTION

Aspirin and some related medicines, such as Arthropan and Disalcid, can lower blood sugar by themselves. In combination with the diabetes drugs, they may lower blood sugar more than expected. *This interaction could be troublesome.*

If you need aspirin or another salicylate as well as one of these diabetes drugs, monitor blood sugar and be alert for symptoms of hypoglycemia. If you notice any, your doctor may wish to adjust the dose of the diabetes drug.

Symptoms of Hypoglycemia (Low Blood Sugar)

Shaking, sweating, tiredness, low temperature, faintness, palpitations, hunger, headache, confusion, irritability, visual disturbances, and coma. Close observation (preferably in the hospital) is recommended for two or three days after such a reaction.

Never take or stop medication without your doctor's advice.

INTERACTION

TROUBLESOME

Diabetes Drug   Cholesterol Drug

BRAND NAME   GENERIC NAME

**DiaBeta, Glynase,
   Micronase**   glyburide

DESCRIPTION

These oral medications are prescribed for non-insulin-dependent diabetics. They help control blood sugar by increasing the amount of insulin the pancreas makes and by making body tissues more sensitive to insulin. When combined with a proper diet, exercise, and blood sugar monitoring, they may reduce the risk of complications of diabetes. Low blood sugar (hypoglycemia) is the most common serious side effect. These medications interact with many other drugs; check with your doctor or pharmacist before adding another medication.

INSTRUCTIONS

DiaBeta, Glynase, and Micronase should be taken 15 minutes to half an hour before meals. Daily blood glucose monitoring is important. Notify the doctor immediately if you experience rash, fever, sore throat, or unusual bleeding or bruising.

BRAND NAME   GENERIC NAME

Lopid   gemfibrozil

DESCRIPTION

Lopid lowers the level of triglycerides and raises the level of beneficial HDL (high-density lipoprotein) in the blood. It is used alone or in conjunction with other cholesterol-lowering drugs to normalize blood cholesterol levels. Lopid may cause digestive distress, headache, and rash.

INSTRUCTIONS

Lopid is to be taken one-half hour before morning and evening meals. It works best in conjunction with a heart-healthy diet and sensible exercise.

INTERACTION

Diabetics are at higher risk of heart disease than the population in general, and many non-insulin-dependent diabetics have high cholesterol levels. It is certainly logical that such a person might end up taking both DiaBeta (or another brand of glyburide) and Lopid. The cholesterol drug can increase the blood-sugar-lowering power of DiaBeta, and the result may be hypoglycemia. *This interaction could be troublesome.*

If you must take both medications, monitor your blood sugar carefully and notify your doctor if it is low. The dose of DiaBeta may need to be adjusted.

Symptoms of Hypoglycemia (Low Blood Sugar)

Shaking, sweating, tiredness, low temperature, faintness, palpitations, hunger, headache, confusion, irritability, visual disturbances, and coma. Close observation (preferably in the hospital) is recommended for two or three days after such a reaction.

Never take or stop medication without your doctor's advice.

INTERACTION

TROUBLESOME

Diabetes Drugs Cortisonelike Drugs

BRAND NAME	GENERIC NAME
DiaBeta, Glynase, Micronase	glyburide
Diabinese	chlorpropamide
Glucotrol	glipizide
Orinase	tolbutamide
Tolinase	tolazamide

DESCRIPTION

These pills are prescribed for non-insulin-dependent diabetics. They help control blood sugar by increasing the amount of insulin the pancreas makes and by making body tissues more sensitive to insulin. With diet, exercise, and blood sugar monitoring, they may reduce the risk of complications of diabetes. Low blood sugar (hypoglycemia) is the most common serious side effect. These medications interact with many others; check with your doctor or pharmacist before taking another drug.

INSTRUCTIONS

DiaBeta, Glucotrol, and Micronase should be taken 15 minutes to half an hour before meals. The others may be taken with food if they upset the stomach. Blood glucose monitoring is important. Notify the doctor immediately if you experience rash, fever, sore throat, or unusual bleeding or bruising.

BRAND NAME	GENERIC NAME
Aristocort, Kenacort	triamcinolone
Celestone	betamethasone
Cortef	hydrocortisone
Cortisone	cortisone
Decadron	dexamethasone
Deltasone	prednisone
etc.	

DESCRIPTION

Cortisonelike drugs have powerful anti-inflammatory action and are used to treat disorders such as rheumatoid arthritis. They are also prescribed for allergies, asthma, connective tissue conditions such as lupus, and skin diseases such as psoriasis, as well as many other diseases. Long-term use has potentially serious side effects, however, so risk must be balanced against benefit. Corticosteroids can cause digestive distress, behavior changes, blood pressure problems, and menstrual irregularities. Longer-term problems include ulcers, muscle and bone loss, and cataracts. Contact your doctor about any unusual symptoms.

INSTRUCTIONS

Any of these medicines could upset the stomach, so they should be taken with food. These medications should not be stopped suddenly, but rather tapered off with gradually decreasing doses as the doctor instructs.

INTERACTION

Cortisone and other drugs in its class can raise blood sugar noticeably. As many as 14 percent of patients taking these drugs for several weeks or more will experience this side effect.

As a consequence, blood sugar control may be affected. Monitor blood sugar carefully when starting or stopping any cortisonelike drug so that the dose of the diabetes medicine can be adjusted if necessary.

Never take or stop medication without your doctor's advice.

INTERACTION

TROUBLESOME

Diabetes Drugs

Diuretics

BRAND NAME	GENERIC NAME
DiaBeta, Glynase, Micronase	glyburide
Diabinese	chlorpropamide
Glucotrol	glipizide
Orinase	tolbutamide
Tolinase	tolazamide

DESCRIPTION

These pills are prescribed for non-insulin-dependent diabetics. They help control blood sugar by increasing the amount of insulin the pancreas makes and by making body tissues more sensitive to insulin. With diet, exercise, and blood sugar monitoring, they may reduce the risk of complications of diabetes. Low blood sugar (hypoglycemia) is the most common serious side effect. These medications interact with many others; check with your doctor or pharmacist before taking another drug.

INSTRUCTIONS

DiaBeta, Glucotrol, and Micronase should be taken 15 minutes to half an hour before meals. The others may be taken with food if they upset the stomach. Blood glucose monitoring is important. Notify the doctor immediately if you experience rash, fever, sore throat, or unusual bleeding or bruising.

BRAND NAME	GENERIC NAME
Aquatensen, Enduron	methyclothiazide
Diachlor, Diuril	chlorothiazide
Diucardin, Saluron	hydroflumethiazide
Dyazide, Maxzide	hydrochlorothiazide and triamterene
Dyrenium	triamterene
Esidrix, HydroDIURIL	hydrochlorothiazide
Hygroton, Hylidone	chlorthalidone
Lozol	indapamide
etc.	

DESCRIPTION

Diuretics, or "water pills," rid the body of excess fluid buildup due to congestive heart failure or kidney trouble, or as a side effect of other drugs. They are, however, most often prescribed to lower blood pressure. They are usually well tolerated, but side effects include stomach upset, sexual difficulties, and gout. Probably the most serious problem associated with these medications is a gradual depletion of potassium or magnesium. Blood levels of these minerals should be monitored.

INSTRUCTIONS

Diuretics should be taken early in the day to reduce the number of times you have to get up at night to urinate. They may be taken with food or milk if they cause stomach upset.

INTERACTION

Diuretics can raise blood sugar in susceptible people, especially diabetics. Such medicine can also make oral diabetes drugs less effective. *This interaction could be troublesome, leading to hyperglycemia.*

The interaction may become noticeable within a few days of taking the two drugs together, or it may not show up for a few months. If both drugs are needed, blood sugar levels should be monitored so that the the doctor can adjust the dose of the diabetes medicine appropriately. Electrolyte levels and kidney function should also be checked; an excessive loss of potassium or even sodium is possible. The latter is especially problematic if Diabinese is prescribed with triamterene (Dyrenium, Dyazide, Maxzide).

Never take or stop medication without your doctor's advice.

INTERACTION

TROUBLESOME

Diabetes Drugs

Heart/Blood Pressure Drugs
(ACE INHIBITORS)

BRAND NAME	GENERIC NAME
DiaBeta, Glynase, Micronase	glyburide
Diabinese	chlorpropamide
Dymelor	acetohexamide
Glucotrol	glipizide
Orinase	tolbutamide
Tolinase	tolazamide

BRAND NAME	GENERIC NAME
Accupril	quinapril
Altace	ramipril
Capoten	captopril
Lotensin	benazepril
Monopril	fosinopril
Prinivil, Zestril	lisinopril
Vasotec	enalapril

DESCRIPTION

These pills are prescribed for non-insulin-dependent diabetics. They help control blood sugar by increasing the amount of insulin the pancreas makes and by making body tissues more sensitive to insulin. With diet, exercise, and blood sugar monitoring, they may reduce the risk of complications of diabetes. Low blood sugar (hypoglycemia) is the most common serious side effect. These medications interact with many others; check with your doctor or pharmacist before taking another drug.

INSTRUCTIONS

DiaBeta, Glucotrol, and Micronase should be taken 15 minutes to half an hour before meals. The others may be taken with food if they upset the stomach. Blood glucose monitoring is important. Notify the doctor immediately if you experience rash, fever, sore throat, or unusual bleeding or bruising.

DESCRIPTION

These medications are used to treat high blood pressure. They block angiotensin-converting enzyme, or ACE. Capoten and Vasotec can also be helpful in treating congestive heart failure. Capoten also helps conserve kidney function in diabetics. The ACE inhibitors are usually very well tolerated, but blood pressure may be lowered so much that a person starting on one of these medicines becomes dizzy or faints, especially upon standing up. Caution is advised. Some people on these medicines develop a nagging dry cough not helped by cough medicine.

INSTRUCTIONS

Capoten should be taken one hour before meals. High-fat meals may reduce absorption of Accupril. Food does not affect the other drugs in this class.

INTERACTION

Like many other drugs, ACE blood pressure medicines may increase the effectiveness of the oral diabetes medications. This could cause a greater drop in blood sugar than expected, with possible symptoms of hypoglycemia. Check with the doctor if you notice a change in blood sugar after starting Capoten, Vasotec, or one of the other drugs in this class. Stay alert for symptoms of hypoglycemia. *This interaction could be troublesome.*

Symptoms of Hypoglycemia (Low Blood Sugar)

Shaking, sweating, tiredness, low temperature, faintness, palpitations, hunger, headache, confusion, irritability, visual disturbances, and coma. Close observation (preferably in the hospital) is recommended for two or three days after such a reaction.

Never take or stop medication without your doctor's advice.

INTERACTION
TROUBLESOME

Diabetes Drugs Oral Contraceptives

BRAND NAME	GENERIC NAME
DiaBeta, Glynase, Micronase	glyburide
Diabinese	chlorpropamide
Glucotrol	glipizide
Orinase	tolbutamide
Tolinase	tolazamide

DESCRIPTION

These pills are prescribed for non-insulin-dependent diabetics. They help control blood sugar by increasing the amount of insulin the pancreas makes and by making body tissues more sensitive to insulin. With diet, exercise, and blood sugar monitoring, they may reduce the risk of complications of diabetes. Low blood sugar (hypoglycemia) is the most common serious side effect. These medications interact with many others; check with your doctor or pharmacist before taking another drug.

INSTRUCTIONS

DiaBeta, Glucotrol, and Micronase should be taken 15 minutes to half an hour before meals. The others may be taken with food if they upset the stomach. Blood glucose monitoring is important. Notify the doctor immediately if you experience rash, fever, sore throat, or unusual bleeding or bruising.

BRAND NAME		
Brevicon	**Demulen**	**Desogen**
Genora	**Levlen**	**Loestrin**
Lo/Ovral	**Modicon**	**N.E.E.**
Nelova	**Nordette**	**Norethin**
Norinyl	**Norlestrin**	**Ortho-**
Ortho-Novum	**Ovcon**	**Cyclen**
Ovral	**Triphasil**	

DESCRIPTION

Lower doses of estrogen and progestin make these drugs safer today than ever before. But women who smoke and take oral contraceptives still run an increased risk of strokes. These drugs are usually well-tolerated, but side effects may include menstrual changes, nausea, migraine, depression, changes in vision, high blood pressure, liver tumors, gallbladder problems, blood clots, and heart attacks. Weigh the benefits and risks with your doctor when considering this form of contraception. Birth control pills interact with several other medications; check with your doctor or pharmacist before taking another drug in conjunction with oral contraceptives.

INSTRUCTIONS

For maximum effectiveness, oral contraceptives should be taken at the same time every day and precisely according to instructions. Missed doses can lead to an unwelcome pregnancy. Additional contraception is needed for at least the first week.

INTERACTION

Oral contraceptives can raise blood sugar, but this effect is less likely with the lower-dose oral contraceptives. If you use an oral contraceptive together with a diabetes drug, measure your blood sugar regularly to make sure it is well controlled. *This interaction could be troublesome.*

Never take or stop medication without your doctor's advice.

INTERACTION
TROUBLESOME

Diabetes Drugs Tuberculosis Drug
(RIFAMPIN)

BRAND NAME	GENERIC NAME
DiaBeta, Glynase,	
Micronase	glyburide
Diabinese	chlorpropamide
Glucotrol	glipizide
Orinase	tolbutamide
Tolinase	tolazamide

DESCRIPTION

These pills are prescribed for non-insulin-dependent diabetics. They help control blood sugar by increasing the amount of insulin the pancreas makes and by making body tissues more sensitive to insulin. With diet, exercise, and blood sugar monitoring, they may reduce the risk of complications of diabetes. Low blood sugar (hypoglycemia) is the most common serious side effect. These medications interact with many others; check with your doctor or pharmacist before taking another drug.

INSTRUCTIONS

DiaBeta, Glucotrol, and Micronase should be taken 15 minutes to half an hour before meals. The others may be taken with food if they upset the stomach. Blood glucose monitoring is important. Notify the doctor immediately if you experience rash, fever, sore throat, or unusual bleeding or bruising.

BRAND NAME	GENERIC NAME
Rifadin	rifampin
Rifamate	isoniazid/rifampin
Rimactane	rifampin

DESCRIPTION

Rifampin is used in combination with other medications to treat tuberculosis. To be effective, it needs to be taken faithfully for an extended period of time (at least six to nine months), as the doctor prescribes. Side effects may include digestive tract problems, menstrual irregularities, difficulty concentrating, fluid retention, and wheezing or shortness of breath. The orange discoloration of urine, saliva, and tears is not harmful, although it may stain contact lenses.

INSTRUCTIONS

Rifampin should be taken on an empty stomach, at least one hour before or two hours after meals. If you develop fever, chills, unusual tiredness, unusual bleeding or bruising, sore throat, muscle and bone pain, or yellow skin and eyes, contact your physician immediately.

INTERACTION

Rifampin revs up the body's machinery for processing these oral diabetes drugs, so they are eliminated more quickly and circulate at lower levels. Studies in healthy people have established this interaction, although they did not have higher blood sugar as a result. Several case reports concern diabetics who required higher doses of their diabetes drug to keep blood sugar under control after starting on the tuberculosis treatment. Monitor blood sugar carefully when starting or stopping rifampin, because the dose of the diabetes drug may need adjustment. *This interaction could be troublesome.*

Never take or stop medication without your doctor's advice.

INTERACTION

TROUBLESOME

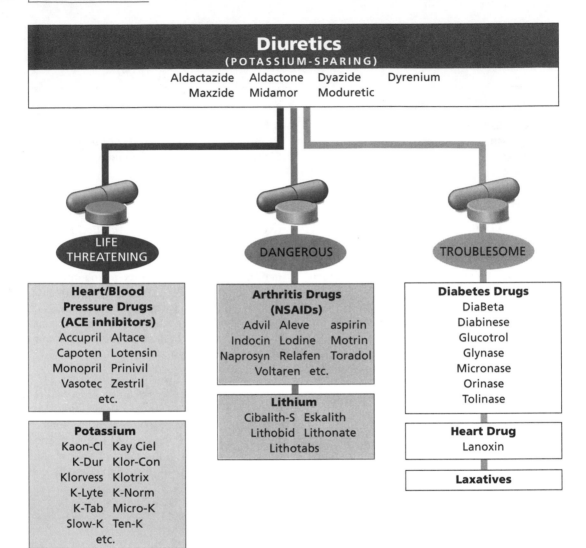

Diuretics
(POTASSIUM-SPARING)

Aldactazide	Aldactone	Dyazide	Dyrenium
Maxzide	Midamor	Moduretic	

LIFE THREATENING

Heart/Blood Pressure Drugs (ACE inhibitors)

Accupril	Altace
Capoten	Lotensin
Monopril	Prinivil
Vasotec	Zestril
etc.	

Potassium

Kaon-Cl	Kay Ciel
K-Dur	Klor-Con
Klorvess	Klotrix
K-Lyte	K-Norm
K-Tab	Micro-K
Slow-K	Ten-K
etc.	

DANGEROUS

Arthritis Drugs (NSAIDs)

Advil	Aleve	aspirin
Indocin	Lodine	Motrin
Naprosyn	Relafen	Toradol
Voltaren	etc.	

Lithium

Cibalith-S	Eskalith
Lithobid	Lithonate
Lithotabs	

TROUBLESOME

Diabetes Drugs
DiaBeta
Diabinese
Glucotrol
Glynase
Micronase
Orinase
Tolinase

Heart Drug
Lanoxin

Laxatives

Not every potassium-saving diuretic interacts with each drug listed on this overview tree. See the individual summaries for details. We have tried to list the most significant interactions, but other medications may also interact. Be sure to check with your physician and pharmacist if you must take other drugs in combination with potassium-sparing diuretics.

LEVELS OF HAZARD: LIFE THREATENING   DANGEROUS   TROUBLESOME

Diuretics
(POTASSIUM-SPARING)

Heart/Blood Pressure Drugs
(ACE INHIBITORS)

BRAND NAME	GENERIC NAME
Aldactazide	spironolactone, HCTZ
Aldactone	spironolactone
Dyazide	triamterene, HCTZ
Dyrenium	triamterene
Maxzide	triamterene, HCTZ
Midamor	amiloride
Moduretic	amiloride, HCTZ

BRAND NAME	GENERIC NAME
Accupril	quinapril
Altace	ramipril
Capoten	captopril
Lotensin	benazepril
Monopril	fosinopril
Prinivil, **Zestril**	lisinopril
Vasotec	enalapril

DESCRIPTION

Diuretics encourage the kidneys to eliminate excess fluid from the body. This can be useful in controlling high blood pressure, congestive heart failure, and certain other conditions. Spironolactone is also used to treat a hormonal condition called hyperaldosteronism. With other diuretics, important minerals (especially potassium and magnesium) are lost along with the fluid. With the above group of drugs, however, potassium is conserved.

INSTRUCTIONS

Midamor and Dyrenium may upset the stomach, so they are best taken right after meals. Maxzide can be taken without regard to meals. Midamor and Aldactone may interfere with the alertness and coordination necessary for driving. Periodic blood tests for magnesium and potassium are advisable.

DESCRIPTION

These medications are used to treat high blood pressure. They block angiotensin-converting enzyme, or ACE. Capoten and Vasotec can also be helpful in treating congestive heart failure. Capoten also helps conserve kidney function in diabetics. The ACE inhibitors are usually very well tolerated, but blood pressure may be lowered so much that a person starting on one of these medicines becomes dizzy or faints, especially upon standing up. Caution is advised. Some people on these medicines develop a nagging dry cough not helped by cough medicine.

INSTRUCTIONS

Capoten should be taken one hour before meals. High-fat meals may reduce absorption of Accupril. Food does not affect the other drugs in this class.

INTERACTION

Capoten, Vasotec, and other drugs in this category may increase potassium levels in susceptible patients. When these drugs are combined with potassium-sparing diuretics, serum potassium levels could rise into the dangerous range. *This situation could be life threatening. Irregular heart rhythms and cardiac arrest might occur.* **Deaths have been reported.** Elderly patients and those with kidney problems appear to be at the highest risk of this interaction. Diabetes may also contribute to the danger. Otherwise healthy patients may have no trouble and some with very low potassium levels may actually benefit from such a combination with careful medical supervision. However, if a potassium-sparing diuretic is prescribed together with an ACE inhibitor blood pressure drug, potassium levels should be monitored very closely. This may also be true of combination diuretics such as Dyazide or Maxzide.

Normal Serum Potassium Levels: 3.5 to 5 mEq/L

Never take or stop medication without your doctor's advice.

INTERACTION

LIFE THREATENING

Diuretics
(POTASSIUM-SPARING)

Potassium

BRAND NAME	GENERIC NAME
Aldactazide	spironolactone, HCTZ
Aldactone	spironolactone
Dyazide	triamterene, HCTZ
Dyrenium	triamterene
Maxzide	triamterene, HCTZ
Midamor	amiloride
Moduretic	amiloride, HCTZ

DESCRIPTION

Diuretics encourage the kidneys to eliminate excess fluid from the body. This can be useful in controlling high blood pressure, congestive heart failure, and certain other conditions. Spironolactone is also used to treat a hormonal condition called hyperaldosteronism. With other diuretics, important minerals (especially potassium and magnesium) are lost along with the fluid. With the above group of drugs, however, potassium is conserved.

INSTRUCTIONS

Midamor and Dyrenium may upset the stomach, so they are best taken right after meals. Maxzide can be taken without regard to meals. Midamor and Aldactone may interfere with the alertness and coordination necessary for driving. Periodic blood tests for magnesium and potassium are advisable.

BRAND NAME

Kaon-Cl	**Kay Ciel**	**K-Dur**
Klor-Con	**Klorvess**	**Klotrix**
K-Lyte	**K-Norm**	**K-Tab**
Micro-K	**Slow-K**	**Ten-K**
etc.		

DESCRIPTION

Potassium is an essential mineral that must be maintained within normal limits for good health. Heart, kidney, muscle, and nerve cells all need it for proper functioning. When potassium levels drop too low, a person may feel weak, tire easily, experience numbness or tingling of hands or feet, and have trouble breathing and abnormal heart rhythms. Too much potassium is equally dangerous, and many of the symptoms are similar: breathing difficulty, heart rhythm disturbances, weakness, tiredness, confusion, slow heart rate, and changes on the electrocardiogram.

INSTRUCTIONS

These supplements may upset the stomach. They are best taken right after meals, with a full glass of water. Tell the doctor immediately if you have nausea, vomiting, abdominal pain, or black stools.

INTERACTION

Potassium-sparing diuretics are capable of increasing potassium levels, particularly in susceptible patients. When these drugs are combined with potassium supplements or salt substitutes that contain potassium, serum potassium levels could rise into the dangerous range. *This situation could be life threatening. Irregular heart rhythms and cardiac arrest might occur.* **Deaths have been reported.**

Elderly patients and those with kidney problems appear to be at the highest risk for this interaction. Diabetes may also contribute to the danger. Patients with very low potassium levels may sometimes be prescribed a potassium-sparing diuretic together with a potassium supplement. In this case potassium levels must be monitored very carefully. *Extreme caution is called for.*

Normal Serum Potassium Levels: 3.5 to 5 mEq/L

Never take or stop medication without your doctor's advice.

INTERACTION

LIFE THREATENING

Diuretics

(POTASSIUM-SPARING)

Arthritis Drugs

(NSAIDS)

BRAND NAME	GENERIC NAME
Aldactazide	spironolactone, HCTZ
Aldactone	spironolactone
Dyazide	triamterene, HCTZ
Dyrenium	triamterene
Maxzide	triamterene, HCTZ
Midamor	amiloride
Moduretic	amiloride, HCTZ

DESCRIPTION

Diuretics encourage the kidney to eliminate excess fluid from the body. This can be useful in controlling high blood pressure, congestive heart failure, and certain other conditions. Spironolactone is also used to treat a hormonal condition called hyperaldosteronism. With other diuretics, important minerals (especially potassium and magnesium) are lost along with the fluid. With this group of drugs, however, potassium is conserved.

INSTRUCTIONS

Midamor and Dyrenium may upset the stomach, so they are best taken right after meals. Maxzide can be taken without regard to meals. Midamor and Aldactone may interfere with the alertness and coordination necessary for driving. Periodic blood tests for magnesium and potassium are advisable.

BRAND NAME	GENERIC NAME
Advil, Motrin, Nuprin	ibuprofen
Aleve, Naprosyn	naproxen
Ansaid	flurbiprofen
Aspirin	aspirin
Indocin	indomethacin
Lodine	etodolac
Relafen	nabumetone
Voltaren	diclofenac
etc.	

DESCRIPTION

Nonsteroidal anti-inflammatory drugs (NSAIDs) can ease pain, lower a fever, and help control inflammation. They are frequently prescribed for arthritis, as well as for muscle strains, headaches, lower back discomfort, menstrual pain, and other conditions. These medications can cause serious digestive tract upset, including heartburn, indigestion, and bleeding or perforated ulcers. Careful medical monitoring is essential.

INSTRUCTIONS

Take with food to reduce the risk of stomach irritation. (See table on pages 59-73.) Aspirin and OTC ibuprofen or naproxen should not be mixed with prescription NSAIDs or each other.

INTERACTION

Some arthritis drugs may reduce the effectiveness of diuretics. Fluid may build up, posing a serious problem for patients with heart trouble. Thiazide diuretics such as hydrochlorothiazide may be less effective in lowering blood pressure. If diuretics and arthritis drugs are taken simultaneously, blood pressure should be monitored carefully. Indocin may raise potassium levels to dangerous levels when combined with potassium-sparing diuretics like Moduretic. Measure potassium levels periodically. Potassium-sparing diuretics containing triamterene (Dyazide, Dyrenium, Maxzide) may interact badly with ibuprofen, Indocin, or Voltaren. Kidney damage has been reported. Other arthritis drugs may also interact.

Symptoms of Heart and Kidney Problems

Notify your doctor of sudden weight gain, swollen legs and feet, change in the color of the urine, unusual back pain, fatigue, cough, or breathlessness. Elevated serum creatinine may mean kidney trouble. Monitor blood pressure frequently.

Never take or stop medication without your doctor's advice.

INTERACTION

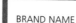

DANGEROUS

Diuretics
(POTASSIUM-SPARING)

Lithium

BRAND NAME	GENERIC NAME
Aldactazide	spironolactone, HCTZ
Aldactone	spironolactone
Dyazide	triamterene, HCTZ
Dyrenium	triamterene
Maxzide	triamterene, HCTZ
Midamor	amiloride
Moduretic	amiloride, HCTZ

DESCRIPTION

Diuretics encourage the kidneys to eliminate excess fluid from the body. This can be useful in controlling high blood pressure, congestive heart failure, and certain other conditions. Spironolactone is also used to treat a hormonal condition called hyperaldosteronism. With other diuretics, important minerals (especially potassium and magnesium) are lost along with the fluid. With the above group of drugs, however, potassium is conserved.

INSTRUCTIONS

Midamor and Dyrenium may upset the stomach, so they are best taken right after meals. Maxzide can be taken without regard to meals. Midamor and Aldactone may interfere with the alertness and coordination necessary for driving. Periodic blood tests for magnesium and potassium are advisable.

BRAND NAME

Cibalith-S
Eskalith
Lithobid
Lithonate
Lithotabs

DESCRIPTION

Lithium is most often used to treat bipolar depression, and seems to be especially helpful in easing the manic phases of this disorder. Regular blood tests are advisable for dose adjustment. The toxic dose is not a great deal higher than the effective dose, so the doctor should be notified of signs such as vomiting, diarrhea, unsteadiness in walking, weakness, or unusual drowsiness. This drug can affect the thyroid gland.

INSTRUCTIONS

Lithium should be taken immediately after meals or with food or milk to reduce stomach upset. It is essential to drink 8 to 12 glasses of water or other fluid each day while on lithium. This medication can affect alertness, so activities such as driving or operating machinery can be dangerous for people on lithium.

INTERACTION

A number of cases have been reported in which diuretics, when taken in conjunction with lithium, have precipitated symptoms of lithium toxicity. Lithium blood levels may be raised into the danger zone. This interaction is somewhat murky and more research is needed to understand the clinical significance. *Nonetheless, this interaction could be dangerous.*

Lithium levels should be monitored periodically. Notify the doctor of any symptoms of lithium toxicity.

Symptoms of Lithium Toxicity

Drowsiness, incoordination, unsteady gait, dizziness, tremor, muscle twitching, blurred vision, ringing in the ears, slurred speech, confusion, seizures, and coma.

INTERACTION

DANGEROUS

Diuretics

(POTASSIUM-SPARING)

Diabetes Drugs

BRAND NAME	GENERIC NAME
Aldactazide	spironolactone, HCTZ
Aldactone	spironolactone
Dyazide	triamterene, HCTZ
Dyrenium	triamterene
Maxzide	triamterene, HCTZ
Midamor	amiloride
Moduretic	amiloride, HCTZ

BRAND NAME	GENERIC NAME
DiaBeta, Glynase,	
Micronase	glyburide
Diabinese	chlorpropamide
Glucotrol	glipizide
Orinase	tolbutamide
Tolinase	tolazamide

DESCRIPTION

Diuretics encourage the kidney to eliminate excess fluid from the body. This can be useful in controlling high blood pressure, congestive heart failure, and certain other conditions. Spironolactone is also used to treat a hormonal condition called hyperaldosteronism. With other diuretics, important minerals (especially potassium and magnesium) are lost along with the fluid. With this group of drugs, however, potassium is conserved.

INSTRUCTIONS

Midamor and Dyrenium may upset the stomach, so they are best taken right after meals. Maxzide can be taken without regard to meals. Midamor and Aldactone may interfere with the alertness and coordination necessary for driving. Periodic blood tests for magnesium and potassium are advisable.

DESCRIPTION

These pills are prescribed for non-insulin-dependent diabetics. They help control blood sugar by increasing the amount of insulin the pancreas makes and by making body tissues more sensitive to insulin. With diet, exercise, and blood sugar monitoring, they may reduce the risk of complications of diabetes. Low blood sugar (hypoglycemia) is the most common serious side effect. These medications interact with many others; check with your doctor or pharmacist before taking another drug.

INSTRUCTIONS

DiaBeta, Glucotrol, and Micronase should be taken 15 minutes to half an hour before meals. The others may be taken with food if they upset the stomach. Blood glucose monitoring is important. Notify your doctor immediately if you experience rash, fever, sore throat, or unusual bleeding or bruising.

INTERACTION

Diuretics can raise blood sugar in susceptible people, especially diabetics. Such medicine can also make oral diabetes drugs less effective. *This interaction could be troublesome, leading to hyperglycemia.*

The interaction may become noticeable within a few days of taking the two drugs together, or it may not show up for a few months. If both drugs are needed, blood sugar levels should be monitored so that the the doctor can adjust the dose of the diabetes medicine appropriately. Electrolyte levels and kidney function should also be checked; an excessive loss of potassium or even sodium is possible. The latter is especially problematic if Diabinese is prescribed with triamterene (Dyrenium, Dyazide, Maxzide).

Never take or stop medication without your doctor's advice.

INTERACTION

TROUBLESOME

Diuretics
(POTASSIUM-SPARING)

Heart Drug
(DIGOXIN)

BRAND NAME | GENERIC NAME

Aldactazide   spironolactone, HCTZ
Aldactone   spironolactone
Midamor   amiloride
Moduretic   amiloride, HCTZ

DESCRIPTION

Diuretics encourage the kidneys to eliminate excess fluid from the body. This can be useful in controlling high blood pressure, congestive heart failure, and certain other conditions. Spironolactone is also used to treat a hormonal condition called hyperaldosteronism. With other diuretics, important minerals (especially potassium and magnesium) are lost along with the fluid. With the above group of drugs, however, potassium is conserved.

INSTRUCTIONS

Midamor may upset the stomach, so it is best taken right after meals. Midamor and Aldactone may interfere with the alertness and coordination necessary for driving. Periodic blood tests for magnesium and potassium are advisable.

BRAND NAME | GENERIC NAME

Lanoxin   digoxin

DESCRIPTION

Digoxin is a heart drug that is often very helpful in treating congestive heart failure. It is also prescribed for certain heart rhythm changes, especially atrial fibrillation, atrial flutter, and paroxysmal atrial tachycardia (PAT). The doctor must monitor the digoxin dose carefully, because the effective dose is not far below the toxic dose. Older people may need dose adjustment.

INSTRUCTIONS

Digoxin should be taken in a consistent fashion, preferably with food but not with a meal high in fiber. Bran may limit the absorption of this drug.

Do not stop this medicine unless your doctor so directs.

INTERACTION

This is an incredibly complicated interaction that could create considerable confusion. Aldactone and Aldactazide may produce falsely elevated readings of standard tests of serum digoxin levels. In other words, because of inaccurate test results, a physician might think patients were getting too much digoxin when in fact they were getting the right amount. But there is also evidence that these diuretics may actually boost digoxin levels, thereby increasing the risk of side effects. Be vigilant for signs of digoxin toxicity.

Midamor and Moduretic may also increase digoxin levels, especially in patients with reduced kidney function. But these diuretics may partially interfere with the effectiveness of digoxin. If such drugs are combined it is very important to monitor digoxin reaction and heart function.

Symptoms of Digoxin Toxicity

Nausea, vomiting, loss of appetite, diarrhea, stomach pain, visual disturbances (green or yellow tint and a halo around lights), weakness, drowsiness, depression, confusion, palpitations, rash, headaches, and hallucinations. Notify the doctor immediately if you experience any of these symptoms.

INTERACTION

TROUBLESOME

Diuretics

(POTASSIUM-SPARING)

Laxatives

BRAND NAME	GENERIC NAME
Dyazide	triamterene, HCTZ
Dyrenium	triamterene
Maxzide	triamterene, HCTZ

(other diuretics also may be affected)

DESCRIPTION

Diuretics encourage the kidneys to eliminate excess fluid from the body. This can be useful in controlling high blood pressure, congestive heart failure, and certain other conditions. With other diuretics, important minerals (especially potassium and magnesium) are lost along with the fluid. With the above group of drugs, however, potassium is conserved.

INSTRUCTIONS

Dyrenium may upset the stomach, so it is best taken right after meals. Maxzide can be taken without regard to meals. Periodic blood tests for magnesium and potassium are advisable.

DESCRIPTION

There is an extraordinary variety of laxatives on the market. They range from relatively mild bulk-forming products that contain methylcellulose and polycarbophil to stimulant cathartics such as castor oil, cascara sagrada, and senna. The regular or routine use of any laxative can create problems and is often referred to as "laxative abuse" by gastroenterologists. It can lead to dehydration, nutritional imbalance, severe diarrhea, and electrolyte imbalance. Potassium loss is considered a very serious consequence, especially for people with heart problems.

INSTRUCTIONS

Try to avoid regular use of any laxative. A high-fiber diet that incorporates bran, fruits, and vegetables and includes lots of liquids can often eliminate the need for laxatives. If a laxative is needed, bulk-forming products are believed to be the safest.

INTERACTION

The manufacturers of Dyazide offer the following caution: "Chronic or overuse of laxatives may reduce serum potassium levels by promoting excessive potassium loss from the intestinal tract; laxatives may interfere with the potassium-retaining effects of triamterene." What this means is that Dyazide, Dyrenium, and Maxzide may not work as well as expected in preserving potassium when they are taken in combination with a laxative. Monitor potassium levels if laxatives are a part of your routine.

Normal Serum Potassium Levels: 3.5 to 5 mEq/L

INTERACTION

TROUBLESOME

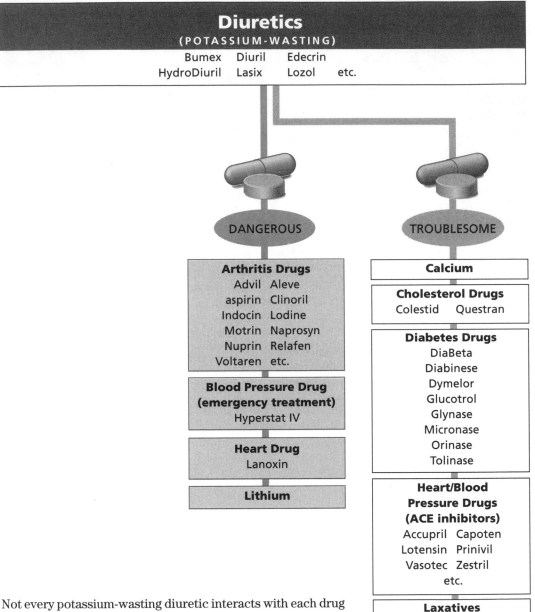

Diuretics
(POTASSIUM-WASTING)

Bumex   Diuril   Edecrin
HydroDiuril   Lasix   Lozol   etc.

DANGEROUS

Arthritis Drugs
Advil   Aleve
aspirin   Clinoril
Indocin   Lodine
Motrin   Naprosyn
Nuprin   Relafen
Voltaren   etc.

**Blood Pressure Drug
(emergency treatment)**
Hyperstat IV

Heart Drug
Lanoxin

Lithium

TROUBLESOME

Calcium

Cholesterol Drugs
Colestid   Questran

Diabetes Drugs
DiaBeta
Diabinese
Dymelor
Glucotrol
Glynase
Micronase
Orinase
Tolinase

**Heart/Blood
Pressure Drugs
(ACE inhibitors)**
Accupril   Capoten
Lotensin   Prinivil
Vasotec   Zestril
etc.

Laxatives

Not every potassium-wasting diuretic interacts with each drug listed on this overview tree. See the descriptions for details. We have tried to list the most significant interactions but other medications may also interact. Be sure to check with your physician and pharmacist if you must take other drugs in combination with potassium-wasting diuretics.

LEVELS OF HAZARD: LIFE THREATENING   DANGEROUS   TROUBLESOME

Diuretics

(POTASSIUM-WASTING)

Arthritis Drugs

(NSAIDS)

BRAND NAME	GENERIC NAME
Bumex	bumetanide
Diachlor, Diuril	chlorothiazide
Diucardin, Saluron	hydroflumethiazide
Edecrin	ethacrynic acid
Enduron	methyclothiazide
Esidrix, HydroDIURIL	hydrochlorothiazide
Hygroton	chlorthalidone
Lasix	furosemide
Lozol	indapamide

BRAND NAME	GENERIC NAME
Advil, Motrin, Nuprin	ibuprofen
Aleve, Naprosyn	naproxen
Aspirin	aspirin
Clinoril	sulindac
Indocin	indomethacin
Lodine	etodolac
Relafen	nabumetone
Voltaren	diclofenac

(Other NSAIDs may also interact.)

DESCRIPTION

Diuretics ("water pills") help the body eliminate excess fluid caused by congestive heart failure or kidney trouble, or as a side effect of other drugs. They are most widely prescribed to lower blood pressure. Side effects may include stomach upset, sexual difficulties, and gout. Probably the most serious side effect is a gradual depletion of potassium or magnesium, which could lead to irregular heart rhythms. Blood levels of these minerals should be monitored.

INSTRUCTIONS

Taking a diuretic early in the day may reduce nighttime urination. If it causes stomach upset, the drug may be taken with food or milk. See the Food and Drug Compatibility Table on pages 59-73 for specifics.

DESCRIPTION

Nonsteroidal anti-inflammatory drugs (NSAIDs) can ease pain, lower a fever, and help control inflammation. They are frequently prescribed for arthritis, as well as for muscle strains, headaches, lower back discomfort, menstrual pain, and other conditions. These medications can cause serious digestive tract upset, including heartburn, indigestion, and bleeding or perforated ulcers. Careful medical monitoring is essential.

INSTRUCTIONS

Take with food to reduce the risk of stomach irritation. (See table on pages 59-73.) Aspirin and OTC ibuprofen or naproxen should not be mixed with prescription NSAIDs or each other.

INTERACTION

NSAIDs such as ibuprofen and Indocin appear to reduce the effectiveness of diuretics such as Bumex and Lasix. (Clinoril may also affect Bumex). Fluid may build up and symptoms of heart failure could become worse. This is a very serious situation for people with heart trouble. Thiazide diuretics such as chlorthalidone, chlorothiazide, and hydrochlorothiazide may be less effective in lowering blood pressure, but this interaction does not seem so serious. Blood pressure should be monitored to make sure adequate control is maintained.

Symptoms of Heart Problems

Fluid retention, fatigue, cough, and breathlessness are possible signs of congestive heart failure. Monitor blood pressure frequently. Notify the physician immediately of symptoms.

Never take or stop medication without your doctor's advice.

INTERACTION

DANGEROUS

Diuretics

(POTASSIUM-WASTING)

Blood Pressure Drug

(EMERGENCY TREATMENT)

BRAND NAME	GENERIC NAME
Bumex	bumetanide
Diachlor, Diuril	chlorothiazide
Diucardin, Saluron	hydroflumethiazide
Edecrin	ethacrynic acid
Enduron	methyclothiazide
Esidrix, HydroDIURIL	hydrochlorothiazide
Hygroton	chlorthalidone
Lasix	furosemide
Lozol	indapamide

DESCRIPTION

Diuretics ("water pills") help the body eliminate excess fluid caused by congestive heart failure or kidney trouble, or as a side effect of other drugs. They are most widely prescribed to lower blood pressure. Side effects may include stomach upset, sexual difficulties, and gout. Probably the most serious side effect is a gradual depletion of potassium or magnesium, which could lead to irregular heart rhythms. Blood levels of these minerals should be monitored.

INSTRUCTIONS

Taking a diuretic early in the day may reduce nighttime urination. If it causes stomach upset, the drug may be taken with food or milk. See the Food and Drug Compatibility Table on pages 59-73 for specifics.

BRAND NAME	GENERIC NAME
Hyperstat I.V.	diazoxide

DESCRIPTION

Diazoxide is used for the emergency treatment of very high blood pressure. It is administered intravenously in a hospital setting. Although not a diuretic, diazoxide is chemically related to thiazide diuretics. When Hyperstat I.V. is injected it dilates blood vessels and produces a rapid and profound drop in blood pressure. Careful monitoring is essential to prevent pressure from going too low. Blood glucose levels can climb, especially in diabetic patients.

INSTRUCTIONS

This drug will be administered by appropriate hospital personnel during an emergency blood pressure situation. If a patient has been taking a thiazide diuretic, make sure health professionals are aware of this potentially serious interaction.

INTERACTION

This combination can lead to very high levels of blood sugar (glucose), creating symptoms of diabetes. Acidosis (a buildup of acid) can have serious consequences. It can take weeks for this effect to wear off. If someone must receive Hyperstat I.V. to control hypertension while they have been on one of these diuretics, it is essential that glucose levels be carefully monitored.
Normal Blood Glucose Levels: 70 to 110 mg/dl

INTERACTION

DANGEROUS

Diuretics
(POTASSIUM-WASTING)

Heart Drug
(DIGOXIN)

BRAND NAME	GENERIC NAME
Bumex	bumetanide
Diachlor, Diuril	chlorothiazide
Diucardin, Saluron	hydroflumethiazide
Edecrin	ethacrynic acid
Enduron	methyclothiazide
Esidrix, HydroDIURIL	hydrochlorothiazide
Hygroton	chlorthalidone
Lasix	furosemide
Lozol	indapamide

DESCRIPTION

Diuretics ("water pills") help the body eliminate excess fluid caused by congestive heart failure or kidney trouble, or as a side effect of other drugs. They are most widely prescribed to lower blood pressure. Side effects may include stomach upset, sexual difficulties, and gout. Probably the most serious side effect is a gradual depletion of potassium or magnesium, which could lead to irregular heart rhythms. Blood levels of these minerals should be monitored.

INSTRUCTIONS

Taking a diuretic early in the day may reduce nighttime urination. If it causes stomach upset, the drug may be taken with food or milk.

BRAND NAME	GENERIC NAME
Lanoxin	digoxin

DESCRIPTION

Digoxin is a heart drug that is often very helpful in treating congestive heart failure. It is also prescribed for certain heart rhythm changes, especially atrial fibrillation, atrial flutter, and paroxysmal atrial tachycardia (PAT). The doctor must monitor the digoxin dose carefully, because the effective dose is not far below the toxic dose. Older people may need dose adjustment.

INSTRUCTIONS

Digoxin should be taken in a consistent fashion, preferably with food but not with a meal high in fiber. Bran may limit the absorption of this drug.

Do not stop this medicine unless your doctor so directs.

INTERACTION

Physicians may prescribe diuretics in combination with digoxin to rid the body of excess fluid. There is rarely a problem, but electrolytes must be monitored carefully to avoid the danger of loss of potassium or magnesium. When these minerals are too low, digoxin might cause dangerous heart rhythm irregularities. *This interaction could be very dangerous.*

Regular blood tests are crucial. If levels of potassium and magnesium drop below the normal range, the doctor will probably prescribe supplements. Keep a diary of your potassium and magnesium levels.

Symptoms of Too Little Potassium: Muscle cramps, weakness, difficulty breathing, lethargy, and irregular heart rhythms.

Symptoms of Low Magnesium: Hard to diagnose. Be alert for loss of appetite, nausea, vomiting, weakness, fatigue, personality change, tremor, and muscle twitches.

Normal Electrolyte Values: Potassium: 3.5 to 5 mEq/L. Magnesium: 1.8 to 3 mEq/L

Never take or stop medication without your doctor's advice.

INTERACTION

DANGEROUS

Diuretics

(POTASSIUM-WASTING)

Lithium

BRAND NAME	GENERIC NAME
Bumex	bumetanide
Diachlor, Diuril	chlorothiazide
Diucardin, Saluron	hydroflumethiazide
Edecrin	ethacrynic acid
Enduron	methyclothiazide
Esidrix, HydroDIURIL	hydrochlorothiazide
Hygroton	chlorthalidone
Lasix	furosemide
Lozol	indapamide

BRAND NAME

Cibalith-S
Eskalith
Lithobid
Lithonate
Lithotabs

DESCRIPTION

Diuretics ("water pills") help the body eliminate excess fluid caused by congestive heart failure or kidney trouble, or as a side effect of other drugs. They are most widely prescribed to lower blood pressure. Side effects may include stomach upset, sexual difficulties, and gout. Probably the most serious side effect is a gradual depletion of potassium or magnesium, which could lead to irregular heart rhythms. Blood levels of these minerals should be monitored.

DESCRIPTION

Lithium is most often used to treat bipolar depression, and seems to be especially helpful in easing the manic phases of this disorder. Regular blood tests are advisable for dose adjustment. The toxic dose is not a great deal higher than the effective dose, so the doctor should be notified of signs such as vomiting, diarrhea, unsteadiness in walking, weakness, or unusual drowsiness. This drug can affect the thyroid gland.

INSTRUCTIONS

Taking a diuretic early in the day may reduce nighttime urination. If it causes stomach upset, the drug may be taken with food or milk. See the Food and Drug Interaction Table on pages 59-73 for specifics.

INSTRUCTIONS

Lithium should be taken immediately after meals or with food or milk to reduce stomach upset. It is essential to drink 8 to 12 glasses of water or other fluid each day while on lithium. This medication can affect alertness, so activities such as driving or operating machinery can be dangerous for people on lithium.

INTERACTION

A number of cases have been reported in which diuretics, when taken in combination with lithium, have precipitated symptoms of lithium toxicity. Lithium blood levels may be raised into the danger zone. This interaction is somewhat murky and more research is needed to understand the clinical significance. Lithium may be taken with diuretics as long as potassium levels are carefully monitored. *Nonetheless, this interaction could be dangerous.* Notify your doctor of any symptoms of lithium toxicity.

Symptoms of Lithium Toxicity

Drowsiness, incoordination, unsteady gait, dizziness, tremor, muscle twitching, blurred vision, ringing in the ears, slurred speech, confusion, seizures, and coma.

Never take or stop medication without your doctor's advice.

INTERACTION

DANGEROUS

Diuretics

(POTASSIUM-WASTING)

Calcium

BRAND NAME	GENERIC NAME
Diachlor, Diuril	chlorothiazide
Diucardin, Saluron	hydroflumethiazide
Diulo, Zaroxolyn	metolazone
Enduron	methyclothiazide
Esidrix	hydrochlorothiazide
HydroDIURIL	hydrochlorothiazide
Hygroton	chlorthalidone
Lozol	indapamide
Naqua	trichlormethiazide
Naturetin	bendroflumethiazide

DESCRIPTION

Diuretics ("water pills") help the body eliminate excess fluid caused by congestive heart failure or kidney trouble, or as a side effect of other drugs. They are most widely prescribed to lower blood pressure. Side effects may include stomach upset, sexual difficulties, and gout. Probably the most serious side effect is a gradual depletion of potassium or magnesium, which could lead to irregular heart rhythms. Blood levels of these minerals should be monitored.

INSTRUCTIONS

Taking a diuretic early in the day may reduce nighttime urination. If it causes stomach upset, the drug may be taken with food or milk. See the Food and Drug Compatibility Table on pages 59-73.

BRAND NAME	GENERIC NAME
Citracal	calcium citrate
Caltrate 600	calcium carbonate
Os-Cal	calcium carbonate
Posture	calcium phosphate
Rolaids Calcium Rich	calcium carbonate
Titralac	calcium carbonate
Tums	calcium carbonate
etc.	

DESCRIPTION

Calcium salts are often taken as a nutritional supplement. They have little toxicity and may help to preserve bone strength and possibly reduce the risk of colon cancer. People who have had kidney stones should not take calcium without supervision, because it might increase the likelihood of a recurrence.

INSTRUCTIONS

Generally, calcium supplements should be taken with meals for best absorption, but not with iron supplements. Calcium carbonate may be constipating in some people, but other calcium salts are less likely to cause this problem.

INTERACTION

Thiazide diuretics such as those listed on this page conserve calcium by modifying the way the kidneys eliminate this mineral. This action might be beneficial against osteoporosis and fractures. A problem may arise, however, if someone also took large amounts of calcium and vitamin D. Too much calcium could build up in the bloodstream, leading to toxicity. If this condition is allowed to progress, it can lead to kidney damage. *This troublesome interaction, if ignored, could become dangerous.*

Symptoms of Calcium Toxicity

Nausea, vomiting, loss of appetite, constipation, pain in the lower stomach, weakness, and headache. Notify the physician of any symptoms. Serum calcium should be monitored.

Normal Serum Calcium Values: 8.8 to 10.3 mg/dl.

Never take or stop medication without your doctor's advice.

INTERACTION

TROUBLESOME

Diuretics
(POTASSIUM-WASTING)

Cholesterol Drugs

BRAND NAME	GENERIC NAME
Diachlor, Diuril	chlorothiazide
Diucardin, Saluron	hydroflumethiazide
Diulo, Zaroxolyn	metolazone
Enduron	methyclothiazide
Esidrix	hydrochlorothiazide
HydroDIURIL	hydrochlorothiazide
Hygroton	chlorthalidone
Lozol	indapamide
Naqua	trichlormethiazide
Naturetin	bendroflumethiazide

DESCRIPTION

Diuretics ("water pills") help the body eliminate excess fluid caused by congestive heart failure or kidney trouble, or as a side effect of other drugs. They are most widely prescribed to lower blood pressure. Side effects may include stomach upset, sexual difficulties, and gout. Probably the most serious side effect is a gradual depletion of potassium or magnesium, which could lead to irregular heart rhythms. Blood levels of these minerals should be monitored.

INSTRUCTIONS

Taking a diuretic early in the day may reduce nighttime urination. If it causes stomach upset, the drug may be taken with food or milk. See the Food and Drug Interaction Table on pages 59-73.

BRAND NAME	GENERIC NAME
Colestid	colestipol
Questran	cholestyramine

DESCRIPTION

Questran and Colestid are effective drugs for lowering total cholesterol and the particularly dangerous LDL (low-density lipoprotein) cholesterol, which is thought to contribute to coronary artery disease. They do this by binding to bile acids in the intestinal tract and removing them from circulation. Bile is made in the liver and used by the body to digest fats in food. When bile acids are reduced, the body has to work harder to convert cholesterol to make more bile. This is thought to reduce the amount of cholesterol circulating in the bloodstream.

INSTRUCTIONS

Questran and Colestid come in powder form and need to be mixed with a glassful of water. Questran should not be taken with carbonated beverages. These medications are usually taken before meals, but check with a physician or pharmacist for specific instructions.

INTERACTION

These cholesterol-lowering drugs may interfere with proper absorption of diuretics. Some studies have shown that Questran can reduce hydrochlorothiazide levels by roughly one third. This could decrease the effectiveness of diuretics. For people with high blood pressure or congestive heart failure such a reaction could be quite serious. If one of these cholesterol-lowering drugs must be used in conjunction with a thiazide diuretic, they should be taken at least four hours apart. This is no guarantee of safety, though, so careful monitoring is essential.

Symptoms of Too Little Diuretic: Blood pressure may increase, fluid could be retained, and symptoms of heart failure might get worse. Measure blood pressure and heart function frequently. Notify the physician of any symptoms.

INTERACTION

TROUBLESOME

Diuretics

(POTASSIUM-WASTING)

Diabetes Drugs

BRAND NAME	GENERIC NAME
Diachlor, Diuril	chlorothiazide
Diucardin, Saluron	hydroflumethiazide
Diulo, Zaroxolyn	metolazone
Enduron	methyclothiazide
Esidrix	hydrochlorothiazide
HCTZ	hydrochlorothiazide
HydroDIURIL	hydrochlorothiazide
Hygroton, Hylidone	chlorthalidone
Lozol	indapamide
Naturetin	bendroflumethiazide
etc.	

DESCRIPTION

Diuretics ("water pills") help eliminate excess fluid due to congestive heart failure or kidney trouble, or as a side effect of other drugs. They are most often prescribed to lower blood pressure. Side effects may include stomach upset, sexual difficulties, and gout. The most serious problem associated with these medications is depletion of potassium or magnesium, which could lead to irregular heart rhythms. Blood levels of these minerals should be monitored.

INSTRUCTIONS

Taking a diuretic early in the day may reduce nighttime urination. If it upsets the stomach, it may be taken with food or milk. See the Food and Drug Compatibility Table on pages 59-73.

BRAND NAME	GENERIC NAME
DiaBeta, Glynase, Micronase	glyburide
Diabinese	chlorpropamide
Glucotrol	glipizide
Orinase	tolbutamide
Tolinase	tolazamide

DESCRIPTION

These pills are prescribed for non-insulin-dependent diabetics. They help control blood sugar by increasing the amount of insulin the pancreas makes and by making body tissues more sensitive to insulin. With diet, exercise, and blood sugar monitoring, they may reduce the risk of complications of diabetes. Low blood sugar (hypoglycemia) is the most common serious side effect. These medications interact with many others; check with your doctor or pharmacist before taking another drug.

INSTRUCTIONS

DiaBeta, Glucotrol, and Micronase should be taken 15 minutes to half an hour before meals. The others may be taken with food if they upset the stomach. Blood glucose monitoring is important. Notify the doctor immediately if you experience rash, fever, sore throat, or unusual bleeding or bruising.

INTERACTION

Diuretics can raise blood sugar in susceptible people, especially diabetics. Such medicine can also make oral diabetes drugs less effective. *This interaction could be troublesome, leading to hyperglycemia.*

The interaction may become noticeable within a few days of taking the two drugs together, or it may not show up for a few months. If both drugs are needed, blood sugar levels should be monitored so that the doctor can adjust the dose of the diabetes medicine appropriately. Electrolyte levels and kidney function should also be checked; an excessive loss of potassium or even sodium is possible.

Never take or stop medication without your doctor's advice.

INTERACTION

TROUBLESOME

Diuretics
(LOOP)

Heart/Blood Pressure Drugs
(ACE INHIBITORS)

BRAND NAME	GENERIC NAME
Bumex	bumetanide
Edecrin	ethacrynic acid
Lasix	furosemide

DESCRIPTION

Diuretics ("water pills") help the body eliminate excess fluid caused by congestive heart failure or kidney trouble, or as a side effect of other drugs. They are, however, most widely prescribed to lower blood pressure. While well tolerated, they may cause side effects, including stomach upset, sexual difficulties, and gout. Probably the most serious problem associated with these medications is a gradual depletion of potassium or magnesium, which could lead to irregular heart rhythms. Blood levels of these minerals should be monitored.

INSTRUCTIONS

Taking a diuretic early in the day may reduce nighttime urination. If it causes stomach upset, the drug may be taken with food or milk. See the Food and Drug Compatibility Table on pages 59-73 for specifics.

BRAND NAME	GENERIC NAME
Accupril	quinapril
Altace	ramipril
Capoten	captopril
Lotensin	benazepril
Monopril	fosinopril
Prinivil, Zestril	lisinopril
Vasotec	enalapril

DESCRIPTION

These medications are used to treat high blood pressure. They block angiotensin-converting enzyme, or ACE. Capoten and Vasotec can also be helpful in treating congestive heart failure. Capoten also helps conserve kidney function in diabetics. The ACE inhibitors are usually very well tolerated, but blood pressure may be lowered so much that a person starting on one of these medicines becomes dizzy or faints, especially upon standing up. Caution is advised. Some people on these medicines develop a nagging dry cough not helped by cough medicine.

INSTRUCTIONS

Capoten should be taken one hour before meals. High-fat meals may reduce absorption of Accupril. Food does not affect the other drugs in this class.

INTERACTION

Often when blood pressure is not completely controlled by the initial medication, the doctor will prescribe a second medicine in addition. As a result, a patient may need to take both an ACE inhibitor blood pressure drug and a strong diuretic. Some patients have experienced problems when ACE inhibitor drugs were added to a high-dose loop diuretic regimen. Starting either Capoten and Vasotec in conjunction with high doses of diuretics may contribute to excessively low blood pressure. People may feel faint. There also have been a few cases reported in which this combination resulted in serious kidney problems. *Blood pressure and kidney function should be monitored in people on a loop diuretic together with an ACE blood pressure drug.* Serum electrolytes (sodium, potassium, etc.) should also be monitored.

Never take or stop medication without your doctor's advice.

INTERACTION

TROUBLESOME

Diuretics

(POTASSIUM-WASTING)

Laxatives

BRAND NAME	GENERIC NAME
Aquatensen, Enduron	methyclothiazide
Bumex	bumetanide
Diachlor, Diuril	chlorothiazide
Diucardin, Saluron	hydroflumethiazide
Edecrin	ethacrynic acid
Esidrix, HydroDIURIL	hydrochlorothiazide
Hygroton, Hylidone	chlorthalidone
Lasix	furosemide
Lozol	indapamide
etc.	

DESCRIPTION

Diuretics ("water pills") help eliminate excess fluid due to congestive heart failure or kidney trouble, or as a side effect of other drugs. They are most often prescribed to lower blood pressure. Side effects may include stomach upset, sexual difficulties, and gout. The most serious problem associated with these medications is depletion of potassium or magnesium, which may lead to irregular heart rhythms. Blood levels of these minerals should be monitored.

INSTRUCTIONS

Taking a diuretic early in the day may reduce nighttime urination. If it upsets the stomach, it may be taken with food or milk. See the Food and Drug Compatibility Table on pages 59-73.

DESCRIPTION

There is an extraordinary variety of laxatives on the market. They range from relatively mild bulk-forming products that contain methylcellulose and polycarbophil to stimulant cathartics such as castor oil, cascara sagrada, and senna. The regular or routine use of any laxative can create problems and is often referred to as "laxative abuse" by gastroenterologists. It can lead to dehydration, nutritional imbalance, severe diarrhea, and electrolyte imbalance. Potassium loss is considered a very serious consequence, especially for people with heart problems.

INSTRUCTIONS

Try to avoid regular use of any laxative. A high-fiber diet that incorporates bran, fruits, and vegetables and includes lots of liquids can often eliminate the need for laxatives. If a laxative is needed, bulk-forming products are believed to be the safest.

INTERACTION

Regular use of laxatives can lead to loss of potassium from the body. Since diuretics can also deplete the body of potassium, such a combination can create serious potassium disturbances. This could be life threatening, especially if a person were also taking a digitalis-type heart medicine (see page 321). DO NOT make laxatives a part of your routine if you are also on a potassium-wasting diuretic!

Normal Serum Potassium Levels: 3.5 to 5 mEq/L

Never take or stop medication without your doctor's advice.

INTERACTION

TROUBLESOME

Heart Drugs
(DIGOXIN)
Lanoxin

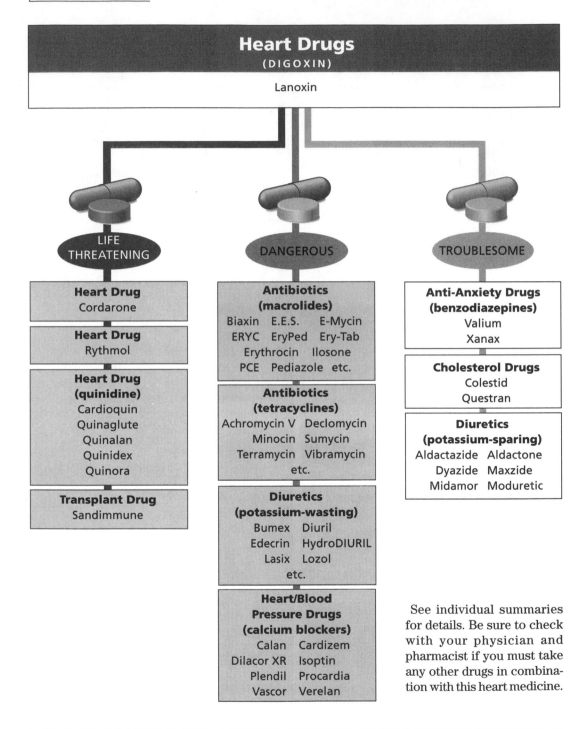

LIFE THREATENING

Heart Drug
Cordarone

Heart Drug
Rythmol

Heart Drug (quinidine)
Cardioquin
Quinaglute
Quinalan
Quinidex
Quinora

Transplant Drug
Sandimmune

DANGEROUS

Antibiotics (macrolides)
Biaxin   E.E.S.   E-Mycin
ERYC   EryPed   Ery-Tab
Erythrocin   Ilosone
PCE   Pediazole etc.

Antibiotics (tetracyclines)
Achromycin V   Declomycin
Minocin   Sumycin
Terramycin   Vibramycin
etc.

Diuretics (potassium-wasting)
Bumex   Diuril
Edecrin   HydroDIURIL
Lasix   Lozol
etc.

Heart/Blood Pressure Drugs (calcium blockers)
Calan   Cardizem
Dilacor XR   Isoptin
Plendil   Procardia
Vascor   Verelan

TROUBLESOME

Anti-Anxiety Drugs (benzodiazepines)
Valium
Xanax

Cholesterol Drugs
Colestid
Questran

Diuretics (potassium-sparing)
Aldactazide   Aldactone
Dyazide   Maxzide
Midamor   Moduretic

See individual summaries for details. Be sure to check with your physician and pharmacist if you must take any other drugs in combination with this heart medicine.

Heart Drug

(DIGOXIN)

Heart Drug

(AMIODARONE)

BRAND NAME	GENERIC NAME
Lanoxin	digoxin

DESCRIPTION

Digoxin is a heart drug that is often very helpful in treating congestive heart failure. It is also prescribed for certain heart rhythm changes, especially atrial fibrillation, atrial flutter, and paroxysmal atrial tachycardia (PAT). The doctor must monitor the digoxin dose carefully, because the effective dose is not far below the toxic dose. Older people may need dose adjustment.

INSTRUCTIONS

Digoxin should be taken in a consistent fashion, preferably with food but not with a meal high in fiber. Bran may limit the absorption of this drug.

Do not stop this medicine unless your doctor so directs.

BRAND NAME	GENERIC NAME
Cordarone	amiodarone

DESCRIPTION

Cordarone is used to treat life-threatening heart rhythm problems affecting the ventricle, or lower part, of the heart. Some doctors prescribe a lower dose for other rhythm disturbances. This medication has potentially serious side effects, and occasionally may exacerbate heart rhythm problems. Hospitalization is recommended for the first doses, and the doctor should monitor your progress carefully.

INSTRUCTIONS

Follow the physician's directions carefully. Tell your doctor if you notice shortness of breath or changes in vision, or if your skin turns blue.

INTERACTION

A patient who needs both these medications should be under the doctor's watchful eye almost all the time. They would be prescribed together only in the case of very serious heart problems. *The interaction is potentially lethal.*

Cordarone can greatly increase levels of the heart drug digoxin, leading to toxicity. In most studies, digoxin levels doubled when Cordarone was added. In some instances, digoxin levels increased as much as 800 percent. At levels this high, a patient is likely to be feeling very sick. Very close monitoring and dose adjustment is essential.

Because Cordarone can last a long time in the body, the problems may continue for some time even if the drug is discontinued. Digoxin levels will probably need close monitoring during that time until they restabilize. If your doctor prescribes this combination, frequent blood tests to check your digoxin levels are essential. Notify your physician immediately if you experience any of the symptoms of digoxin overdose.

Symptoms of Digoxin Toxicity

Nausea, vomiting, loss of appetite, diarrhea, stomach pain, visual disturbances (green or yellow tint and a halo around lights), weakness, drowsiness, depression, confusion, palpitations, rash, headaches, and hallucinations. Notify your doctor immediately if you experience any of these symptoms.

Never take or stop medication without your doctor's advice.

INTERACTION

LIFE THREATENING

Heart Drug

(DIGOXIN)

Heart Drug

(PROPAFENONE)

BRAND NAME	GENERIC NAME
Lanoxin	digoxin

DESCRIPTION

Digoxin is a heart drug that is often very helpful in treating congestive heart failure. It is also prescribed for certain heart rhythm changes, especially atrial fibrillation, atrial flutter, and paroxysmal atrial tachycardia (PAT). The doctor must monitor the digoxin dose carefully, because the effective dose is not far below the toxic dose. Older people may need dose adjustment.

INSTRUCTIONS

Digoxin should be taken in a consistent fashion, preferably with food but not with a meal high in fiber. Bran may limit the absorption of this drug.

Do not stop this medicine unless your doctor so directs.

BRAND NAME	GENERIC NAME
Rythmol	propafenone

DESCRIPTION

Rythmol is used to treat severe, life-threatening heartbeat disturbances affecting the lower part of the heart, called the ventricle. Some doctors have prescribed it for other serious arrhythmias. Older people may need lower doses.

INSTRUCTIONS

These tablets are best taken with food every eight hours. Alert the doctor if you develop symptoms of toxicity such as unusual sleepiness, low blood pressure, slower heart rate, or abnormal heartbeats. Do not stop this medicine unless your doctor tells you to.

INTERACTION

A patient with complicated heart problems may require this combination of potent medications together with very careful monitoring. Both of these heart medicines are used to control irregular heartbeats. This is a relatively new interaction, but it seems well documented. Digoxin levels may become dangerously high. *This situation could be lethal.*

To avoid digoxin toxicity, make sure your physician monitors your serum digoxin levels very closely. The dose may have to be adjusted to keep the digoxin level normal. Notify your physician instantly if you experience any symptoms of toxicity.

Symptoms of Digoxin Toxicity

Nausea, vomiting, loss of appetite, diarrhea, stomach pain, visual disturbances (green or yellow tint and a halo around lights), weakness, drowsiness, depression, confusion, palpitations, rash, headaches, and hallucinations. Notify your doctor immediately if you experience any of these symptoms.

Never take or stop medication without your doctor's advice.

INTERACTION

LIFE THREATENING

Heart Drug

(DIGOXIN)

Heart Drug

(QUINIDINE)

BRAND NAME	GENERIC NAME
Lanoxin	digoxin

DESCRIPTION

Digoxin is a heart drug that is often very helpful in treating congestive heart failure. It is also prescribed for certain heart rhythm changes, especially atrial fibrillation, atrial flutter, and paroxysmal atrial tachycardia (PAT). The doctor must monitor the digoxin dose carefully, because the effective dose is not far below the toxic dose. Older people may need dose adjustment.

INSTRUCTIONS

Digoxin should be taken in a consistent fashion, preferably with food but not with a meal high in fiber. Bran may limit the absorption of this drug.

Do not stop this medicine unless your doctor so directs.

BRAND NAME	GENERIC NAME
Cardioquin	quinidine
Quinaglute	quinidine
Quinalan	quinidine
Quinidex	quinidine
Quinora	quinidine

DESCRIPTION

Quinidine is prescribed for a variety of heart rhythm disturbances. The first dose is considered a test to see if the patient will have a dangerous reaction. People with heart failure, or with liver or kidney disease, need close monitoring.

INSTRUCTIONS

Quinidine may upset the stomach. Taking it with food may help alleviate this problem. Sustained-release tablets (Quinaglute Dura-Tabs, Quinalan, Quinidex Extentabs) should not be chewed or crushed.

Quinidine may provoke visual disturbances, ringing in the ears, headache, dizziness, nausea, skin rash, or breathing difficulties. Notify your doctor if you develop any of these symptoms. Do not stop this medicine unless your doctor so directs.

INTERACTION

These drugs may both be needed for treating atrial flutter or atrial fibrillation, or in some other situations. Unfortunately, quinidine increases and may even double blood levels of digoxin. *This interaction could result in serious or life-threatening digitalis toxicity.*

It took 60 years before doctors discovered how dangerous these two heart drugs can be in combination. If both drugs are needed, the cardiologist should monitor you closely so the dose can be adjusted properly. Measuring serum levels of digoxin may not be enough to ensure safety. It is necessary but not sufficient, since electrocardiogram changes may occur even when blood levels of digoxin are within the "normal" range (0.5 to 2 ng/ml). Stay in close touch with your doctor and let him or her know of any symptoms.

Symptoms of Digoxin Toxicity

Nausea, vomiting, loss of appetite, diarrhea, stomach pain, visual disturbances (green or yellow tint and a halo around lights), weakness, drowsiness, depression, confusion, palpitations, rash, headaches, and hallucinations. Notify your doctor immediately if you experience any of these symptoms.

Never take or stop medication without your doctor's advice.

INTERACTION

LIFE THREATENING

Heart Drug
(DIGOXIN)

Transplant Drug
(CYCLOSPORINE)

BRAND NAME | GENERIC NAME
Lanoxin | digoxin

DESCRIPTION

Digoxin is a heart drug that is often very helpful in treating congestive heart failure. It is also prescribed for certain heart rhythm changes, especially atrial fibrillation, atrial flutter, and paroxysmal atrial tachycardia (PAT). The doctor must monitor the digoxin dose carefully, because the effective dose is not far below the toxic dose. Older people may need dose adjustment.

INSTRUCTIONS

Digoxin should be taken in a consistent fashion, preferably with food but not with a meal high in fiber. Bran may limit the absorption of this drug.

Do not stop this medicine unless your doctor so directs.

BRAND NAME | GENERIC NAME
Sandimmune | cyclosporine

DESCRIPTION

Sandimmune suppresses the immune system so that a person receiving a transplant does not reject this lifesaving organ. Doctors have also tried using it in treating autoimmune diseases, in which the immune system attacks a person's own tissues. Multiple sclerosis is an example.

INSTRUCTIONS

Sandimmune comes as an oral solution with a taste reminiscent of castor oil. It should be mixed in a glass with milk, chocolate milk, or orange juice at room temperature and drunk at once. Then the glass (no plastic) should be rinsed and the rinsing fluid drunk to get the full dose. Do not take Sandimmune with grapefruit juice unless the physician is monitoring blood levels of the drug closely. (See page 43.) Due to a possible interaction between cyclosporine and oral contraceptives, barrier methods of contraception should be used while taking this drug.

Regular monitoring is important. Do not stop this medicine unless your doctor so directs.

INTERACTION

This interaction could be life threatening. It was discovered when people awaiting heart transplant were given the immune-suppressing drug Sandimmune in addition to the heart drug digoxin. The result was a significant rise in digoxin levels and severe digoxin toxicity. When patients require both these medications, they are usually seriously ill and under close medical supervision. Physicians will need to monitor digoxin blood levels closely and adjust the dose carefully. *Be alert for signs of toxicity and notify your doctor if you experience any.*

Symptoms of Digoxin Toxicity

Nausea, vomiting, loss of appetite, diarrhea, stomach pain, visual disturbances (green or yellow tint and a halo around lights), weakness, drowsiness, depression, confusion, palpitations, rash, headaches, and hallucinations. Notify the doctor immediately if you experience any of these symptoms.

INTERACTION

LIFE THREATENING

Heart Drug

(DIGOXIN)

Antibiotics

(MACROLIDES)

BRAND NAME | GENERIC NAME

Lanoxin | digoxin

DESCRIPTION

Digoxin is a heart drug that is often very helpful in treating congestive heart failure. It is also prescribed for certain heart rhythm changes, especially atrial fibrillation, atrial flutter, and paroxysmal atrial tachycardia (PAT). The doctor must monitor the digoxin dose carefully, because the effective dose is not far below the toxic dose. Older people may need dose adjustment.

INSTRUCTIONS

Digoxin should be taken in a consistent fashion, preferably with food but not with a meal high in fiber. Bran may limit the absorption of this drug.

Do not stop this medicine unless your doctor so directs.

E.E.S.	**E-Mycin**
ERYC	**EryPed**
Ery-Tab	**Erythrocin**
Eryzole	**Ilosone**
Ilotycin	**Pediazole**
PCE	**Robimycin**

DESCRIPTION

The antibiotic erythromycin is widely prescribed for upper respiratory tract infections, ear infections, *Chlamydia*, and other infections of the reproductive tract (nongonococcal urethritis in men, some pelvic inflammations in women), Legionnaires' disease, intestinal amoebas, and certain other infections.

INSTRUCTIONS

Some forms of erythromycin must be taken on an empty stomach; others may be taken with food. See pages 59-73 for specifics. Liquid suspensions should be stored in the refrigerator and shaken well before each dose. Finish the entire prescription unless your doctor tells you to stop.

INTERACTION

This is a strange interaction that affects only a small percentage of those who take the heart medicine digoxin. No one knows why one in ten people reacts differently to digoxin than the rest of us. These individuals depend on bacteria in their digestive tract to help eliminate this heart medicine from their system. If bacteria in the gut are killed off by the antibiotic erythromycin, digoxin levels can climb, possibly to toxic levels. *In susceptible people, erythromycin boosts blood levels of digoxin; this interaction could prove dangerous.*

There is no simple way to tell if you are among the 10 percent who depend on bacteria in the GI tract to metabolize digoxin. To avoid toxicity, ask your physician to monitor your serum digoxin levels carefully and adjust the dose accordingly. This reaction can persist for weeks or months after erythromycin has been stopped. That is because it can take a long time for the good bacteria in your gut to reestablish a normal balance. Tell your doctor if you have symptoms of digoxin overdose.

Symptoms of Digoxin Toxicity

Nausea, vomiting, loss of appetite, diarrhea, stomach pain, visual disturbances (green or yellow tint and a halo around lights), weakness, drowsiness, depression, confusion, palpitations, rash, headaches, and hallucinations. Notify your doctor immediately if you experience any of these symptoms.

Never take or stop medication without your doctor's advice.

INTERACTION

DANGEROUS

Heart Drug
(DIGOXIN)

Antibiotics
(TETRACYCLINES)

BRAND NAME	GENERIC NAME
Lanoxin	digoxin

DESCRIPTION

Digoxin is a heart drug that is often very helpful in treating congestive heart failure. It is also prescribed for certain heart rhythm changes, especially atrial fibrillation, atrial flutter, and paroxysmal atrial tachycardia (PAT). The doctor must monitor the digoxin dose carefully, because the effective dose is not far below the toxic dose. Older people may need dose adjustment.

INSTRUCTIONS

Digoxin should be taken in a consistent fashion, preferably with food but not with a meal high in fiber. Bran may limit the absorption of this drug.

Do not stop this medicine unless your doctor so directs.

BRAND NAME	GENERIC NAME
Achromycin V	tetracycline
Declomycin	demeclocycline
Doryx	doxycycline
Minocin	minocycline
Rondomycin	methacycline
Sumycin	tetracycline
Terramycin	oxytetracycline
Uri-Tet	oxytetracycline
Vibramycin	doxycycline

DESCRIPTION

Tetracycline antibiotics are prescribed for a wide variety of infections, from Rocky Mountain spotted fever to common problems such as acne. Tetracycline is generally inappropriate for pregnant women and young children, because it may stain permanent teeth.

INSTRUCTIONS

Take most forms of tetracycline on an empty stomach. See pages 59-73 for specifics. Do not take these drugs with antacids, calcium or iron supplements, or dairy products. Never take outdated tetracycline, which may be toxic to the kidneys.

INTERACTION

This strange interaction affects only a small portion of those who take the heart medicine digoxin. No one knows why one in ten people depends on bacteria in their digestive tracts to help eliminate this heart medicine. If bacteria in the gut are killed off by tetracycline antibiotics, digoxin levels can climb, possibly to toxic levels. *In susceptible people, tetracycline boosts blood levels of digoxin; this interaction could prove dangerous.*

It's hard to tell if you are among the 10 percent who depend on bacteria to metabolize digoxin. To avoid toxicity, ask your physician to monitor your serum digoxin levels carefully and adjust the dose accordingly. It can take a long time for the bacteria in your gut to reestablish a normal balance after tetracycline has been stopped, so this reaction can persist for weeks or months. Tell your doctor if you have symptoms of digoxin toxicity.

Symptoms of Digoxin Toxicity

Nausea, vomiting, loss of appetite, diarrhea, stomach pain, visual disturbances (green or yellow tint and a halo around lights), weakness, drowsiness, depression, confusion, palpitations, rash, headaches, and hallucinations. Notify the doctor immediately if you experience any of these symptoms.

INTERACTION

DANGEROUS

Heart Drug

(DIGOXIN)

Diuretics

(POTASSIUM-WASTING)

BRAND NAME	GENERIC NAME
Lanoxin	digoxin

DESCRIPTION

Digoxin is a heart drug that is often very helpful in treating congestive heart failure. It is also prescribed for certain heart rhythm changes, especially atrial fibrillation, atrial flutter, and paroxysmal atrial tachycardia (PAT). The doctor must monitor the digoxin dose carefully, because the effective dose is not far below the toxic dose. Older people may need dose adjustment.

INSTRUCTIONS

Digoxin should be taken in a consistent fashion, preferably with food but not with a meal high in fiber. Bran may limit the absorption of this drug.

Do not stop this medicine unless your doctor so directs.

BRAND NAME	GENERIC NAME
Bumex	bumetanide
Diachlor, Diuril	chlorothiazide
Diucardin, Saluron	hydroflumethiazide
Edecrin	ethacrynic acid
Enduron	methyclothiazide
Esidrix, HydroDIURIL	hydrochlorothiazide
Hygroton	chlorthalidone
Lasix	furosemide
Lozol	indapamide

DESCRIPTION

Diuretics ("water pills") help the body eliminate excess fluid caused by congestive heart failure or kidney trouble, or as a side effect of other drugs. They are most widely prescribed to lower blood pressure. Side effects may include stomach upset, sexual difficulties, and gout. Probably the most serious side effect is a gradual depletion of potassium or magnesium, which could lead to irregular heart rhythms. Blood levels of these minerals should be monitored.

INSTRUCTIONS

Taking a diuretic early in the day may reduce nighttime urination. If it causes stomach upset, the drug may be taken with food or milk.

INTERACTION

Physicians may prescribe diuretics in combination with digoxin to rid the body of excess fluid. There is rarely a problem, but electrolytes must be monitored carefully to avoid the danger of loss of potassium or magnesium. When these minerals are too low, digoxin might cause dangerous heart rhythm irregularities. *This interaction could be very dangerous.*

Regular blood tests are crucial. If levels of potassium and magnesium drop below the normal range, your doctor will probably prescribe supplements. Keep a diary of your potassium and magnesium levels.

Symptoms of Too Little Potassium: Muscle cramps, weakness, difficulty breathing, lethargy, and irregular heart rhythms.

Symptoms of Low Magnesium: Hard to diagnose. Be alert for loss of appetite, nausea, vomiting, weakness, fatigue, personality change, tremor, and muscle twitches.

Normal Electrolyte Values: Potassium: 3.5 to 5 mEq/L . Magnesium: 1.8 to 3 mEq/L

INTERACTION

DANGEROUS

Heart Drug
(DIGOXIN)

Heart/Blood Pressure Drugs
(CALCIUM CHANNEL BLOCKERS)

BRAND NAME	GENERIC NAME
Lanoxin	digoxin

DESCRIPTION

Digoxin is a heart drug that is often very helpful in treating congestive heart failure. It is also prescribed for certain heart rhythm changes, especially atrial fibrillation, atrial flutter, and paroxysmal atrial tachycardia (PAT). The doctor must monitor the digoxin dose carefully, because the effective dose is not far below the toxic dose. Older people may need dose adjustment.

INSTRUCTIONS

Digoxin should be taken in a consistent fashion, preferably with food but not with a meal high in fiber. Bran may limit the absorption of this drug.

Do not stop this medicine unless your doctor so directs.

BRAND NAME	GENERIC NAME
Adalat, Procardia	nifedipine
Calan, Isoptin, Verelan	verapamil
Cardizem, Dilacor XR	diltiazem
Plendil	felodipine
Vascor	bepridil

DESCRIPTION

Calcium channel blockers are popular drugs for lowering blood pressure, treating angina, and, in the case of verapamil, stabilizing irregular heart rhythms. Some of these drugs are prescribed to prevent migraine or cluster headaches, ward off exercise-induced asthma, or treat congestive heart failure.

INSTRUCTIONS

These drugs come in a variety of doses; follow the doctor's directions. Sustained-release forms should not be chewed or crushed. Taking Adalat, Plendil, or Procardia with grapefruit juice could boost blood levels of the drug unexpectedly. See the table of Food and Drug Compatibility on pages 59-73. If the drug must be discontinued, follow the doctor's instructions for gradual tapering.

INTERACTION

Patients with certain heart rhythm problems may require this combination of medicines. Others might be taking both drugs to treat different conditions. In either event, this interaction could be a problem, resulting in higher than expected digoxin levels. Be alert for signs of toxicity. The doctor should monitor blood levels of digoxin and also the electrocardiogram. Verapamil can raise serum digoxin levels as much as 75 percent, enough to result in toxicity in some cases. Diltiazem also seems to raise digoxin levels in the blood, although the studies do not agree on this effect. Bepridil, a relatively new blood pressure medicine, interacts with digoxin to slow heartbeat and modify the electrocardiogram. *This interaction could be dangerous.*

Symptoms of Digoxin Toxicity

Nausea, vomiting, loss of appetite, diarrhea, stomach pain, visual disturbances (green or yellow tint and a halo around lights), weakness, drowsiness, depression, confusion, palpitations, rash, headaches, and hallucinations. Notify your doctor immediately if you experience any of these symptoms.

INTERACTION

DANGEROUS

Heart Drug

(DIGOXIN)

Anti-Anxiety Drugs

(BENZODIAZEPINES)

BRAND NAME	GENERIC NAME
Lanoxin	digoxin

DESCRIPTION

Digoxin is a heart drug that is often very helpful in treating congestive heart failure. It is also prescribed for certain heart rhythm changes, especially atrial fibrillation, atrial flutter, and paroxysmal atrial tachycardia (PAT). The doctor must monitor the digoxin dose carefully, because the effective dose is not far below the toxic dose. Older people may need dose adjustment.

INSTRUCTIONS

Digoxin should be taken in a consistent fashion, preferably with food but not with a meal high in fiber. Bran may limit the absorption of this drug.

Do not stop this medicine unless your doctor so directs.

BRAND NAME	GENERIC NAME
Valium	diazepam
Xanax	alprazolam

DESCRIPTION

Benzodiazepines are used to treat anxiety disorders and insomnia. Some are employed to relieve panic attacks, seizures, and muscle cramps. Anesthesiologists use such medications before certain surgical procedures.

Prolonged use may lead to dependence. Withdrawal should always be supervised by your physician.

INSTRUCTIONS

These drugs may be taken with food, especially if they upset the digestive tract.

INTERACTION

Valium (diazepam) has been shown to raise the blood levels of digoxin. One woman had a dramatic jump in digoxin after she started taking Xanax at bedtime for insomnia. She experienced symptoms of digoxin toxicity, including digestive tract upset, fatigue, and "head pressure." This Xanax and digoxin interaction remains unconfirmed in a more scientific study, however. Other benzodiazepines have not been adequately tested. Until such research is completed, people should have their digoxin levels monitored frequently if they need to take a benzodiazepine-type drug simultaneously.

Symptoms of Digoxin Toxicity

Nausea, vomiting, loss of appetite, diarrhea, stomach pain, visual disturbances (green or yellow tint and a halo around lights), weakness, drowsiness, depression, confusion, palpitations, rash, headaches, and hallucinations. Notify your doctor immediately if you experience any of these symptoms.

Never take or stop medication without your doctor's advice.

INTERACTION

TROUBLESOME

Heart Drug
(DIGOXIN)

Cholesterol Drugs

BRAND NAME | GENERIC NAME
Lanoxin | digoxin

DESCRIPTION

Digoxin is a heart drug that is often very helpful in treating congestive heart failure. It is also prescribed for certain heart rhythm changes, especially atrial fibrillation, atrial flutter, and paroxysmal atrial tachycardia (PAT). The doctor must monitor the digoxin dose carefully, because the effective dose is not far below the toxic dose. Older people may need dose adjustment.

INSTRUCTIONS

Digoxin should be taken in a consistent fashion, preferably with food but not with a meal high in fiber. Bran may limit the absorption of this drug.

Do not stop this medicine unless your doctor so directs.

BRAND NAME | GENERIC NAME
Colestid | colestipol
Questran | cholestyramine

DESCRIPTION

These medicines are used to lower blood cholesterol and thus reduce the risk of heart attack. They work by binding to cholesterol-rich bile acids in the intestine and removing them from the circulation. For best effectiveness, they should be used together with a heart-healthy, low-fat diet.

INSTRUCTIONS

These drugs are to be taken before meals and washed down with plenty of fluids. Vitamin supplements may be advisable. If used, the supplements should be taken at least one hour before or six hours after the cholesterol medicine.

INTERACTION

It is entirely possible a person could have irregular heartbeats and high cholesterol, and so need both these medicines. Unfortunately, Colestid and Questran bind not only to bile acids, but also to other drugs. They can reduce the absorption of digoxin by 20 to 40 percent, leading to lowered digoxin levels. *For patients with irregular heart rhythms or congestive heart failure who depend on digoxin, this interaction is worrisome.*

It is usually possible to overcome this drug interaction by taking the cholesterol-lowering drugs at a different time of day from digoxin. Allow at least eight hours either before or after taking digoxin to prevent interference with its absorption.

The best way to determine if this interaction is causing trouble is to monitor serum digoxin levels carefully. Ask your physician for periodic tests. If digoxin levels drop too low, your doctor will want to adjust the dosage.

Never take or stop medication without your doctor's advice.

INTERACTION

TROUBLESOME

Heart Drug

(DIGOXIN)

Diuretics

(POTASSIUM-SPARING)

BRAND NAME	GENERIC NAME
Lanoxin	digoxin

DESCRIPTION

Digoxin is a heart drug that is often very helpful in treating congestive heart failure. It is also prescribed for certain heart rhythm changes, especially atrial fibrillation, atrial flutter, and paroxysmal atrial tachycardia (PAT). The doctor must monitor the digoxin dose carefully, because the effective dose is not far below the toxic dose. Older people may need dose adjustment.

INSTRUCTIONS

Digoxin should be taken in a consistent fashion, preferably with food but not with a meal high in fiber. Bran may limit the absorption of this drug.

Do not stop this medicine unless your doctor so directs.

BRAND NAME	GENERIC NAME
Aldactazide	spironolactone, HCTZ
Aldactone	spironolactone
Dyazide	triamterene, HCTZ
Maxzide	triamterene, HCTZ
Midamor	amiloride
Moduretic	amiloride, HCTZ

DESCRIPTION

Diuretics encourage the kidneys to eliminate excess fluid from the body. This can be useful in controlling high blood pressure, congestive heart failure, and certain other conditions. Spironolactone is also used to treat a hormonal condition called hyperaldosteronism. With other diuretics, important minerals (especially potassium and magnesium) are lost along with the fluid. With the above group of drugs, however, potassium is conserved.

INSTRUCTIONS

Midamor may upset the stomach, so it is best taken right after meals. Midamor and Aldactone may interfere with the alertness and coordination necessary for driving. Periodic blood tests for magnesium and potassium are advisable.

INTERACTION

This is an incredibly complicated interaction that could create considerable confusion. Aldactone and Aldactazide may produce falsely elevated readings of standard tests of serum digoxin levels. In other words, because of inaccurate test results, a physician might think patients were getting too much digoxin when in fact they were getting the right amount of digoxin. But there is also evidence that these diuretics may actually boost digoxin levels, thereby increasing the risk of side effects. Be vigilant for signs of digoxin toxicity.

Midamor and Moduretic may also increase digoxin levels, especially in patients with reduced kidney function. But these diuretics may partially interfere with the effectiveness of digoxin. If such drugs are combined, it is very important to monitor digoxin reaction and heart function.

Symptoms of Digoxin Toxicity

Nausea, vomiting, loss of appetite, diarrhea, stomach pain, visual disturbances (green or yellow tint and a halo around lights), weakness, drowsiness, depression, confusion, palpitations, rash, headaches, and hallucinations. Notify your doctor immediately if you experience any of these symptoms.

Never take or stop medication without your doctor's advice.

INTERACTION

TROUBLESOME

Heart/Blood Pressure Drugs
(ACE INHIBITORS)

| Accupril | Altace | Capoten | Lotensin |
| Monopril | Prinivil | Vasotec | Zestril |

LIFE THREATENING

Diuretics (potassium-sparing)
Aldactazide   Aldactone
Dyazide   Dyrenium
Maxzide   Midamor
Moduretic

Potassium
Kaon-Cl   Kay Ciel
K-Dur   Klor-Con
Klorvess   Klotrix
K-Lyte   K-Norm
K-Tab   Micro-K
Slow-K   Ten-K
etc.

DANGEROUS

Arthritis Drugs and Aspirin

Gout Medicine
Zyloprim

Lithium
Cibalith-S   Eskalith
Lithobid   Lithonate
Lithotabs

Transplant Drug
Sandimmune

TROUBLESOME

Diabetes Drugs
DiaBeta
Diabinese
Dymelor
Glucotrol
Glynase
Micronase
Orinase
Tolinase

Diuretics (loop)
Bumex
Edecrin
Lasix

Tuberculosis Drug (rifampin)
Rifadin
Rifamate
Rimactane

Not every ACE inhibitor blood pressure drug interacts with each drug listed on this overview tree. See individual descriptions for details. Be sure to check with your physician and pharmacist if you must take any other drugs in combination with any of these blood pressure pills.

LEVELS OF HAZARD: LIFE THREATENING   DANGEROUS   TROUBLESOME

Heart/Blood Pressure Drugs
(ACE INHIBITORS)

Diuretics
(POTASSIUM-SPARING)

BRAND NAME	GENERIC NAME
Accupril	quinapril
Altace	ramipril
Capoten	captopril
Lotensin	benazepril
Monopril	fosinopril
Prinivil, Zestril	lisinopril
Vasotec	enalapril

BRAND NAME	GENERIC NAME
Aldactazide	spironolactone, HCTZ
Aldactone	spironolactone
Dyazide	triamterene, HCTZ
Dyrenium	triamterene
Maxzide	triamterene, HCTZ
Midamor	amiloride
Moduretic	amiloride, HCTZ

DESCRIPTION

These medications are used to treat high blood pressure. They block angiotensin-converting enzyme, or ACE. Capoten and Vasotec can also be helpful in treating congestive heart failure. Capoten also helps conserve kidney function in diabetics. The ACE inhibitors are usually very well tolerated, but blood pressure may be lowered so much that a person starting on one of these medicines becomes dizzy or faints, especially upon standing up. Caution is advised. Some people on these medicines develop a nagging dry cough not helped by cough medicine.

INSTRUCTIONS

Capoten should be taken one hour before meals. High-fat meals may reduce absorption of Accupril. Food does not affect the other drugs in this class.

DESCRIPTION

Diuretics encourage the kidneys to eliminate excess fluid from the body. This can be useful in controlling high blood pressure, congestive heart failure, and certain other conditions. Spironolactone is also used to treat a hormonal condition called hyperaldosteronism. With other diuretics, important minerals (especially potassium and magnesium) are lost along with the fluid. With the above group of drugs, however, potassium is conserved.

INSTRUCTIONS

Midamor and Dyrenium may upset the stomach, so they are best taken right after meals. Maxzide can be taken without regard to meals. Midamor and Aldactone may interfere with the alertness and coordination necessary for driving. Periodic blood tests for magnesium and potassium are advisable.

INTERACTION

Capoten, Vasotec, and other drugs in this category may increase potassium levels in susceptible patients. When these drugs are combined with potassium-sparing diuretics, serum potassium levels could rise into the dangerous range. *This situation could be life threatening. Irregular heart rhythms and cardiac arrest might occur.* **Deaths have been reported.** Elderly patients and those with kidney problems appear to be at the highest risk of this interaction. Diabetes may also contribute to the danger. Otherwise healthy patients may have no trouble and some with very low potassium levels may actually benefit from such a combination with careful medical supervision. However, if a potassium-sparing diuretic is prescribed together with an ACE inhibitor blood pressure drug, potassium levels should be monitored very closely. This may also be true of combination diuretics such as Dyazide and Maxzide.

Normal Serum Potassium Levels: 3.5 to 5 mEq/L

Never take or stop medication without your doctor's advice.

INTERACTION

LIFE THREATENING

Heart/Blood Pressure Drugs
(ACE INHIBITORS)

Potassium

BRAND NAME	GENERIC NAME
Accupril	quinapril
Altace	ramipril
Capoten	captopril
Lotensin	benazepril
Monopril	fosinopril
Prinivil, Zestril	lisinopril
Vasotec	enalapril

DESCRIPTION

These medications are used to treat high blood pressure. They block angiotensin-converting enzyme, or ACE. Capoten and Vasotec are helpful in treating congestive heart failure. Capoten also helps conserve kidney function in diabetics. The ACE inhibitors are usually very well tolerated, but blood pressure may be lowered so much that a person starting on one of these medicines becomes dizzy or faints upon standing up. Caution is advised. Some people on these medicines develop a nagging dry cough.

INSTRUCTIONS

Capoten should be taken one hour before meals. High-fat meals may reduce absorption of Accupril. Food does not affect the other drugs in this class.

BRAND NAME		
Kaon-Cl	**Kay Ciel**	**K-Dur**
Klor-Con	**Klorvess**	**Klotrix**
K-Lyte	**K-Norm**	**K-Tab**
Micro-K	**Slow-K**	**Ten-K**
etc.		

DESCRIPTION

Potassium is an essential mineral that must be maintained within normal limits for good health. Heart, kidney, muscle, and nerve cells all need it for proper functioning. When potassium levels drop too low, a person may feel weak, tire easily, experience numbness or tingling of hands or feet, and have trouble breathing and abnormal heart rhythms. Too much potassium is equally dangerous, and many of the symptoms are similar: breathing difficulty, heart rhythm disturbances, weakness, tiredness, confusion, slow heart rate, and changes on the electrocardiogram.

INSTRUCTIONS

These supplements may upset the stomach. They are best taken right after meals, with a full glass of water. Tell your doctor immediately if you have nausea, vomiting, abdominal pain, or black stools.

INTERACTION

Capoten, Vasotec, and other drugs in this category may increase potassium levels, particularly in susceptible patients. Without frequent blood tests to monitor serum potassium levels, the combination of potassium supplements and one of these ACE inhibitors can lead to excessive levels of the mineral (over 5.5 mEq/L). *This interaction could lead to irregular heart rhythms and cardiac arrest.* **Deaths have been reported.**

Elderly patients and those with kidney problems appear at highest risk from this interaction. Diabetes may also contribute to the danger. Otherwise healthy patients may have no trouble. However, if a potassium supplement is prescribed together with an ACE blood pressure drug, potassium levels should be monitored closely.

Salt substitutes, many containing potassium, are often recommended for people with high blood pressure. If you are taking one of these blood pressure medicines, do not use a commercial salt substitute unless you have regular blood tests for serum potassium.

Normal Serum Potassium Levels: 3.5 to 5 mEq/L

INTERACTION

LIFE THREATENING

Heart/Blood Pressure Drugs
(ACE INHIBITORS)

Arthritis Drugs
(NSAIDS)

BRAND NAME	GENERIC NAME
Accupril	quinapril
Altace	ramipril
Capoten	captopril
Lotensin	benazepril
Monopril	fosinopril
Prinivil, Zestril	lisinopril
Vasotec	enalapril

BRAND NAME	GENERIC NAME
Advil, Motrin, Nuprin	ibuprofen
Aleve, Naprosyn	naproxen
Ansaid	flurbiprofen
Aspirin	aspirin
Indocin	indomethacin
Lodine	etodolac
Relafen	nabumetone
Toradol	ketorolac
etc.	

DESCRIPTION

These medications are used to treat high blood pressure. They block angiotensin-converting enzyme, or ACE. Capoten and Vasotec can also be helpful in treating congestive heart failure. Capoten also helps conserve kidney function in diabetics. The ACE inhibitors are usually very well tolerated, but blood pressure may be lowered so much that a person starting on one of these medicines becomes dizzy or faints, especially upon standing up. Caution is advised. Some people on these medicines develop a nagging dry cough not helped by cough medicine.

INSTRUCTIONS

Capoten should be taken one hour before meals. High-fat meals may reduce absorption of Accupril. Food does not affect the other drugs in this class.

DESCRIPTION

Nonsteroidal anti-inflammatory drugs (NSAIDs) can ease pain, lower a fever, and help control inflammation. They are frequently prescribed for arthritis, as well as for muscle strains, headaches, lower back discomfort, menstrual pain, and other conditions. These medications can cause serious digestive tract upset, including heartburn, indigestion, and bleeding or perforated ulcers. Careful medical monitoring is essential.

INSTRUCTIONS

Take with food to reduce the risk of stomach irritation. (See table on pages 59-73.) Aspirin and OTC ibuprofen or naproxen should not be mixed with prescription NSAIDs or each other.

INTERACTION

Some of the arthritis drugs on this list can drastically diminish the effectiveness of blood pressure medicines such as Capoten or Vasotec. Indocin can wipe out the blood-pressure-lowering power of these drugs; ibuprofen can interact similarly with Capoten. Even aspirin given with or before Vasotec can reduce that drug's benefit for treating congestive heart failure. Although some people do not react badly to this combination, it makes sense to assume that any arthritis medicine could interfere with any ACE medication, and keep careful tabs on blood pressure and cardiac function if both drugs are needed. *This interaction could be dangerous.*

Kidney problems are a rare but serious reaction to both these classes of drugs. Taking them in combination may increase the risk of this problem. *Notify the doctor immediately of sudden weight gain, swollen legs and feet, change in the color of the urine, or unusual back pain.* A kidney function test may be in order. **Monitor blood pressure regularly.**

Never take or stop medication without your doctor's advice.

INTERACTION

DANGEROUS

Heart/Blood Pressure Drugs
(ACE INHIBITORS)

Gout Medicine
(ALLOPURINOL)

BRAND NAME	GENERIC NAME
Accupril	quinapril
Altace	ramipril
Capoten	captopril
Lotensin	benazepril
Monopril	fosinopril
Prinivil, Zestril	lisinopril
Vasotec	enalapril

DESCRIPTION

These medications are used to treat high blood pressure. They block angiotensin-converting enzyme, or ACE. Capoten and Vasotec can also be helpful in treating congestive heart failure. Capoten also helps conserve kidney function in diabetics. The ACE inhibitors are usually very well tolerated, but blood pressure may be lowered so much that a person starting on one of these medicines becomes dizzy or faints, especially upon standing up. Caution is advised. Some people on these medicines develop a nagging dry cough not helped by cough medicine.

INSTRUCTIONS

Capoten should be taken one hour before meals. High-fat meals may reduce absorption of Accupril. Food does not affect the other drugs in this class.

BRAND NAME	GENERIC NAME
Lopurin	allopurinol
Zurinol	allopurinol
Zyloprim	allopurinol

DESCRIPTION

Gout occurs when high blood levels of uric acid lead to a buildup of uric acid crystals in the joints. Allopurinol blocks the enzyme that leads to uric acid formation, and thereby keeps levels of uric acid in the body and in the joints under control. It is sometimes prescribed for other conditions in which uric acid levels may be high, such as leukemia and lymphoma, and is helpful in preventing the formation of calcium oxalate kidney stones. Rash, fever, unusual bleeding or bruising, muscle aches, or yellow skin and eyes could indicate a serious reaction to allopurinol. Contact your doctor immediately if you notice any of these symptoms.

INSTRUCTIONS

Allopurinol may upset the stomach less if it is taken with food or milk. While on this drug, drink at least ten full glasses of fluid daily. Because allopurinol may cause drowsiness, try to avoid driving or other complex tasks while taking this medicine.

INTERACTION

If gout and high blood pressure are both problems, the doctor may want to prescribe both these medications. There are several cases reported of serious hypersensitivity reactions when Zyloprim and Capoten are combined. This reaction may begin as a rash and progress to a potentially fatal syndrome called Stevens-Johnson. Joint pain and fever may accompany this reaction. Although researchers cannot be sure that the cases were due to the interaction rather than to either drug alone, it is suspected that a person on both medicines may be more susceptible. *This interaction could be dangerous. At least one death has been reported.*

Patients with kidney failure are likely to be at greatest risk of this problem. There are no reports of Zyloprim interacting with other ACE medications, and experts speculate that an interaction with Vasotec may be unlikely. If you take both allopurinol and an ACE inhibitor, notify your doctor at the earliest hint of a rash.
Symptoms to notice: Rash, joint pain, fever.

Never take or stop medication without your doctor's advice.

INTERACTION

DANGEROUS

Heart/Blood Pressure Drugs
(ACE INHIBITORS)

Lithium

BRAND NAME	GENERIC NAME
Accupril	quinapril
Altace	ramipril
Capoten	captopril
Lotensin	benazepril
Monopril	fosinopril
Prinivil, Zestril	lisinopril
Vasotec	enalapril

DESCRIPTION

These medications are used to treat high blood pressure. They block angiotensin-converting enzyme, or ACE. Capoten and Vasotec can also be helpful in treating congestive heart failure. Capoten also helps conserve kidney function in diabetics. The ACE inhibitors are usually very well tolerated, but blood pressure may be lowered so much that a person starting on one of these medicines becomes dizzy or faints, especially upon standing up. Caution is advised. Some people on these medicines develop a nagging dry cough not helped by cough medicine.

INSTRUCTIONS

Capoten should be taken one hour before meals. High-fat meals may reduce absorption of Accupril. Food does not affect the other drugs in this class.

BRAND NAME
Cibalith-S
Eskalith
Lithobid
Lithonate
Lithotabs

DESCRIPTION

Lithium is most often used to treat bipolar depression, and seems to be especially helpful in easing the manic phases of this disorder. Regular blood tests are advisable for dose adjustment. The toxic dose is not a great deal higher than the effective dose, so the doctor should be notified of signs such as vomiting, diarrhea, unsteadiness in walking, weakness, or unusual drowsiness. This drug can affect the thyroid gland.

INSTRUCTIONS

Lithium should be taken immediately after meals or with food or milk to reduce stomach upset. It is essential to drink 8 to 12 glasses of water or other fluid each day while on lithium. This medication can affect alertness, so activities such as driving or operating machinery can be dangerous for people on lithium.

INTERACTION

A number of cases have been reported in which one of these blood pressure drugs added to a previously stable lithium regimen precipitated symptoms of lithium toxicity. Lithium blood levels were raised into the danger zone. This interaction did not occur in an experiment with ten healthy volunteers, so there may be other factors at play. *Nonetheless, this interaction could be dangerous.*

If both lithium and an ACE blood pressure drug are needed, lithium levels should be monitored.

Symptoms of Lithium Toxicity

Nausea, diarrhea, incoordination, muscle weakness, and difficulty walking may be signs of toxicity. Ringing in the ears, visual problems, dizziness, slurred speech, confusion, agitation, and incontinence are more serious. Notify the physician promptly of any such symptoms.

Never take or stop medication without your doctor's advice.

INTERACTION

DANGEROUS

Heart/Blood Pressure Drugs
(ACE INHIBITORS)

Transplant Drug
(CYCLOSPORINE)

BRAND NAME	GENERIC NAME
Accupril	quinapril
Altace	ramipril
Capoten	captopril
Lotensin	benazepril
Monopril	fosinopril
Prinivil, Zestril	lisinopril
Vasotec	enalapril

DESCRIPTION

These medications are used to treat high blood pressure. They block angiotensin-converting enzyme, or ACE. Capoten and Vasotec can also be helpful in treating congestive heart failure. Capoten also helps conserve kidney function in diabetics. The ACE inhibitors are usually very well tolerated, but blood pressure may be lowered so much that a person starting on one of these medicines becomes dizzy or faints, especially upon standing up. Caution is advised. Some people on these medicines develop a nagging dry cough not helped by cough medicine.

INSTRUCTIONS

Capoten should be taken one hour before meals. High-fat meals may reduce absorption of Accupril. Food does not affect the other drugs in this class.

BRAND NAME	GENERIC NAME
Sandimmune	cyclosporine

DESCRIPTION

Sandimmune suppresses the immune system so that a person receiving a transplant does not reject this lifesaving organ. Doctors have also tried using it in treating autoimmune diseases, in which the immune system attacks a person's own tissues. Multiple sclerosis is an example.

INSTRUCTIONS

Sandimmune comes as an oral solution with a taste reminiscent of castor oil. It should be mixed in a glass with milk, chocolate milk, or orange juice at room temperature and drunk at once. Then the glass (no plastic) should be rinsed and the rinsing fluid drunk to get the full dose. Do not take Sandimmune with grapefruit juice unless the physician is monitoring blood levels of the drug closely. (See page 43.)

Due to a possible interaction between cyclosporine and oral contraceptives, barrier methods of contraception should be used while taking this drug.

Regular monitoring is important. Do not stop this medicine unless your doctor so directs.

INTERACTION

Experts are not sure if Sandimmune really interacts with the ACE blood pressure medicines, but at least two cases have been reported. In these cases, kidney failure developed after Vasotec was added to the patients' medications, and cleared up when Vasotec was withdrawn. There is no reason to believe that Vasotec would be different from other ACE inhibitor drugs in this respect. If one of these medications is needed for a patient taking Sandimmune, kidney function should be monitored closely for at least the first several months. *This interaction could be dangerous.*

INTERACTION

DANGEROUS

Heart/Blood Pressure Drugs
(ACE INHIBITORS)

Diabetes Drugs

BRAND NAME	GENERIC NAME
Accupril	quinapril
Altace	ramipril
Capoten	captopril
Lotensin	benazepril
Monopril	fosinopril
Prinivil, **Zestril**	lisinopril
Vasotec	enalapril

BRAND NAME	GENERIC NAME
DiaBeta, Glynase,	
Micronase	glyburide
Diabinese	chlorpropamide
Dymelor	acetohexamide
Glucotrol	glipizide
Orinase	tolbutamide
Tolinase	tolazamide

DESCRIPTION

These medications are used to treat high blood pressure. They block angiotensin-converting enzyme, or ACE. Capoten and Vasotec can also be helpful in treating congestive heart failure. Capoten also helps conserve kidney function in diabetics. The ACE inhibitors are usually very well tolerated, but blood pressure may be lowered so much that a person starting on one of these medicines becomes dizzy or faints, especially upon standing up. Caution is advised. Some people on these medicines develop a nagging dry cough not helped by cough medicine.

INSTRUCTIONS

Capoten should be taken one hour before meals. High-fat meals may reduce absorption of Accupril. Food does not affect the other drugs in this class.

DESCRIPTION

These pills are prescribed for non-insulin-dependent diabetics. They help control blood sugar by increasing the amount of insulin the pancreas makes and by making body tissues more sensitive to insulin. With diet, exercise, and blood sugar monitoring, they may reduce the risk of complications of diabetes. Low blood sugar (hypoglycemia) is the most common serious side effect. These medications interact with many others; check with your doctor or pharmacist before taking another drug.

INSTRUCTIONS

DiaBeta, Glucotrol, and Micronase should be taken 15 minutes to half an hour before meals. The others may be taken with food if they upset the stomach. Blood glucose monitoring is important. Notify your doctor immediately if you experience rash, fever, sore throat, or unusual bleeding or bruising.

INTERACTION

Like many other drugs, ACE blood pressure medicines may increase the effectiveness of the oral diabetes medications. This could cause a greater drop in blood sugar than expected, with possible symptoms of hypoglycemia. Check with your doctor if you notice a change in blood sugar after starting Capoten, Vasotec, or one of the other drugs in this class. Stay alert for symptoms of hypoglycemia. *This interaction could be troublesome.*

Symptoms of Hypoglycemia (Low Blood Sugar)

Shaking, sweating, tiredness, low temperature, faintness, palpitations, hunger, headache, confusion, irritability, visual disturbances, coma. Close observation (preferably in the hospital) is recommended for two or three days after such a reaction.

Never take or stop medication without your doctor's advice.

INTERACTION

TROUBLESOME

Heart/Blood Pressure Drugs
(ACE INHIBITORS)

BRAND NAME	GENERIC NAME
Accupril	quinapril
Altace	ramipril
Capoten	captopril
Lotensin	benazepril
Monopril	fosinopril
Prinivil, Zestril	lisinopril
Vasotec	enalapril

DESCRIPTION

These medications are used to treat high blood pressure. They block angiotensin-converting enzyme, or ACE. Capoten and Vasotec can also be helpful in treating congestive heart failure. Capoten also helps conserve kidney function in diabetics. The ACE inhibitors are usually very well tolerated, but blood pressure may be lowered so much that a person starting on one of these medicines becomes dizzy or faints, especially upon standing up. Caution is advised. Some people on these medicines develop a nagging dry cough not helped by cough medicine.

INSTRUCTIONS

Capoten should be taken one hour before meals. High-fat meals may reduce absorption of Accupril. Food does not affect the other drugs in this class.

Diuretics
(LOOP)

BRAND NAME	GENERIC NAME
Bumex	bumetanide
Edecrin	ethacrynic acid
Lasix	furosemide

DESCRIPTION

Diuretics ("water pills") help the body eliminate excess fluid caused by congestive heart failure or kidney trouble, or as a side effect of other drugs. They are, however, most widely prescribed to lower blood pressure. While well tolerated, they may cause side effects, including stomach upset, sexual difficulties, and gout. Probably the most serious problem associated with these medications is a gradual depletion of potassium or magnesium, which could lead to irregular heart rhythms. Blood levels of these minerals should be monitored.

INSTRUCTIONS

Taking a diuretic early in the day may reduce nighttime urination. If it causes stomach upset, the drug may be taken with food or milk. See the Food and Drug Compatibility Table on pages 59-73 for specifics.

INTERACTION

Often when blood pressure is not completely controlled by the initial medication, the doctor will prescribe a second medicine in addition. As a result, a patient may need to take both an ACE inhibitor blood pressure drug and a strong diuretic. Some patients have experienced problems when ACE inhibitor drugs are added to a high-dose loop diuretic regimen. Starting either Capoten and Vasotec in conjunction with high doses of diuretics may contribute to excessively low blood pressure. People may feel faint. There are also a few cases reported in which this combination resulted in serious kidney problems. *Blood pressure and kidney function should be monitored in people on a loop diuretic together with an ACE blood pressure drug.* Serum electrolytes (sodium, potassium, etc.) should also be monitored.

Never take or stop medication without your doctor's advice.

INTERACTION

TROUBLESOME

Heart/Blood Pressure Drugs
(ACE INHIBITORS)

Tuberculosis Drug
(RIFAMPIN)

BRAND NAME	GENERIC NAME
Accupril	quinapril
Altace	ramipril
Capoten	captopril
Lotensin	benazepril
Monopril	fosinopril
Prinivil, Zestril	lisinopril
Vasotec	enalapril

DESCRIPTION

These medications are used to treat high blood pressure. They block angiotensin-converting enzyme, or ACE. Capoten and Vasotec can also be helpful in treating congestive heart failure. Capoten also helps conserve kidney function in diabetics. The ACE inhibitors are usually very well tolerated, but blood pressure may be lowered so much that a person starting on one of these medicines becomes dizzy or faints, especially upon standing up. Caution is advised. Some people on these medicines develop a nagging dry cough not helped by cough medicine.

INSTRUCTIONS

Capoten should be taken one hour before meals. High-fat meals may reduce absorption of Accupril. Food does not affect the other drugs in this class.

BRAND NAME	GENERIC NAME
Rifadin	rifampin
Rifamate	isoniazid/rifampin
Rimactane	rifampin

DESCRIPTION

Rifampin is used in combination with other medications to treat tuberculosis. To be effective, it needs to be taken faithfully for an extended period of time (at least six to nine months), as the doctor prescribes. Side effects may include digestive tract problems, menstrual irregularities, difficulty concentrating, fluid retention, and wheezing or shortness of breath. The orange discoloration of urine, saliva, and tears is not harmful, although it may stain contact lenses.

INSTRUCTIONS

Rifampin should be taken on an empty stomach, at least one hour before or two hours after meals. If you develop fever, chills, unusual tiredness, unusual bleeding or bruising, sore throat, muscle and bone pain, or yellow skin and eyes, contact your physician immediately.

INTERACTION

The tuberculosis medication may counteract the ACE blood pressure drugs, although evidence for this interaction is weak. One 35-year-old man with high blood pressure and tuberculosis was treated with this combination of medicines (together with several others). Vasotec was controlling his blood pressure well, but when rifampin was added, his blood pressure rose. Rifampin was discontinued, and his blood pressure returned to normal. When the antituberculosis agent was given again, his blood pressure soared again.

No one knows if the interaction was peculiar to this individual, or if it may occur more commonly. If both rifampin and an ACE inhibitor drug are needed, blood pressure should be monitored carefully. *This interaction could be troublesome.*
Monitor blood pressure regularly.

INTERACTION

TROUBLESOME

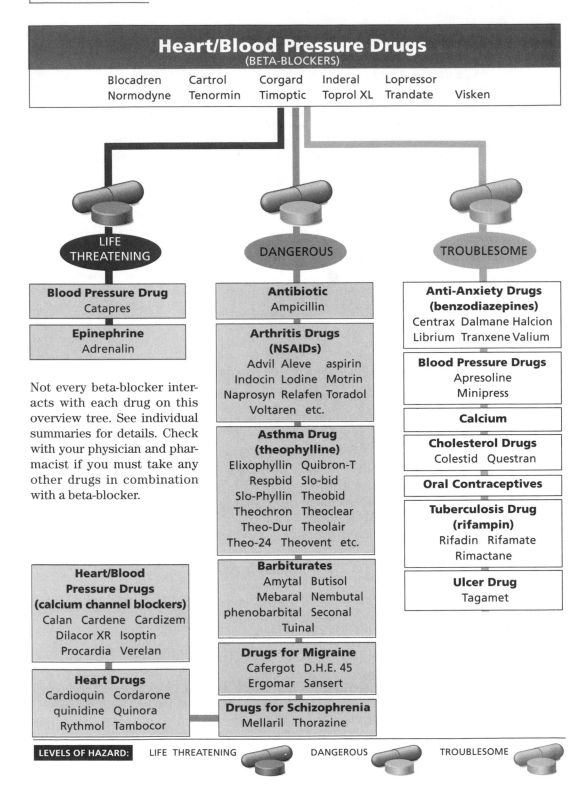

Heart/Blood Pressure Drugs
(BETA-BLOCKERS)

Blocadren	Cartrol	Corgard	Inderal	Lopressor	
Normodyne	Tenormin	Timoptic	Toprol XL	Trandate	Visken

LIFE THREATENING

Blood Pressure Drug
Catapres

Epinephrine
Adrenalin

Not every beta-blocker interacts with each drug on this overview tree. See individual summaries for details. Check with your physician and pharmacist if you must take any other drugs in combination with a beta-blocker.

**Heart/Blood Pressure Drugs
(calcium channel blockers)**
Calan Cardene Cardizem
Dilacor XR Isoptin
Procardia Verelan

Heart Drugs
Cardioquin Cordarone
quinidine Quinora
Rythmol Tambocor

DANGEROUS

Antibiotic
Ampicillin

**Arthritis Drugs
(NSAIDs)**
Advil Aleve aspirin
Indocin Lodine Motrin
Naprosyn Relafen Toradol
Voltaren etc.

**Asthma Drug
(theophylline)**
Elixophyllin Quibron-T
Respbid Slo-bid
Slo-Phyllin Theobid
Theochron Theoclear
Theo-Dur Theolair
Theo-24 Theovent etc.

Barbiturates
Amytal Butisol
Mebaral Nembutal
phenobarbital Seconal
Tuinal

Drugs for Migraine
Cafergot D.H.E. 45
Ergomar Sansert

Drugs for Schizophrenia
Mellaril Thorazine

TROUBLESOME

**Anti-Anxiety Drugs
(benzodiazepines)**
Centrax Dalmane Halcion
Librium Tranxene Valium

Blood Pressure Drugs
Apresoline
Minipress

Calcium

Cholesterol Drugs
Colestid Questran

Oral Contraceptives

**Tuberculosis Drug
(rifampin)**
Rifadin Rifamate
Rimactane

Ulcer Drug
Tagamet

LEVELS OF HAZARD: LIFE THREATENING   DANGEROUS   TROUBLESOME

Heart/Blood Pressure Drugs
(BETA-BLOCKERS)

Blood Pressure Drug
(CLONIDINE)

BRAND NAME	GENERIC NAME
Blocadren	timolol
Inderal	propranolol
Tenormin	atenolol
(other beta-blockers may also interact)	

DESCRIPTION

Beta-blockers such as these are often used to lower blood pressure, stabilize irregular heartbeats, relieve angina, or prevent migraines. Despite the great usefulness and versatility of these medicines, in general they are not appropriate for people with chronic breathing problems, because they can trigger airway tightening. Other side effects include changes in heart rate, cold hands and feet, and depression.

INSTRUCTIONS

Propranolol is best absorbed with meals, but consistency is the most important factor. These drugs should be taken at about the same time every day. Do not stop any of these medicines suddenly except on doctor's orders. Serious side effects could result.

BRAND NAME	GENERIC NAME
Catapres	clonidine

DESCRIPTION

Catapres is used primarily to control high blood pressure. Although the FDA has not approved its use for other indications, this drug has been employed to relieve withdrawal symptoms associated with stopping narcotics, nicotine, and alcohol. It has also been used to treat the flushing of menopause and the nerve pain left after an attack of shingles.

INSTRUCTIONS

The dose of clonidine must be individualized. There are no recommendations about taking it with food or on an empty stomach. A morning and bedtime dose represents the usual regimen. Catapres should never be discontinued abruptly because it may cause jitteriness, agitation, headache, rapid pulse, palpitations, and a sudden rise in blood pressure. If this drug must be stopped, the dose should be gradually reduced over two to four days under careful medical supervision.

INTERACTION

There are confusing reports that simultaneous administration of Inderal and Catapres may reduce the antihypertensive action of one or both drugs. This has not been confirmed. What does appear clear, however, is that no one who is taking both a beta-blocker and clonidine should ever discontinue either drug suddenly. There have been life-threatening sudden increases in blood pressure when Catapres was stopped while someone was also taking a beta-blocker. *This situation is potentially lethal.*

The manufacturer recommends that "if therapy is to be discontinued in patients receiving beta-blockers and clonidine concurrently, beta-blockers should be discontinued several days before the gradual withdrawal of Catapres."

Symptoms of Rebound Hypertension

Sudden discontinuation of Catapres could lead to anxiety, agitation, headache, palpitations, rapid pulse, nausea, flushing, vomiting, or rapid increase in blood pressure. Notify the physician immediately of any of these symptoms.

Never take or stop medication without your doctor's advice.

INTERACTION

LIFE THREATENING

Heart/Blood Pressure Drugs
(BETA-BLOCKERS)

Epinephrine

BRAND NAME	GENERIC NAME
Blocadren	timolol
Corgard	nadolol
Inderal	propranolol

(other beta-blockers may also interact)

DESCRIPTION

Beta-blockers such as these are often used to lower blood pressure, stabilize irregular heartbeats, relieve angina, or prevent migraines. Despite the great usefulness and versatility of these medicines, in general they are not appropriate for people with chronic breathing problems, because they can trigger airway tightening. Other side effects include changes in heart rate, cold hands and feet, and depression.

INSTRUCTIONS

Propranolol is best absorbed with meals, but consistency is the most important factor. These drugs should be taken at about the same time every day. Do not stop any of these medicines suddenly except on doctor's orders. Serious side effects could result.

BRAND NAME	
Adrenalin	**Ana-Guard**
Ana-Kit	**Bronitin Mist**
Emergent-Ez Kit	**EpiPen**
Primatene Mist	**Sus-Phrine**
etc.	

DESCRIPTION

Epinephrine (Adrenalin) is used either in an aerosol inhaler or by injection to relieve acute asthma attacks. It is also the first step in the emergency treatment of severe allergic reactions (anaphylaxis) to drugs (such as penicillin) or insect stings (wasps, yellow jackets, etc.). Epinephrine is often included with injectable local anesthetics (lidocaine, Xylocaine, etc.) to constrict blood vessels, prevent bleeding, and delay absorption of the local anesthetic as used during plastic surgery, dentistry, and minor surgical procedures.

INSTRUCTIONS

Injectable epinephrine is often administered by a physician or nurse. Patients may carry emergency sting kits (Ana-Kit, EpiPen) for use against a life-threatening allergic reaction.

INTERACTION

People taking a beta-blocker may experience an extremely dangerous elevation in blood pressure if epinephrine is injected. There are a number of cases in the medical literature of people who went in for plastic surgery while taking propranolol. Shortly after an injection of the local anesthetic Xylocaine combined with epinephrine, systolic blood pressure skyrocketed—in some cases to over 200. One woman went to the emergency room with a bad case of hives. When she arrived her blood pressure was 120/70. Two minutes after an injection of epinephrine she complained of a bad headache and her blood pressure zoomed to 220/110. She experienced a stroke. *This interaction can be life threatening.*

We have found no cases of hypertensive crisis due to the aerosol form of epinephrine interacting with beta-blockers, but a physician should supervise such a combination.

Symptoms of Hypertensive Crisis

Headache, rapid increase in blood pressure, palpitations, chest pain, chills, nausea, anxiety, and perspiration. Stroke is a risk. Notify your physician immediately of any of these symptoms.

Never take or stop medication without your doctor's advice.

INTERACTION

LIFE THREATENING

Heart/Blood Pressure Drugs
(BETA-BLOCKERS)

Antibiotic
(PENICILLIN-TYPE)

BRAND NAME	GENERIC NAME
Tenormin	atenolol

(other beta-blockers may also interact)

DESCRIPTION

Beta-blockers are often used to lower blood pressure, stabilize irregular heartbeats, relieve angina, or prevent migraines. Despite the great usefulness and versatility of these medicines, in general they are not appropriate for people with chronic breathing problems, because they can trigger airway tightening. Other side effects include changes in heart rate, cold hands and feet, and depression. These adverse reactions may be less common with Tenormin, but careful monitoring is essential.

INSTRUCTIONS

Tenormin is probably best taken with meals, but consistency is the most important factor. Tenormin should be taken at roughly the same time every day. Do not stop any beta-blocker suddenly except on doctor's orders. Serious side effects could result.

BRAND NAME	GENERIC NAME
Omnipen	ampicillin
Polycillin	ampicillin
Principen	ampicillin
Totacillin	ampicillin

DESCRIPTION

Ampicillin is a penicillin-type broad-spectrum antibiotic. It is effective against a wide range of bacterial infections, including those caused by staph, strep, *Salmonella*, and *Shigella*. It is prescribed for conditions such as strep throat, ear infections, pneumonia, sinusitis, urinary tract infections, and gonorrhea. People who are allergic to penicillin cannot take ampicillin. Such reactions can be life threatening. Skin rash, itching, breathing difficulty, anxiety, and agitation are symptoms of an allergic reaction and require immediate emergency treatment.

INSTRUCTIONS

Ampicillin, like most penicillin-type antibiotics, is best taken with a full eight-ounce glass of water on an empty stomach (one hour before meals or two hours after eating). Successful therapy requires completing all pills to prevent reinfection.

INTERACTION

Ampicillin may reduce the absorption of Tenormin. Blood levels of this beta-blocker may reach only one fourth to one half of those expected when the antihypertensive agent is taken by itself. This might diminish the blood-pressure-lowering and anti-anginal benefits of the beta-blocker. Such an effect could be disastrous for certain patients. If an antibiotic such as penicillin must be given to someone taking a beta-blocker such as Tenormin, it is critical to monitor blood pressure and heart function frequently.

People allergic to penicillin may be in far greater danger if they are also taking a beta-blocker. Deaths are reported in cases in which people taking Inderal or Corgard developed anaphylactic shock after exposure to penicillin. Beta-blockers may make severe allergic reactions (anaphylactic shock) worse and may make treatment more difficult (see epinephrine, page 338).

Symptoms of Beta-Blocker Undertreatment

Blood pressure may climb and heart symptoms might appear. Notify your physician promptly of any symptoms such as chest pain or palpitations.

INTERACTION

DANGEROUS

Heart/Blood Pressure Drugs
(BETA-BLOCKERS)

Arthritis Drugs
(NSAIDS)

BRAND NAME	GENERIC NAME
Blocadren	timolol
Corgard	nadolol
Inderal	propranolol
Lopressor, Toprol XL	metoprolol
Tenormin	atenolol
Visken	pindolol

(Other beta-blockers may also interact.)

DESCRIPTION

Beta-blockers such as these are often used to lower blood pressure, stabilize irregular heartbeats, relieve angina, or prevent migraines. Despite the usefulness of these medicines, in general they are not appropriate for people with chronic breathing problems, because they can trigger airway tightening. Other side effects include changes in heart rate, cold hands and feet, and depression.

INSTRUCTIONS

Inderal and Lopressor are best taken with meals, but consistency is the most important factor. These drugs should be taken at about the same time every day. Do not stop any of these medicines suddenly except on doctor's orders. Serious side effects could result.

BRAND NAME	GENERIC NAME
Advil, Motrin, Nuprin	ibuprofen
Aleve, Naprosyn	naproxen
Ansaid	flurbiprofen
Aspirin	aspirin
Indocin	indomethacin
Lodine	etodolac
Relafen	nabumetone
Toradol	ketorolac
etc.	

DESCRIPTION

Nonsteroidal anti-inflammatory drugs (NSAIDs) can ease pain, lower a fever, and help control inflammation. They are prescribed for arthritis, muscle strains, headaches, and other conditions. These medications can cause serious digestive tract upset, including heartburn, indigestion, and bleeding or perforated ulcers. Careful medical monitoring is essential.

INSTRUCTIONS

Take with food to reduce the risk of stomach irritation. (See table on pages 59-73.) Aspirin and OTC ibuprofen or naproxen should not be mixed with prescription NSAIDs or each other.

INTERACTION

This combination is of concern because so many people take beta-blockers for high blood pressure and heart problems. Millions rely on NSAIDs for pain relief. And people also consume huge quantities of over-the-counter aspirin, ibuprofen, and naproxen. Some interactions are likely to occur. NSAIDs may reduce the effectiveness of blood-pressure-lowering beta-blockers. Physicians and patients may not realize a beta-blocker is not working as efficiently as it should to control hypertension. Experts warn doctors to avoid this combination if possible. The arthritis drug Clinoril (sulindac) may be less likely to interact with beta-blockers, but no matter which arthritis drug is used, people taking an arthritis drug in combination with a beta-blocker will need to have blood pressure monitored frequently. If hypertension becomes a problem, the physician should adjust the dose of beta-blocker or reconsider treatment options.

Symptoms of Beta-Blocker Undertreatment

Blood pressure may climb and heart symptoms might appear. Be alert for chest pain or palpitations and notify your doctor immediately. Monitor blood pressure carefully.

INTERACTION

DANGEROUS

Heart/Blood Pressure Drugs
(BETA-BLOCKERS)

Asthma Drug
(THEOPHYLLINE)

BRAND NAME	GENERIC NAME
Blocadren	timolol
Cartrol	carteolol
Inderal	propranolol
Levatol	penbutolol
Timoptic	timolol
Visken	pindolol

BRAND NAME

Aerolate	**Aquaphyllin**	**Asmalix**
Bronkodyl	**Elixomin**	**Elixophyllin**
Quibron-T	**Respbid**	**Slo-bid**
Slo-Phyllin	**Theobid**	**Theochron**
Theoclear	**Theo-Dur**	**Theolair**
Theo-24	**Theovent**	**Theo-X**
T-Phyl	**Uniphyl**	

DESCRIPTION

Beta-blockers are prescribed to lower blood pressure, stabilize irregular heartbeats, or prevent migraines. Timoptic eye drops help control glaucoma. Despite the usefulness and versatility of these medicines, in general they are not appropriate for people with chronic breathing problems, because they can trigger airway tightening. Other side effects include changes in heart rate, cold hands and feet, and depression.

INSTRUCTIONS

Cartrol, Levatol, and Visken are taken with or without food. Inderal is best absorbed with meals, but consistency is more important. It should be taken at roughly the same time every day. Ask your eye doctor to show you how to administer Timoptic drops so that their absorption is minimized. Do not stop any of these medicines suddenly except on doctor's orders. Serious side effects could result.

DESCRIPTION

Theophylline helps to open airways, so it is generally used to treat and prevent asthma attacks. It may also be prescribed for people with emphysema or other chronic breathing problems. Babies and elderly men may need lower doses. The dose is monitored with regular blood tests to ensure that levels are less than 20 mcg/ml.

INSTRUCTIONS

Theophylline interacts with food in complex ways, so discuss this issue thoroughly with your doctor and pharmacist. Theophylline may upset the stomach. In some cases this problem can be alleviated by taking the drug with food. See the table of Food and Drug Interactions on pages 59-73 for more information.

INTERACTION

Because beta-blockers can make breathing difficult, they are not often prescribed for people with asthma. The beta-blockers named above can reduce the body's ability to clear theophylline, resulting in increased blood levels of theophylline, with the potential for theophylline toxicity. *This interaction could be dangerous.*

Neither Corgard nor Tenormin interferes with theophylline clearance. It is uncommon but certainly not unknown for eye drops such as Timoptic to be absorbed into the body and produce systemic side effects. In that case, Timoptic could interact with theophylline.

Symptoms of Theophylline Toxicity

Nausea, diarrhea, stomach pain, headache, insomnia, restlessness, and irritability. Severe toxicity (convulsions, heart rhythm changes, or death) may occur with no warning symptoms. Notify your doctor immediately if you suspect a problem.

Never take or stop medication without your doctor's advice.

INTERACTION

DANGEROUS

Heart/Blood Pressure Drugs
(BETA-BLOCKERS)

Barbiturates

BRAND NAME	GENERIC NAME
Inderal	propranolol
Lopressor, Toprol XL	metoprolol
(other beta-blockers may also interact)	

DESCRIPTION

Beta-blockers such as these are often used to lower blood pressure, stabilize irregular heartbeats, relieve angina, or prevent migraines. Despite the great usefulness and versatility of these medicines, in general they are not appropriate for people with chronic breathing problems, because they can trigger airway tightening. Other side effects include changes in heart rate, cold hands and feet, and depression.

INSTRUCTIONS

Propranolol and metoprolol are best taken with meals, but consistency is the most important factor. These drugs should be taken at about the same time every day. Do not stop any of these medicines suddenly except on doctor's orders. Serious side effects could result.

BRAND NAME	GENERIC NAME
Alurate	aprobarbital
Amytal	amobarbital
Butisol	butabarbital
Fiorinal	butalbital/aspirin/ caffeine
Lotusate	talbutal
Mebaral	mephobarbital
Nembutal	pentobarbital
Seconal	secobarbital
Solfoton	phenobarbital
Tuinal	combination

DESCRIPTION

Barbiturates were once used as sedatives, but some are prescribed more frequently now to prevent seizures. Fiorinal is used to treat tension headaches. These medications can cause dependence if used for an extended period of time. Stopping suddenly could trigger severe withdrawal symptoms. Barbiturates interact with many other drugs, so check with your pharmacist or physician before taking any other medications.

INSTRUCTIONS

Any of these medications can cause drowsiness and should not be used if you must drive or operate machinery. Never drink alcohol if you are taking a barbiturate.

INTERACTION

Because barbiturates accelerate drug metabolism, many medications become less effective if they are taken in combination with barbiturates. Birth control pills, acetaminophen (Tylenol, etc.), and beta-blockers are just some of the drugs that are affected. Physicians and patients may not realize a beta-blocker is not working as efficiently as it should to control hypertension or maintain heart health. Anyone taking a beta-blocker such as Inderal or Lopressor should have blood pressure and heart function monitored carefully. If problems develop, a physician may need to change the dose of the beta-blocker or reevaluate treatment options.

Symptoms of Beta-Blocker Undertreatment

Blood pressure may climb and heart symptoms might appear. Be alert for chest pain or palpitations. Monitor blood pressure carefully. Notify the physician promptly of any symptoms.

INTERACTION

DANGEROUS

Heart/Blood Pressure Drugs

(BETA-BLOCKERS)

Drugs for Migraine

(ERGOT-BASED)

BRAND NAME	GENERIC NAME
Blocadren	timolol
Corgard	nadolol
Inderal	propranolol
Levatol	penbutolol
Visken	pindolol

(other beta-blockers may also interact)

BRAND NAME	GENERIC NAME
Cafergot	ergotamine
Cafetrate	ergotamine
D.H.E. 45	dihydroergotamine
Ercaf	ergotamine
Ergomar	ergotamine
Ergostat	ergotamine
Sansert	methysergide

DESCRIPTION

These beta-blockers are used to lower blood pressure, stabilize irregular heartbeats, relieve angina, or prevent migraines. Timoptic eye drops treat glaucoma. Despite their usefulness, in general these medicines are not appropriate for people with chronic breathing problems, because they can make airways tighten. Other side effects include changes in heart rate, cold hands and feet, and depression.

INSTRUCTIONS

Inderal is best absorbed with meals, but consistency is most important. Take these drugs at approximately the same time every day. Do not stop any of these medicines suddenly because serious side effects could result.

DESCRIPTION

The precise mechanism of migraine medicine remains elusive. Ergotamine may modify neurochemicals responsible for pain. Sansert affects serotonin, a key neurotransmitter in migraine attacks. Ergotamine can constrict blood vessels throughout the body, especially in the hands and feet. Patients should NEVER take more medicine than recommended by a physician! Circulatory problems could result.

INSTRUCTIONS

Sansert is best taken with food to reduce digestive upset. Ergotamine is to be taken at the very first signs of a migraine attack. Never take more than three tablets per 24 hours, or more than 10 mg per week.

INTERACTION

This interaction is quite controversial. Physicians have been arguing about its likelihood and significance for more than 20 years. We do worry about it, though, because beta-blockers such as propranolol are often prescribed to prevent migraine headaches. Such patients may also take ergotamine to treat a severe migraine attack. Consequently, this interaction could occur quite frequently. The fear is that such a combination may increase constriction in blood vessels in the extremities. This could lead to reduced blood flow and even gangrene. One person had his leg amputated below the knee because of such a reaction. Physicians should be very cautious about prescribing beta-blockers and ergotamine simultaneously. Dosage should be adjusted carefully and people monitored for adequate circulation.

Symptoms of Ergotamine Toxicity

Pale, cold fingers or toes; a feeling of numbness, tingling, or pain in extremities; weakness in arms or legs, especially after exercise. Such symptoms require emergency treatment.

Never take or stop medication without your doctor's advice.

INTERACTION

DANGEROUS

Heart/Blood Pressure Drugs
(BETA-BLOCKERS)

BRAND NAME	GENERIC NAME
Inderal	propranolol
Visken	pindolol

(other beta-blockers may also interact)

DESCRIPTION

Beta-blockers such as these are often used to lower blood pressure, stabilize irregular heartbeats, relieve angina, or prevent migraines. Despite the great usefulness and versatility of these medicines, in general they are not appropriate for people with chronic breathing problems, as they can trigger airway tightening. Other side effects include changes in heart rate, cold hands and feet, and depression.

INSTRUCTIONS

Inderal is best absorbed with meals, but consistency is the most important factor. These drugs should be taken at the same time and in the same way every day. Do not stop any of these medicines suddenly except on doctor's orders. Serious side effects could result.

Drugs for Schizophrenia

BRAND NAME	GENERIC NAME
Mellaril	thioridazine
Thorazine	chlorpromazine

DESCRIPTION

Mellaril and Thorazine are prescribed primarily for serious mental illness, agitation, and anxiety disorders. Such drugs can help control hallucinations and disorganized thinking. These antipsychotic medications have a range of serious side effects and may affect the electrocardiogram. Muscle spasms and uncontrollable movements (tardive dyskinesia) may appear, particularly after long-term use.

INSTRUCTIONS

Mellaril and Thorazine are best taken with food. The dose is highly variable and must be individualized for each patient. These drugs can make skin more sensitive to sunburn; avoid exposure or use appropriate protection. Notify your doctor of vision problems, yellow skin or eyes, or muscle twitching.

INTERACTION

This is a very complex interaction. Each drug may affect metabolism of the other to increase blood levels. This could lead to increased side effects from either or both. In one study, blood levels of Thorazine were five times higher in many patients while they also took propranolol.

Other beta-blockers may also interact with the drugs for schizophrenia. For example, Visken (pindolol) boosted Mellaril levels by more than one-third.

Mellaril and Thorazine can also increase blood levels of beta-blockers. Be alert for increased side effects. Anyone on such a combination should be monitored carefully. *This interaction could be dangerous.*

Symptoms of Beta-Blocker Toxicity

If beta-blocker blood levels get too high, people may experience side effects such as low blood pressure, very slow heart rate, breathing difficulties, or heart failure.

Symptoms of Chlorpromazine Toxicity

Delirium, agitation, drowsiness, low blood pressure, supersensitivity to sun, grand mal seizure. Notify the physician promptly of any symptoms of toxicity of either drug.

Never take or stop medication without your doctor's advice.

INTERACTION

DANGEROUS

Heart/Blood Pressure Drugs
(BETA-BLOCKERS)

Heart Drugs

BRAND NAME	GENERIC NAME
Inderal	propranolol
Lopressor, Toprol XL	metoprolol
Tenormin	atenolol

DESCRIPTION

Beta-blockers such as these are often used to lower blood pressure, stabilize irregular heartbeats, relieve angina, or prevent migraines. Despite the great usefulness and versatility of these medicines, in general they are not appropriate for people with chronic breathing problems, because they can trigger airway tightening. Other side effects include changes in heart rate, cold hands and feet, and depression.

INSTRUCTIONS

Propranolol and metoprolol are best taken with meals, but consistency is the most important factor. These drugs should be taken at about the same time every day. Do not stop any of these medicines suddenly except on doctor's orders. Serious side effects could result.

BRAND NAME	GENERIC NAME
Cardioquin	quinidine
Cordarone	amiodarone
Quinaglute	quinidine
Quinidex	quinidine
Quinora	quinidine
Rythmol	propafenone
Tambocor	flecaininde

DESCRIPTION

Cordarone, quinidine, Rythmol, and Tambocor are prescribed to control serious arrhythmias (irregular heart rhythms). Unfortunately, these drugs can also promote arrhythmias. Cardiologists are cautious about prescribing such medications because of the possibility of causing more harm than good. Consequently, they are often reserved for life-threatening arrhythmias. Hospitalization is recommended for the first doses of Cordarone, and the doctor should monitor the patient's progress carefully.

INSTRUCTIONS

Quinidine is best taken with food to reduce stomach upset. Tambocor can also be taken with meals. Check with your physician and pharmacist on proper dosing for all these drugs because the dose must be individualized and timed carefully.

INTERACTION

Cordarone, quinidine, Rythmol, and Tambocor may alter the metabolism of some beta-blockers. Blood levels of propranolol, metoprolol, and atenolol have been increased, sometimes substantially. This has occasionally lead to an exaggerated effect of the beta-blocker and produced symptoms such as dizziness, low blood pressure, nightmares, and cardiac failure. If such drugs are prescribed together, it is important that a physician monitor cardiac function quite carefully and modify dosage if side effects become a problem. Cordarone may not interact with Tenormin.

Symptoms of Beta-Blocker Toxicity

If beta-blocker blood levels get too high, people may experience side effects such as low blood pressure, dizziness, very slow heart rate, breathing difficulties, or heart failure. Notify your physician promptly of any symptoms.

INTERACTION

DANGEROUS

Heart/Blood Pressure Drugs

(BETA-BLOCKERS)

Heart/Blood Pressure Drugs

(CALCIUM CHANNEL BLOCKERS)

BRAND NAME	GENERIC NAME
Blocadren	timolol
Inderal	propranolol
Lopressor, Toprol XL	metoprolol
Tenormin	atenolol
Timoptic	timolol
Visken	pindolol

BRAND NAME	GENERIC NAME
Adalat, Procardia	nifedipine
Calan, Isoptin,	
Verelan	verapamil
Cardene	nicardipine
Cardizem, Dilacor XR	diltiazem
DynaCirc	isradipine
Plendil	felodipine

DESCRIPTION

These beta-blockers are used to lower blood pressure, stabilize irregular heartbeats, relieve angina, or prevent migraines. Timoptic eye drops treat glaucoma. Despite their usefulness, in general these medicines are not appropriate for people with chronic breathing problems, as they can make airways tighten. Other side effects include changes in heart rate, cold hands and feet, and depression.

INSTRUCTIONS

Inderal and Lopressor are best taken with meals, but consistency is most important. Take these drugs at roughly the same time every day. Ask your eye doctor to show you how to instill Timoptic drops to minimize absorption. Do not stop any of these medicines suddenly because serious side effects could result.

DESCRIPTION

Calcium channel blockers such as Calan and Cardizem are popular drugs for lowering blood pressure, treating angina, and, in the case of verapamil, stabilizing irregular heart rhythms. Some of these drugs have been prescribed to prevent migraine or cluster headaches, ward off exercise-induced asthma, or treat congestive heart failure.

INSTRUCTIONS

These drugs come in a variety of doses; follow the doctor's directions. Sustained-release forms, such as Calan SR and Dilacor XR, should not be chewed or crushed. Taking Adalat, Plendil, or Procardia with grapefruit juice could boost blood levels of the drug unexpectedly. See the table of Food and Drug Compatibility on pages 59-73. If the drug must be discontinued, follow your doctor's instructions for gradual tapering.

INTERACTION

Many people with high blood pressure or unstable angina need a combination of drugs to control their symptoms. Often, a calcium channel blocker and a beta-blocker will work together. Some people, however, experience serious heart problems as a result of an interaction. *This interaction could be dangerous.*

A person who needs both a beta-blocker and a calcium channel blocker should have cardiac function monitored carefully. The doctor may need to adjust the dose of one or both drugs. Nifedipine may be somewhat less likely than other calcium channel blockers to interact with beta-blockers, but serious problems have been reported. Even Timoptic eye drops are capable of interacting with verapamil and, presumably, other calcium blockers. *Notify the doctor if you experience* irregular heartbeat or palpitations, worsening of angina, swelling of hands and feet, shortness of breath, hives, rash, or unusual bleeding.

INTERACTION

DANGEROUS

Heart/Blood Pressure Drugs
(BETA-BLOCKERS)

Anti-Anxiety Drugs
(BENZODIAZEPINES)

BRAND NAME	GENERIC NAME
Inderal	propranolol
Lopressor, Toprol XL	metoprolol

DESCRIPTION

Beta-blockers such as these are often used to lower blood pressure, stabilize irregular heartbeats, relieve angina, or prevent migraines. Despite the great usefulness and versatility of these medicines, in general they are not appropriate for people with chronic breathing problems because they can trigger airway tightening. Other side effects include changes in heart rate, cold hands and feet, and depression.

INSTRUCTIONS

Propranolol and metoprolol are best absorbed with meals, but consistency is the most important factor. These drugs should be taken at about the same time every day. Do not stop any of these medicines suddenly except on doctor's orders. Serious side effects could result.

BRAND NAME	GENERIC NAME
Dalmane	flurazepam
Halcion	triazolam
Librium	chlordiazepoxide
Tranxene	clorazepate
Valium	diazepam

DESCRIPTION

Benzodiazepines are used primarily to treat anxiety disorders and insomnia. Some have also been employed to relieve panic attacks, seizures, muscle cramps, and contractions. Anesthesiologists often use such medications before certain surgical procedures. Xanax has also been prescribed for agoraphobia (fear of crowds or open spaces), premenstrual tension, and psychological depression.

Prolonged use may lead to dependence. Sudden withdrawal can produce unpleasant side effects and should always be supervised by a physician.

INSTRUCTIONS

These drugs may be taken with food, especially if they upset the digestive tract.

INTERACTION

Blood levels of diazepam may be slightly increased by beta-blockers such as metoprolol and propranolol. The anti-anxiety agent also appears to persist longer in the body. People may find they are less alert when on such a combination and their visual acuity and reaction time might be affected. Serax does not seem to be impacted by propranolol. Be sensitive for any change in consciousness.

Symptoms of Benzodiazepine Overdose:

This interaction could lead to symptoms of overdose such as disorientation, unsteadiness, confusion, slurred speech, drowsiness, dizziness, amnesia, and loss of motor coordination. Contact your physician if such symptoms occur.

Never take or stop medication without your doctor's advice.

INTERACTION

TROUBLESOME

Heart/Blood Pressure Drugs
(BETA-BLOCKERS)

Blood Pressure Drugs

BRAND NAME	GENERIC NAME
Inderal	propranolol
Lopressor, Toprol XL	metoprolol

(other beta-blockers may also interact)

DESCRIPTION

Beta-blockers such as these are often used to lower blood pressure, stabilize irregular heartbeats, relieve angina, or prevent migraines. Despite the great usefulness and versatility of these medicines, in general they are not appropriate for people with chronic breathing problems, because they can trigger airway tightening. Other side effects include changes in heart rate, cold hands and feet, and depression.

INSTRUCTIONS

Propranolol and metoprolol are best taken with meals, but consistency is the most important factor. These drugs should be taken at about the same time every day. Do not stop any of these medicines suddenly except on doctor's orders. Serious side effects could result.

BRAND NAME	GENERIC NAME
Alazine	hydralazine
Apresoline	hydralazine
Apresazide	hydralazine, HCTZ
Minipress	prazosin

DESCRIPTION

Hydralazine works to lower blood pressure by dilating blood vessels. It is also used to treat certain heart conditions, such as congestive heart failure. Prazosin is also effective in the treatment of hypertension in part by dilating vessels. Prazosin has been used to improve urinary flow when the prostate gland is enlarged. It may also improve symptoms of Raynaud's disease, a circulatory condition in which the hands and fingers become numb and painful. Side effects of these drugs include dizziness, nausea, and palpitations. When beginning treatment with prazosin, be especially careful because the drug can cause severe dizziness.

INSTRUCTIONS

Hydralazine is best taken with meals. Food will enhance absorption and reduce stomach upset.

INTERACTION

Physicians prescribe beta-blockers and hydralazine with some regularity so this is not an interaction that causes great concern. Nevertheless, the potential exists for each of these drugs to increase blood levels of the other compound and magnify the antihypertensive effect. Beta-blockers also seem to exaggerate the dizziness that occurs when people stand up suddenly while taking prazosin. Blood pressure response should be carefully monitored for people combining beta-blockers and hydralazine or prazosin. If dizziness or low blood pressure becomes a problem, the doctor may need to modify the dose.

Symptoms of Hydralazine Toxicity

Be vigilant for low blood pressure, dizziness, rapid pulse, headache, flushing, and palpitations. With prazosin, be very careful about standing suddenly, as this may lead to dizziness or fainting. Notify your physician of any symptoms.

INTERACTION

TROUBLESOME

Heart/Blood Pressure Drugs
(BETA-BLOCKERS)

Calcium

BRAND NAME	GENERIC NAME
Tenormin	atenolol

(other beta-blockers may also interact)

DESCRIPTION

Beta-blockers are often used to lower blood pressure, stabilize irregular heartbeats, relieve angina, or prevent migraines. Despite the great usefulness and versatility of these medicines, in general they are not appropriate for people with chronic breathing problems, because they can trigger airway tightening. Other side effects include changes in heart rate, cold hands and feet, and depression. These adverse reactions may be less common with Tenormin, but careful monitoring is essential.

INSTRUCTIONS

Tenormin is probably best taken with meals, but consistency is the most important factor. Tenormin should be taken at roughly the same time every day. Do not stop any beta-blocker suddenly except on doctor's orders. Serious side effects could result.

BRAND NAME	GENERIC NAME
Caltrate 600	calcium carbonate
Citracal	calcium citrate
Os-Cal	calcium carbonate
Posture	calcium phosphate
Rolaids Calcium Rich	calcium carbonate
Titralac	calcium carbonate
Tums	calcium carbonate
etc.	

DESCRIPTION

Calcium carbonate is a common antacid found in such popular products as Alkets, Di-Gel Advanced Formula, Dicarbosil, Maalox Caplets, Mylanta Gelcaps, Rolaids Calcium Rich, Titralac, and Tums. It effectively neutralizes stomach acid. Calcium is also used as a dietary supplement to provide nutritional support against osteoporosis. Physicians generally recommend 800 to 1,200 mg of pure calcium daily either from the diet or from mineral supplements. Vitamin D and magnesium enhance the benefits of calcium.

INSTRUCTIONS

Experts recommend that calcium be taken with meals to improve absorption.

INTERACTION

This is probably not a particularly dangerous interaction, but because Tenormin is prescribed so frequently and because so many people are taking calcium-based antacids or supplements, it is an interaction that may occur more frequently than physicians or pharmacists realize. There is data to suggest that calcium reduces blood levels of Tenormin by 30 to 50 percent. Whether this is clinically significant is yet to be determined. There is no agreement in this regard. At the very least people who take atenolol should monitor blood pressure before and after the addition of calcium to their regimen. That way they should be able to determine if calcium supplementation in any way reduces the antihypertensive benefits of this beta-blocker.

Symptoms of Beta-Blocker Undertreatment

Blood pressure may climb and heart symptoms might appear. Be alert for chest pain or palpitations. Monitor blood pressure carefully. Notify your physician of any symptoms.

Never take or stop medication without your doctor's advice.

INTERACTION

TROUBLESOME

Heart/Blood Pressure Drugs
(BETA-BLOCKERS)

Cholesterol Drugs

BRAND NAME	GENERIC NAME
Inderal	propranolol

DESCRIPTION

Beta-blockers such as propranolol are often used to lower blood pressure, stabilize irregular heartbeats, relieve angina, or prevent migraines. Despite the great usefulness and versatility of propranolol, in general it is not appropriate for people with chronic breathing problems, because it can trigger airway tightening. Other side effects include changes in heart rate, cold hands and feet, and depression.

INSTRUCTIONS

Inderal is best absorbed with meals, but consistency is the most important factor. This drug should be taken at approximately the same time every day. Do not stop propranolol or any beta-blocker suddenly except on doctor's orders. Serious side effects could result, including angina, irregular heartbeats, and heart attack.

BRAND NAME	GENERIC NAME
Colestid	colestipol
Questran	cholestyramine

DESCRIPTION

Questran and Colestid are effective drugs for lowering total cholesterol and the particularly dangerous LDL (low-density lipoprotein) cholesterol, which is thought to contribute to coronary artery disease. They do this by binding to bile acids in the intestinal tract and removing them from circulation. Bile is made in the liver and used by the body to digest fats in food. When bile acids are reduced, the body has to work harder to convert cholesterol to make more bile. This is thought to reduce the amount of cholesterol circulating in the bloodstream.

INSTRUCTIONS

Questran and Colestid come in powder form and need to be mixed with a glassful of water. Questran should not be taken with carbonated beverages. These medications are usually taken before meals, but check with your physician or pharmacist for specific instructions.

INTERACTION

The absorption of many drugs may be reduced by these common cholesterol-lowering agents. Acetaminophen (Tylenol, etc.), cortisone-type medications, Coumadin, digitalis drugs, arthritis compounds, diuretics, thyroid hormone, and propranolol seem to be affected. Levels of propranolol could be reduced substantially but experts are still debating the significance of this effect. There is some contradictory data with regard to Colestid; one study actually showed an increase in the blood levels of propranolol when it was taken in combination with Colestid. The recommendation is to monitor blood pressure to see if there is lowered effectiveness. An added precaution to reduce the likelihood of an interaction would be to take propranolol at least one hour before—or four to five hours after—swallowing this cholesterol-lowering drink.

Symptoms of Beta-Blocker Undertreatment

Blood pressure may climb and heart symptoms might appear. Be alert for chest pain or palpitations. Monitor blood pressure carefully. Notify your physician of any symptoms.

INTERACTION

TROUBLESOME

Heart/Blood Pressure Drugs
(BETA-BLOCKERS)

Oral Contraceptives

BRAND NAME	GENERIC NAME
Inderal	propranolol
Lopressor, Toprol XL	metoprolol

(other beta-blockers may also interact)

DESCRIPTION

Beta-blockers such as these are often used to lower blood pressure, stabilize irregular heartbeats, relieve angina, or prevent migraines. Despite the great usefulness and versatility of these medicines, in general they are not appropriate for people with chronic breathing problems, because they can trigger airway tightening. Other side effects include changes in heart rate, cold hands and feet, and depression.

INSTRUCTIONS

Propranolol and metoprolol are best taken with meals, but consistency is the most important factor. These drugs should be taken at about the same time every day. Do not stop any of these medicines suddenly except on doctor's orders. Serious side effects could result.

BRAND NAME

Brevicon	**Demulen**	**Desogen**
Genora	**Levlen**	**Loestrin**
Lo/Ovral	**Modicon**	**N.E.E.**
Nelova	**Nordette**	**Norethin**
Norinyl	**Norlestrin**	**Ortho-**
Ortho-Novum	**Ovcon**	**Cyclen**
Ovral	**Triphasil**	

DESCRIPTION

Lower doses of estrogen and progestin make these drugs safer today than ever before. But women who smoke and take oral contraceptives still run an increased risk of strokes. These drugs are usually well tolerated, but side effects may include menstrual changes, nausea, migraine, depression, changes in vision, high blood pressure, liver tumors, gallbladder problems, blood clots, and heart attacks. Weigh the benefits and risks with your doctor when considering this form of contraception. Birth control pills interact with several other medications; check with your doctor or pharmacist before taking another drug in conjunction with oral contraceptives.

INSTRUCTIONS

For maximum effectiveness, oral contraceptives should be taken at the same time every day and precisely according to instructions. Missed doses can lead to an unwelcome pregnancy. Additional contraception is needed for at least the first week.

INTERACTION

There are several reports that birth control pills can increase blood levels of metoprolol and propranolol. The significance of this interaction is somewhat murky. There may be no cause for concern, but the possibility exists that the effects of these beta-blockers could be magnified. Blood pressure and pulse should be monitored carefully and if the drugs produce side effects, the prescribing physician may choose to reevaluate the dose of beta-blocker.

Symptoms of Beta-Blocker Toxicity

Low blood pressure, dizziness, very slow heart rate, breathing difficulties, and heart failure. Notify your physician of any symptoms.

INTERACTION

TROUBLESOME

Heart/Blood Pressure Drugs
(BETA-BLOCKERS)

Tuberculosis Drug
(RIFAMPIN)

BRAND NAME	GENERIC NAME
Inderal	propranolol
Lopressor, Toprol XL	metoprolol
(other beta-blockers may also interact)	

BRAND NAME	GENERIC NAME
Rifadin	rifampin
Rifamate	isoniazid/rifampin
Rimactane	rifampin

DESCRIPTION

Beta-blockers such as these are often used to lower blood pressure, stabilize irregular heartbeats, relieve angina, or prevent migraines. Despite the great usefulness and versatility of these medicines, in general they are not appropriate for people with chronic breathing problems, because they can trigger airway tightening. Other side effects include changes in heart rate, cold hands and feet, and depression.

INSTRUCTIONS

Propranolol and metoprolol are best taken with meals, but consistency is the most important factor. These drugs should be taken at about the same time every day. Do not stop any of these medicines suddenly except on doctor's orders. Serious side effects could result.

DESCRIPTION

Rifampin is used in combination with other medications to treat tuberculosis. To be effective, it needs to be taken faithfully for an extended period of time (at least six to nine months), as the doctor prescribes. Side effects may include digestive tract problems, menstrual irregularities, difficulty concentrating, fluid retention, and wheezing or shortness of breath. The orange discoloration of urine, saliva, and tears is not harmful, although it may stain contact lenses.

INSTRUCTIONS

Rifampin should be taken on an empty stomach, at least one hour before or two hours after meals. If you develop fever, chills, unusual tiredness, unusual bleeding or bruising, sore throat, muscle and bone pain, or yellow skin and eyes, contact your physician immediately.

INTERACTION

Rifampin stimulates the liver to metabolize other drugs more efficiently. This means that blood levels of other medications may be reduced along with their effectiveness. Acetaminophen (Tylenol, etc.), oral contraceptives, and beta-blockers are just some of the compounds that can be affected. The clinical significance of this interaction remains controversial. At the time of this writing all we can say is that careful monitoring of blood pressure before and after initiation of tuberculosis treatment is crucial. If blood pressure climbs, your physician will have to reevaluate the beta-blocker dosage or treatment regimen.

Symptoms of Beta-Blocker Undertreatment

Blood pressure may climb and heart symptoms might appear. Be alert for chest pain or palpitations. Monitor blood pressure carefully. Notify your physician of any symptoms.

INTERACTION

TROUBLESOME

Heart/Blood Pressure Drugs

(BETA-BLOCKERS)

Ulcer Drug

(H₂ ANTAGONIST)

BRAND NAME	GENERIC NAME
Inderal	propranolol
Lopressor	metoprolol
Normodyne	labetalol
Trandate	labetalol

DESCRIPTION

Beta-blockers such as these are often used to lower blood pressure, stabilize irregular heartbeats, relieve angina, or prevent migraines. Despite the great usefulness and versatility of these medicines, in general they are not appropriate for people with chronic breathing problems, because they can trigger airway tightening. Other side effects include changes in heart rate, cold hands and feet, and depression.

INSTRUCTIONS

Inderal and Lopressor are best taken with meals, but consistency is the most important factor. They should be taken at roughly the same time every day. Do not stop these medicines suddenly except on doctor's orders. Serious side effects could result.

BRAND NAME	GENERIC NAME
Tagamet	cimetidine

DESCRIPTION

Tagamet revolutionized the treatment of ulcers and serious heartburn by blocking special receptors, thereby reducing the acid environment of the stomach. Cimetidine usually has few side effects, although headaches, dizziness, and mild diarrhea are potential reactions. Some men complain of antitestosterone effects. At higher doses, this may lead to enlarged breasts or sexual problems. Older people and those who are very ill may experience depression, mental confusion, or disorientation. The dose may need to be adjusted for them. Tagamet may modify the metabolism of a number of medications, so check with your doctor and pharmacist if you take cimetidine with another medicine.

INSTRUCTIONS

Tagamet is usually taken with meals and/or at bedtime. Antacids may reduce absorption of Tagamet; do not take one for at least two hours after taking Tagamet.

INTERACTION

Tagamet appears to affect the liver's ability to metabolize certain beta-blockers such as Inderal and Lopressor. These drugs may not be eliminated as efficiently as expected, leading to increased blood levels. One study noted a doubling or even tripling impact on propranolol. The effect on metoprolol is more complicated. Some research has shown increased blood levels while other data show there is no problem. With such contradictory information, all we can suggest is prudent caution.

When blood levels of beta-blockers are substantially increased, there could be unwanted side effects. There have been reports of very slow heart rate and low blood pressure. If there is a compelling reason to take both Tagamet and Inderal or Lopressor simultaneously, blood pressure and pulse should be closely monitored. A physician may wish to reevaluate the standard dose of beta-blocker as well.

Symptoms of Beta-Blocker Toxicity

If beta-blocker blood levels get too high, people may experience side effects such as low blood pressure, dizziness, very slow heart rate, breathing difficulties, or heart failure. Notify your physician promptly of any symptoms.

Never take or stop medication without your doctor's advice.

INTERACTION

TROUBLESOME

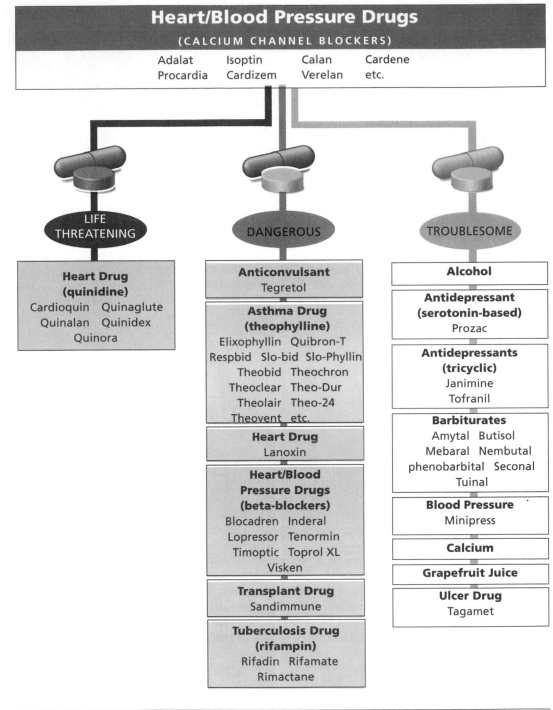

Heart/Blood Pressure Drugs
(CALCIUM CHANNEL BLOCKERS)

Adalat	Isoptin	Calan	Cardene
Procardia	Cardizem	Verelan	etc.

LIFE THREATENING

Heart Drug (quinidine)
Cardioquin   Quinaglute
Quinalan   Quinidex
Quinora

DANGEROUS

Anticonvulsant
Tegretol

Asthma Drug (theophylline)
Elixophyllin   Quibron-T
Respbid   Slo-bid   Slo-Phyllin
Theobid   Theochron
Theoclear   Theo-Dur
Theolair   Theo-24
Theovent   etc.

Heart Drug
Lanoxin

Heart/Blood Pressure Drugs (beta-blockers)
Blocadren   Inderal
Lopressor   Tenormin
Timoptic   Toprol XL
Visken

Transplant Drug
Sandimmune

Tuberculosis Drug (rifampin)
Rifadin   Rifamate
Rimactane

TROUBLESOME

Alcohol

Antidepressant (serotonin-based)
Prozac

Antidepressants (tricyclic)
Janimine
Tofranil

Barbiturates
Amytal   Butisol
Mebaral   Nembutal
phenobarbital   Seconal
Tuinal

Blood Pressure
Minipress

Calcium

Grapefruit Juice

Ulcer Drug
Tagamet

LEVELS OF HAZARD: LIFE THREATENING   DANGEROUS   TROUBLESOME

Heart/Blood Pressure Drugs
(CALCIUM CHANNEL BLOCKERS)

Heart Drug
(QUINIDINE)

BRAND NAME	GENERIC NAME
Adalat, Procardia	nifedipine
Calan, Isoptin,	
Verelan	verapamil

DESCRIPTION
Calcium channel blockers are popular drugs for lowering blood pressure, treating angina, and, in the case of verapamil, stabilizing irregular heart rhythms. Some of these drugs are prescribed to prevent migraine or cluster headaches, ward off exercise-induced asthma, or treat congestive heart failure.

INSTRUCTIONS
These drugs come in a variety of doses; follow the doctor's directions. Sustained-release forms such as Calan SR should not be chewed or crushed. Taking Adalat or Procardia with grapefruit juice could boost blood levels of the drug unexpectedly. See the table of Food and Drug Compatibility, pages 59-73. If the drug must be discontinued, follow the doctor's instructions for gradual tapering.

BRAND NAME	GENERIC NAME
Cardioquin	quinidine
Quinaglute	quinidine
Quinalan	quinidine
Quinidex	quinidine
Quinora	quinidine

DESCRIPTION
Quinidine is prescribed for a variety of heart rhythm disturbances. The first dose is considered a test to see if the patient will have a dangerous reaction. People with heart failure or with liver or kidney disease need close monitoring.

INSTRUCTIONS
This drug may upset the stomach and should be taken with food. Sustained-release tablets should not be chewed or crushed.

Quinidine may provoke visual disturbances, ringing in the ears, headache, dizziness, nausea, skin rash, or breathing difficulties. Notify your doctor if you develop any of these symptoms. Do not stop this medicine unless your doctor so directs.

INTERACTION

This interaction is extremely complicated. Both of these medicines are used to control irregular heartbeats, and some patients do well on this combination. Others may experience very low blood pressure, very slow heart rate, or serious changes in heart rhythm. *Although no deaths have been reported, in theory this interaction could be lethal.* Verapamil can apparently lead to higher quinidine levels and potentially to toxicity.

Nifedipine, on the other hand, has been reported to lower quinidine levels, although this seems to be rare. Quinidine, however, may increase circulating nifedipine. Evidence on other calcium channel blockers is lacking.

The doctor should probably monitor cardiac function carefully for at least several months after a patient starts taking quinidine together with any calcium channel blocker.

Symptoms of Quinidine Toxicity
Nausea, diarrhea, vomiting, headache, lethargy, confusion, palpitations, blurred vision, ringing in the ears, slowed breathing. Notify your doctor immediately of such symptoms.

Symptoms of Calcium Channel Blocker Toxicity
Headaches, facial flushing, low blood pressure, dizziness, fluid retention, nervousness, weakness, sleep problems, rapid or irregular heartbeat, palpitations. Notify the doctor promptly.

INTERACTION

LIFE THREATENING

Heart/Blood Pressure Drugs
(CALCIUM CHANNEL BLOCKERS)

Anticonvulsant
(CARBAMAZEPINE)

BRAND NAME	GENERIC NAME
Calan, Isoptin, Verelan	verapamil
Cardizem, Dilacor XR	diltiazem
Plendil	felodipine

DESCRIPTION

Calcium channel blockers such as Calan and Cardizem are popular drugs for lowering blood pressure, treating angina, and, in the case of verapamil, stabilizing irregular heart rhythms. Some of these drugs have been prescribed to prevent migraine or cluster headaches, ward off exercise-induced asthma, or treat congestive heart failure.

INSTRUCTIONS

These drugs come in a variety of doses; follow the doctor's directions. Sustained-release forms, such as Calan SR and Dilacor XR, should not be chewed or crushed. Taking Plendil with grapefruit juice could boost blood levels of the drug unexpectedly. See the table of Food and Drug Compatibility on pages 59-73. If the drug must be discontinued, follow the doctor's instructions for gradual tapering.

BRAND NAME	GENERIC NAME
Tegretol	carbamazepine

DESCRIPTION

Carbamazepine is often prescribed to people for whom other anticonvulsants have not worked well. It is also used to control severe facial pain related to the trigeminal nerve. Carbamazepine may trigger a potentially lethal blood abnormality, so regular monitoring is critical, particularly during the first two months. This drug can cause drowsiness or dizziness; driving may be impaired. Contact your doctor if you experience drowsiness, dizziness, confusion, mood or behavior changes, nausea, swollen legs and feet, pale stools, yellow skin or eyes, unusual bleeding or bruising, dark urine, sore throat, mouth sores, fever, or chills.

INSTRUCTIONS

Carbamazepine may upset the stomach; if so, take it with food or milk. Do not stop this drug suddenly; seizures could result. To maintain its strength, it must be stored away from humidity and heat in a tightly closed container.

INTERACTION

Both verapamil and diltiazem have been associated with elevated blood levels of carbamazepine, with the possibility of toxicity. *This interaction could be dangerous.*

Carbamazepine concentrations should be monitored closely if this drug is taken with a calcium channel blocker. Nifedipine may not interact, but the dose of carbamazepine may need to be reduced by as much as 50 percent when combined with verapamil. Monitoring is crucial if a patient on Tegretol stops taking a calcium channel blocker.

If a patient on Plendil takes carbamazepine, blood pressure may not be controlled with the normal dose of Plendil. One study found that patients on Tegretol had only about 6 percent the amount of Plendil in their bloodstreams as people taking Plendil alone. In such a case, the doctor may want to adjust the dose of Plendil.

Symptoms of Carbamazepine Toxicity

Nausea, vomiting, drowsiness, unsteadiness, incoordination, dizziness, muscle twitching or tremor, irregular breathing, rapid heartbeat, changes in blood pressure, changes in urination, and impaired consciousness. Notify the physician immediately of any such symptoms.

INTERACTION

DANGEROUS

Heart/Blood Pressure Drugs
(CALCIUM CHANNEL BLOCKERS)

Asthma Drug
(THEOPHYLLINE)

BRAND NAME	GENERIC NAME
Adalat, Procardia	nifedipine
Calan, Isoptin, Verelan	verapamil
Cardizem, Dilacor XR	diltiazem

DESCRIPTION

These medications are prescribed primarily to treat angina, lower high blood pressure, or, in the case of verapamil, stabilize irregular heart rhythms. They are usually well tolerated and are among the most popular cardiovascular drugs, but can cause gastrointestinal upset, dizziness, fluid retention, and other side effects. Elderly patients may require dosage adjustment.

INSTRUCTIONS

These drugs come in a variety of doses; follow the doctor's directions carefully. Sustained-release forms, such as Calan SR and Dilacor XR, should not be chewed or crushed and are best taken with food. Avoid taking Adalat or Procardia with grapefruit juice, as this could boost blood levels unexpectedly. See the table on pages 59-73 for specific instructions. Withdrawal symptoms, especially chest pain, may occur if these drugs are stopped suddenly. Follow your doctor's instructions for tapering slowly if the medicine must be discontinued.

BRAND NAME

Aerolate	**Aquaphyllin**	**Asmalix**
Bronkodyl	**Elixomin**	**Elixophyllin**
Quibron-T	**Respbid**	**Slo-bid**
Slo-Phyllin	**Theobid**	**Theochron**
Theoclear	**Theo-Dur**	**Theolair**
Theo-24	**Theovent**	**Theo-X**
T-Phyl	**Uniphyl**	

DESCRIPTION

Theophylline helps to open airways, so it is generally used to treat and prevent asthma attacks. It may also be prescribed for people with emphysema or other chronic breathing problems. Babies and elderly men may need lower doses. The dose is monitored with regular blood tests to ensure that levels are less than 20 mcg/ml.

INSTRUCTIONS

Theophylline interacts with food in complex ways, so discuss this issue thoroughly with your doctor and pharmacist. Theophylline may upset the stomach. In some cases this problem can be alleviated by taking the drug with food. See the table of Food and Drug Compatibility on pages 59-73 for more information.

INTERACTION

Many medicines, including diltiazem and verapamil, are capable of elevating blood levels of theophylline by interfering with metabolism of the drug. People seem to vary in the degree to which they react to this interaction. *Although the documented increase in circulating theophylline is not large, it could be dangerous for someone whose blood levels were already high.*

Most studies indicate that Procardia has little effect on serum theophylline levels, but there are a few cases of patients who developed toxicity as a result of this interaction.

Symptoms of Theophylline Toxicity

Nausea, diarrhea, stomach pain, headache, insomnia, restlessness, and irritability. Severe toxicity (convulsions, heart rhythm changes, or death) may occur with no warning symptoms. Notify your doctor immediately if you suspect a problem.

Never take or stop medication without your doctor's advice.

INTERACTION

DANGEROUS

Heart/Blood Pressure Drugs
(CALCIUM CHANNEL BLOCKERS)

BRAND NAME	GENERIC NAME
Adalat, Procardia	nifedipine
Calan, Isoptin, Verelan	verapamil
Cardizem, Dilacor XR	diltiazem
Plendil	felodipine
Vascor	bepridil

DESCRIPTION

Calcium channel blockers are popular drugs for lowering blood pressure, treating angina, and, in the case of verapamil, stabilizing irregular heart rhythms. Some of these drugs are prescribed to prevent migraine or cluster headaches, ward off exercise-induced asthma, or treat congestive heart failure.

INSTRUCTIONS

These drugs come in a variety of doses; follow the doctor's directions. Sustained-release forms should not be chewed or crushed. Taking Adalat, Plendil, or Procardia with grapefruit juice could boost blood levels of the drug unexpectedly. See the table of Food and Drug Compatibility on pages 59-73. If the drug must be discontinued, follow your doctor's instructions for gradual tapering.

Heart Drug
(DIGOXIN)

BRAND NAME	GENERIC NAME
Lanoxin	digoxin

DESCRIPTION

Digoxin is a heart drug that is often very helpful in treating congestive heart failure. It is also prescribed for certain heart rhythm changes, especially atrial fibrillation, atrial flutter, and paroxysmal atrial tachycardia (PAT). The doctor must monitor the digoxin dose carefully, because the effective dose is not far below the toxic dose. Older people may need dose adjustment.

INSTRUCTIONS

Digoxin should be taken in a consistent fashion, preferably with food but not with a meal high in fiber. Bran may limit the absorption of this drug.

Do not stop this medicine unless your doctor so directs.

INTERACTION

Patients with certain heart rhythm problems may require this combination of medicines. Others might be taking both drugs to treat different conditions. In either event, this interaction could be a problem, resulting in higher than expected digoxin levels. Be alert for signs of toxicity. The doctor should monitor blood levels of digoxin and also the electrocardiogram. Verapamil can raise serum digoxin levels as much as 75 percent, enough to result in toxicity in some cases. Diltiazem also seems to raise digoxin levels in the blood, although the studies do not agree on this effect. Bepridil, a relatively new blood pressure medicine, interacts with digoxin to slow heart beat and modify the electrocardiogram. *This interaction could be dangerous.*

Symptoms of Digoxin Toxicity

Nausea, vomiting, loss of appetite, diarrhea, stomach pain, visual disturbances (green or yellow tint and a halo around lights), weakness, drowsiness, depression, confusion, palpitations, rash, headaches, and hallucinations. Notify your doctor immediately if you experience any of these symptoms.

INTERACTION

DANGEROUS

Heart/Blood Pressure Drugs
(CALCIUM CHANNEL BLOCKERS)

BRAND NAME	GENERIC NAME
Adalat, Procardia	nifedipine
Calan, Isoptin, Verelan	verapamil
Cardene	nicardipine
Cardizem, Dilacor XR	diltiazem
DynaCirc	isradipine
Plendil	felodipine

DESCRIPTION

Calcium channel blockers such as Calan and Cardizem are popular drugs for lowering blood pressure, treating angina, and, in the case of verapamil, stabilizing irregular heart rhythms. Some of these drugs have been prescribed to prevent migraine or cluster headaches, ward off exercise-induced asthma, or treat congestive heart failure.

INSTRUCTIONS

These drugs come in a variety of doses; follow the doctor's directions. Sustained-release forms, such as Calan SR and Dilacor XR, should not be chewed or crushed. Taking Adalat, Plendil, or Procardia with grapefruit juice could boost blood levels of the drug unexpectedly. See the table of Food and Drug Compatibility on pages 59-73. If the drug must be discontinued, follow your doctor's instructions for gradual tapering.

Heart/Blood Pressure Drugs
(BETA-BLOCKERS)

BRAND NAME	GENERIC NAME
Blocadren	timolol
Inderal	propranolol
Lopressor, Toprol XL	metoprolol
Tenormin	atenolol
Timoptic	timolol
Visken	pindolol

DESCRIPTION

These beta-blockers are used to lower blood pressure, stabilize irregular heartbeats, relieve angina, or prevent migraines. Timoptic eye drops treat glaucoma. Despite their usefulness, in general these medicines are not appropriate for people with chronic breathing problems, as they can make airways tighten. Other side effects include changes in heart rate, cold hands and feet, and depression.

INSTRUCTIONS

Inderal and Lopressor are best taken with meals, but consistency is most important. Take these drugs at roughly the same time every day. Ask your eye doctor to show you how to instill Timoptic drops to minimize absorption. Do not stop any of these medicines suddenly because serious side effects could result.

INTERACTION

Many people with high blood pressure or unstable angina need a combination of drugs to control their symptoms. Often, a calcium channel blocker and a beta-blocker will work together. Some people, however, experience serious heart problems as a result of an interaction. *This interaction could be dangerous.*

A person who needs both a beta-blocker and a calcium channel blocker should have cardiac function monitored carefully. The doctor may need to adjust the dose of one or both drugs. Nifedipine may be somewhat less likely than other calcium channel blockers to interact with beta-blockers, but serious problems have been reported. Even Timoptic eye drops are capable of interacting with verapamil and, presumably, other calcium blockers. ***Notify your doctor if you experience*** irregular heartbeat or palpitations, worsening of angina, swelling of hands and feet, shortness of breath, hives, rash, or unusual bleeding.

Never take or stop medication without your doctor's advice.

INTERACTION

DANGEROUS

Heart/Blood Pressure Drugs

(CALCIUM CHANNEL BLOCKERS)

Transplant Drug

BRAND NAME	GENERIC NAME
Calan, Isoptin, Verelan	verapamil
Cardene	nicardipine
Cardizem, Dilacor XR	diltiazem

DESCRIPTION

Calcium channel blockers are popular drugs for lowering blood pressure, treating angina, and, in the case of verapamil, stabilizing irregular heart rhythms. Some of these drugs are prescribed to prevent migraine or cluster headaches, ward off exercise-induced asthma, or treat congestive heart failure.

INSTRUCTIONS

These drugs come in a variety of doses; follow the doctor's directions. Sustained-release forms such as Calan SR should not be chewed or crushed. See the table of Food and Drug Compatibility on pages 59-73. If the drug must be discontinued, follow your doctor's instructions for gradual tapering.

BRAND NAME	GENERIC NAME
Sandimmune	cyclosporine

DESCRIPTION

Sandimmune suppresses the immune system so that a person receiving a transplant does not reject this lifesaving organ. Doctors have also tried using it in treating autoimmune diseases, in which the immune system attacks a person's own tissues.

INSTRUCTIONS

Sandimmune comes as an oral solution with a taste reminiscent of castor oil. It should be mixed in a glass with milk, chocolate milk, or orange juice at room temperature and drunk at once. Then the glass (no plastic) should be rinsed and the rinsing fluid drunk to get the full dose. Do not take Sandimmune with grapefruit juice unless the physician is monitoring blood levels of the drug closely. (See page 43.)

Due to a possible interaction between cyclosporine and oral contraceptives, barrier methods of contraception should be used while taking this drug.

Regular monitoring is important. Do not stop this medicine unless your doctor so directs.

INTERACTION

The potential interaction is complicated, because patients receiving a kidney or heart transplant may be given a calcium channel blocker such as diltiazem or verapamil first before Sandimmune. When given in this manner, these medications seem to help protect the kidney from possible damage due to Sandimmune.

If Sandimmune is already being taken, however, both verapamil and diltiazem can raise blood levels of this transplant drug to potentially toxic levels, usually within a week. Whenever the dose of one of these drugs is changed, cyclosporine levels should be monitored carefully so that the dose may be adjusted if necessary. *This interaction could be dangerous.*

Cardene has also been reported to interact with Sandimmune, while the calcium channel blocker Procardia does not seem to.

Signs of Cyclosporine Toxicity

Kidney problems, changes in liver or kidney function. Close monitoring of blood and urine is essential.

Never take or stop medication without your doctor's advice.

INTERACTION

DANGEROUS

Heart/Blood Pressure Drugs
(CALCIUM CHANNEL BLOCKERS)

BRAND NAME	GENERIC NAME
Calan, Isoptin, Verelan	verapamil
Cardene	nicardipine
Cardizem, Dilacor XR	diltiazem

DESCRIPTION

Calcium channel blockers are popular drugs for lowering blood pressure, treating angina, and, in the case of verapamil, stabilizing irregular heart rhythms. Some of these drugs are prescribed to prevent migraine or cluster headaches, ward off exercise-induced asthma, or treat congestive heart failure.

INSTRUCTIONS

These drugs come in a variety of doses; follow your doctor's directions. Sustained-release forms such as Calan SR should not be chewed or crushed. See the table of Food and Drug Compatibility on pages 59-73. If the drug must be discontinued, follow your doctor's instructions for gradual tapering.

Tuberculosis Drug
(RIFAMPIN)

BRAND NAME	GENERIC NAME
Rifadin	rifampin
Rifamate	isoniazid/rifampin
Rimactane	rifampin

DESCRIPTION

Rifampin is used in combination with other medications to treat tuberculosis. To be effective, it needs to be taken faithfully for an extended period of time (at least six to nine months), as the doctor prescribes. Side effects may include digestive tract problems, menstrual irregularities, difficulty concentrating, fluid retention, and wheezing or shortness of breath. The orange discoloration of urine, saliva, and tears is not harmful, although it may stain contact lenses.

INSTRUCTIONS

Rifampin should be taken on an empty stomach, at least one hour before or two hours after meals. If you develop fever, chills, unusual tiredness, unusual bleeding or bruising, sore throat, muscle and bone pain, or yellow skin and eyes, contact your physician immediately.

INTERACTION

Tuberculosis medicines containing rifampin can dramatically reduce the effectiveness of verapamil, leading to a potentially dangerous rise in blood pressure or increase in angina symptoms. A similar interaction has been reported with nifedipine and may be expected with Cardene. Injected (IV) verapamil does not appear to be much affected by rifampin. If rifampin is needed, the doctor will want to monitor the patient closely to make sure the calcium channel blocker is working properly. In some cases, an alternate medication may be needed.

INTERACTION

DANGEROUS

Heart/Blood Pressure Drugs

(CALCIUM CHANNEL BLOCKERS)

Alcohol

BRAND NAME

Calan, Isoptin, Verelan

GENERIC NAME

verapamil

DESCRIPTION

Calcium channel blockers such as Calan are popular drugs for lowering blood pressure, treating angina, and stabilizing irregular heart rhythms. Calcium channel blockers have been prescribed to prevent migraine or cluster headaches, ward off exercise-induced asthma, or treat congestive heart failure.

INSTRUCTIONS

These drugs come in a variety of doses; it is important to follow your doctor's directions to get the proper dose. Sustained-release forms such as Calan SR should not be chewed or crushed. See the table of Food and Drug Compatibility on pages 59-73. If the drug must be discontinued, follow your doctor's instructions for gradual tapering.

NAME

beer
liquor
wine
medicines that contain alcohol

DESCRIPTION

Alcohol comes in many guises. The obvious ones are liquor, beer, and wine. But you can also find substantial amounts of alcohol in certain medicines. Over-the-counter cough and cold products can contain up to 40 or 50 proof (20 to 25 percent by volume), which is a higher alcohol content than you would find in beer or wine. "Nighttime" remedies like NyQuil, Nytcold Medicine, and Pertussin PM Liquid are as much as 50 proof. This may not be a problem if all you take is a spoonful before bedtime, but some drugs may interact poorly with even modest amounts of alcohol.

INSTRUCTIONS

The absorption and effects of alcohol are magnified if you drink on an empty stomach. Fatty food can delay alcohol absorption. If you drink, do so in moderation, and never drive.

INTERACTION

People taking Calan, Isoptin, or Verelan may get more of a bang from their booze than they bargained for. A study of healthy young men showed that verapamil can increase blood alcohol concentrations by an average of 17 percent, and keep the alcohol in the bloodstream about 30 percent longer. This drug interferes with the body's ability to eliminate alcohol and can prolong the effects of alcohol intoxication. Remember that some liquid medicines contain alcohol (see page 154 in the discussion on alcohol for a list). *This interaction between alcohol and verapamil could be troublesome.*

Symptoms of Alcohol Overdose

This interaction may lead to alcohol toxicity. Disorientation, unsteadiness, or loss of motor coordination would be symptoms to watch for.

INTERACTION
TROUBLESOME

Heart/Blood Pressure Drugs
(CALCIUM CHANNEL BLOCKERS)

BRAND NAME	GENERIC NAME
Adalat, Procardia	nifedipine
Calan, Isoptin, Verelan	verapamil

DESCRIPTION
Calcium channel blockers are popular drugs for lowering blood pressure, treating angina, and, in the case of verapamil, stabilizing irregular heart rhythms. Some of these drugs are prescribed to prevent migraine or cluster headaches, ward off exercise-induced asthma, or treat congestive heart failure.

INSTRUCTIONS
These drugs come in a variety of doses; follow your doctor's directions. Sustained-release forms such as Calan SR should not be chewed or crushed. Taking Adalat or Procardia with grapefruit juice could boost blood levels of the drug unexpectedly. See the table of Food and Drug Compatibility, pages 59-73. If the drug must be discontinued, follow your doctor's instructions for gradual tapering.

Antidepressants
(SEROTONIN-BASED)

BRAND NAME	GENERIC NAME
Prozac	fluoxetine

DESCRIPTION
This antidepressant works by blocking the reuptake into brain cells of serotonin, a chemical messenger. Because it works differently from the older cyclic-type antidepressants, it has a different set of side effects and has become more popular. It may also work against a different array of problems, for instance, bulimia or obsessive-compulsive disorder. Older people and those with kidney or liver problems may need reduced doses. Prozac is cleared from the body very slowly and may linger weeks after discontinuation.

INSTRUCTIONS
Prozac is taken in the morning, or, if a higher dose has been prescribed, in the morning and at noon. It may be taken without regard to meals. Taking it with food may reduce stomach upset. A few patients experience serious weight loss on this medication. If this occurs, your doctor should be notified.

INTERACTION

There are a few case reports of increased toxicity of calcium channel blockers such as Calan and Procardia due to this combination. *This interaction could be troublesome.*
Side Effects of Calcium Channel Blockers
Nausea, constipation, skin rash, dizziness, headache, drowsiness, insomnia, shortness of breath, fluid retention, and changes in heart rate or rhythm. Contact your physician promptly if any such adverse effects appear while you are on Prozac and one of the calcium channel blockers.

Never take or stop medication without your doctor's advice.

INTERACTION

TROUBLESOME

Heart/Blood Pressure Drugs
(CALCIUM CHANNEL BLOCKERS)

Antidepressants
(TRICYCLIC)

BRAND NAME	GENERIC NAME
Calan, Isoptin, Verelan	verapamil
Cardizem, Dilacor XR	diltiazem

DESCRIPTION

Calcium channel blockers are popular drugs for lowering blood pressure, treating angina, and, in the case of verapamil, stabilizing irregular heart rhythms. Some of these drugs are prescribed to prevent migraine or cluster headaches, ward off exercise-induced asthma, or treat congestive heart failure.

INSTRUCTIONS

These drugs come in a variety of doses; follow your doctor's directions. Sustained-release forms such as Calan SR should not be chewed or crushed. See the table of Food and Drug Compatibility on pages 59-73. If the drug must be discontinued, follow your doctor's instructions for gradual tapering.

BRAND NAME	GENERIC NAME
Janimine	imipramine
Tofranil	imipramine

DESCRIPTION

Tricyclic antidepressants became popular during the 1970s and 1980s although they often cause unpleasant side effects (constipation, weight gain, sexual dysfunction, sluggishness, increased sun sensitivity, etc.). While used primarily to treat depression, these drugs have been used occasionally for other purposes (though not approved by the FDA) such as relieving chronic pain, panic disorders, bed-wetting, and hives.

INSTRUCTIONS

Usually imipramine is better taken with food. A high-fiber diet may interfere with absorption, however. Do not stop taking this drug suddenly; if it must be discontinued, your doctor will supervise gradual phaseout.

INTERACTION

Diltiazem and verapamil may raise blood levels of the antidepressant imipramine. The clinical significance of this interaction remains murky. For some people this might lead to imipramine toxicity. It would be a good idea to have serum imipramine levels monitored periodically.

Symptoms of Antidepressant Toxicity

People vary in their response to higher doses of tricyclics. Side effects may include sedation, confusion, dilated pupils, flushing, dry mouth, hallucinations, heart palpitations, and agitation. Older people may be especially vulnerable. Notify your physician of symptoms.

INTERACTION

TROUBLESOME

Heart/Blood Pressure Drugs
(CALCIUM CHANNEL BLOCKERS)

Barbiturates

BRAND NAME	GENERIC NAME
Adalat, Procardia	nifedipine
Calan, Isoptin	
Verelan	verapamil
Cardizem, Dilacor XR	diltiazem

DESCRIPTION

Calcium channel blockers are popular drugs for lowering blood pressure, treating angina, and, in the case of verapamil, stabilizing irregular heart rhythms. Some of these drugs are prescribed to prevent migraine or cluster headaches, ward off exercise-induced asthma, or treat congestive heart failure.

INSTRUCTIONS

These drugs come in a variety of doses; follow your doctor's directions. Sustained-release forms such as Calan SR should not be chewed or crushed. See the table of Food and Drug Compatibility on pages 59-73. If the drug must be discontinued, follow the doctor's instructions for gradual tapering.

BRAND NAME	GENERIC NAME
Amytal	amobarbital
Butisol	butabarbital
Fiorinal	butalbital/aspirin/ caffeine
Lotusate	talbutal
Mebaral	mephobarbital
Nembutal	pentobarbital
Seconal	secobarbital
Solfoton	phenobarbital
Tuinal	amobarbital/ secobarbital

DESCRIPTION

Barbiturates were once used as sedatives, but some are prescribed more frequently now to prevent seizures. Fiorinal is used to treat tension headaches. These medications can cause dependence if used for an extended period of time. Stopping suddenly could trigger severe withdrawal symptoms. Barbiturates interact with many other drugs, so check with your physician or pharmacist before taking any other medications.

INSTRUCTIONS

Any of these medications can cause drowsiness and should not be used if you must drive or operate machinery. Never drink alcohol if you are taking a barbiturate.

INTERACTION

Studies have shown that phenobarbital and other barbiturates speed the body's elimination of both nifedipine and verapamil. If both a calcium channel blocker and a barbiturate are needed, the clinical response to the calcium channel blocker should be monitored; a higher dose could be required. *This interaction could be troublesome.*

Never take or stop medication without your doctor's advice.

INTERACTION

TROUBLESOME

Heart/Blood Pressure Drugs
(CALCIUM CHANNEL BLOCKERS)

Blood Pressure Drug
(PRAZOSIN)

BRAND NAME   GENERIC NAME

Calan, Isoptin, Verelan   verapamil

DESCRIPTION

Calcium channel blockers are popular drugs for lowering blood pressure, treating angina, and, in the case of verapamil, stabilizing irregular heart rhythms. Some of these drugs are prescribed to prevent migraine or cluster headaches, ward off exercise-induced asthma, or treat congestive heart failure.

INSTRUCTIONS

These drugs come in a variety of doses; follow your doctor's directions. Sustained-release forms such as Calan SR should not be chewed or crushed. See the table of Food and Drug Compatibility on pages 59-73. If the drug must be discontinued, follow your doctor's instructions for gradual tapering.

BRAND NAME   GENERIC NAME

Minipress   prazosin

DESCRIPTION

Prazosin is effective in the treatment of hypertension in part by dilating vessels. Prazosin has been used to improve urinary flow when the prostate gland is enlarged. It may also improve symptoms of Raynaud's disease, a circulatory condition in which the hands and fingers become numb and painful. Side effects include dizziness, nausea, and palpitations. When beginning treatment with prazosin, be especially careful; the drug can cause severe dizziness.

INSTRUCTIONS

The first dose of prazosin should be taken at bedtime to reduce the risk of falls. Do not drive or operate machinery the day after the first dose or a dose increase.

INTERACTION

When a person taking Minipress starts taking verapamil as well, blood levels of prazosin may increase by over 100 percent. Increased blood levels of Minipress could result in excessively low blood pressure.

A person starting on this combination should have blood pressure carefully monitored, so that the doctor can adjust the dose if necessary. The precautions for avoiding severe dizziness with the first dose of Minipress are appropriate when verapamil is added to the regimen. Lightheadedness can lead to falls, which may be very serious. *This interaction could be troublesome.*

Symptoms of Prazosin Overdose
Drowsiness, extremely low blood pressure, which may cause dizziness. Notify your physician of any symptoms.

Never take or stop medication without your doctor's advice.

INTERACTION

TROUBLESOME

Heart/Blood Pressure Drugs

(CALCIUM CHANNEL BLOCKERS)

Calcium

BRAND NAME	GENERIC NAME
Calan, Isoptin, Verelan	verapamil

DESCRIPTION

Calcium channel blockers are popular drugs for lowering blood pressure, treating angina, and, in the case of verapamil, stabilizing irregular heart rhythms. Calcium channel blockers have been prescribed to prevent migraine or cluster headaches, ward off exercise-induced asthma, or treat congestive heart failure.

INSTRUCTIONS

These drugs come in a variety of doses; follow your doctor's directions. Sustained-release forms such as Calan SR should not be chewed or crushed. See the table of Food and Drug Compatibility on pages 59-73. If the drug must be discontinued, follow your doctor's instructions for gradual tapering.

Caltrate 600	calcium carbonate
Citracal	calcium citrate
Os-Cal	calcium carbonate
Posture	calcium phosphate
Rolaids Calcium Rich	calcium carbonate
Titralac	calcium carbonate
Tums	calcium carbonate
etc.	

DESCRIPTION

Calcium salts are often taken as a nutritional supplement. They have little toxicity and may help to preserve bone strength and possibly reduce the risk of colon cancer. People who have had kidney stones should not take calcium without supervision, because it might increase the likelihood of a recurrence.

INSTRUCTIONS

Generally, calcium supplements should be taken with meals for best absorption, but not with iron supplements. Calcium carbonate may be constipating in some people, but other calcium salts are less likely to cause this problem.

INTERACTION

Calcium salts have been used in some cases of verapamil overdose or toxicity to reduce the effects of this calcium channel blocker. It is not clear if daily doses of calcium will modify the effectiveness of verapamil.

Tell your doctor if you plan to start or stop calcium supplements so that your clinical response can be monitored. The dose of verapamil may need to be adjusted.

Never take or stop medication without your doctor's advice.

INTERACTION

TROUBLESOME

Heart/Blood Pressure Drugs

(CALCIUM CHANNEL BLOCKERS)

Grapefruit Juice

BRAND NAME	GENERIC NAME
Adalat, Procardia	nifedipine
Plendil	felodipine
Calan, Isoptin,	
Verelan	verapamil

DESCRIPTION

Calcium channel blockers such as Procardia are popular drugs for lowering blood pressure and treating angina. Drugs in this class have been prescribed to prevent migraine or cluster headaches, ward off exercise-induced asthma, or treat congestive heart failure.

INSTRUCTIONS

These drugs come in a variety of doses; follow your doctor's directions. Taking Adalat, Procardia, or Plendil with grapefruit juice could boost blood levels of the drug unexpectedly. See the table of Food and Drug Compatibility on pages 59-73. If the drug must be discontinued, follow your doctor's instructions for gradual tapering.

FLAVONOID INGREDIENTS

kaempferol
naringenin
quercetin

DESCRIPTION

Grapefruit juice contains ingredients called flavonoids that can have a profound effect on drug metabolism. Naringenin is present in highest concentrations and may impart the bitter aftertaste to grapefruit juice. It and other flavonoids can knock out an important enzyme in the liver (CYP-3A4) that is responsible for deactivating many medications. This can cause drug levels to climb and may lead to toxicity.

INSTRUCTIONS

Research on the effects of grapefruit juice on drug metabolism is still in its infancy. No one knows how many medications may be affected. To be on the safe side, do not take your medicines with grapefruit or grapefruit juice unless advised to do so by your physician. Preliminary data suggest that grapefruit is far less likely to affect blood levels if ingested four or more hours after taking medicine (Dr. David Flockhart, personal communication).

INTERACTION

The first warning that grapefruit juice could interact with drugs came during a study of the blood pressure medicine Plendil (felodipine). Investigators were shocked to discover that blood levels of the drug jumped an astonishing 284 percent beyond predicted levels when the medicine was swallowed with grapefruit juice. Side effects were also far more prominent when grapefruit juice was used. Other studies have confirmed that grapefruit juice magnifies the drug's effects and side effects.

The same investigators found that blood levels of Procardia (nifedipine) were also 134 percent higher when the drug was taken with grapefruit juice than when it was taken with water. Apparently the flavonoids in the grapefruit juice slow the metabolism of these calcium channel blockers. *This interaction could be troublesome.*

Symptoms of Plendil or Procardia Toxicity

Headaches, facial flushing, low blood pressure, nausea, dizziness, confusion, fluid retention, nervousness, weakness, sleep problems, changes in heart rate or irregular heartbeat, and palpitations. Notify your physician of any symptoms.

INTERACTION

TROUBLESOME

Heart/Blood Pressure Drugs

(CALCIUM CHANNEL BLOCKERS)

Ulcer Drug

(H₂ ANTAGONIST)

BRAND NAME	GENERIC NAME
Adalat, Procardia	nifedipine

DESCRIPTION

Calcium channel blockers such as Procardia are popular drugs for lowering blood pressure and treating angina. Drugs in this class have been prescribed to prevent migraine or cluster headaches, ward off exercise-induced asthma, or treat congestive heart failure.

INSTRUCTIONS

These drugs come in a variety of doses; follow your doctor's directions. Taking Adalat or Procardia with grapefruit juice could boost blood levels of the drug unexpectedly. See the table of Food and Drug Compatibility on pages 59-73. If the drug must be discontinued, follow your doctor's instructions for gradual tapering.

BRAND NAME	GENERIC NAME
Tagamet	cimetidine

DESCRIPTION

Tagamet has revolutionized the treatment of ulcers and serious heartburn (esophagitis) by blocking special receptors (the histamine H_2 receptors), thereby reducing the acidity of the stomach. Cimetidine is usually well tolerated and has few side effects, although headaches, dizziness, and mild diarrhea are potential reactions. Some men complain of anti-testosterone effects. At higher doses, this may lead to enlarged breasts or sexual problems. Older people and those who are very ill may experience depression, mental confusion, or disorientation. The dose may need to be adjusted for them. Tagamet can affect the liver, modifying the metabolism and elimination of a number of medications. Higher blood levels of such drugs may lead to increased toxicity, so check with your doctor and pharmacist if you take cimetidine with another medicine.

INSTRUCTIONS

Tagamet is usually taken with meals and/or at bedtime. Antacids may reduce absorption of Tagamet; do not take one for at least two hours after taking Tagamet.

INTERACTION

Cimetidine affects the liver's ability to metabolize many drugs. Nifedipine is vulnerable to this interaction. This combination of medications can lead to blood levels of nifedipine that are substantially higher than normal. This could lead to an exaggerated response to the blood pressure medicine. *This interaction could be troublesome.*

Studies on other calcium channel blockers are contradictory. It is possible that Tagamet increases levels of other calcium channel blockers such as verapamil or diltiazem slightly, but it does not appear that the effectiveness of these medications is likely to be affected.

Symptoms of Nifedipine Toxicity

Headaches, facial flushing, low blood pressure, nausea, dizziness, confusion, fluid retention, nervousness, weakness, sleep problems, changes in heart rate or irregular heartbeat, and palpitations. Notify your physician of any symptoms.

Never take or stop medication without your doctor's advice.

INTERACTION

TROUBLESOME

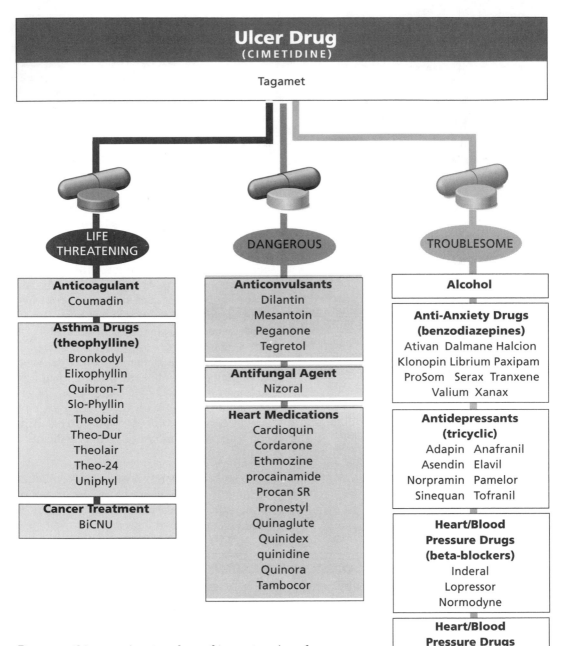

Ulcer Drug
(CIMETIDINE)

Tagamet

LIFE THREATENING

DANGEROUS

TROUBLESOME

| **Anticoagulant**
Coumadin | **Anticonvulsants**
Dilantin
Mesantoin
Peganone
Tegretol | **Alcohol** |

Asthma Drugs (theophylline)
Bronkodyl
Elixophyllin
Quibron-T
Slo-Phyllin
Theobid
Theo-Dur
Theolair
Theo-24
Uniphyl

Cancer Treatment
BiCNU

Antifungal Agent
Nizoral

Heart Medications
Cardioquin
Cordarone
Ethmozine
procainamide
Procan SR
Pronestyl
Quinaglute
Quinidex
quinidine
Quinora
Tambocor

Anti-Anxiety Drugs (benzodiazepines)
Ativan Dalmane Halcion
Klonopin Librium Paxipam
ProSom   Serax Tranxene
Valium Xanax

Antidepressants (tricyclic)
Adapin   Anafranil
Asendin   Elavil
Norpramin   Pamelor
Sinequan   Tofranil

Heart/Blood Pressure Drugs (beta-blockers)
Inderal
Lopressor
Normodyne

Heart/Blood Pressure Drugs (calcium channel blockers)
Adalat
Procardia

Drugs on this overview tree have the most serious known reactions with Tagamet. Not every interaction is listed. Be sure to check with a health professional before you take any other medication together with this ulcer drug.

LEVELS OF HAZARD: LIFE THREATENING   DANGEROUS   TROUBLESOME

Ulcer Drug

(H₂ ANTAGONIST)

Anticoagulant

(WARFARIN)

BRAND NAME

Tagamet

GENERIC NAME

cimetidine

DESCRIPTION

Tagamet has revolutionized the treatment of ulcers and serious heartburn (esophagitis) by blocking special receptors (the histamine H_2 receptors), thereby reducing the acid environment of the stomach. Cimetidine is usually well tolerated, and has few side effects, although headaches, dizziness, and mild diarrhea are potential reactions. Some men complain of antitestosterone effects. At higher doses, this may lead to enlarged breasts or sexual problems. Older people and those who are very ill may experience depression, mental confusion, or disorientation. The dose may need to be adjusted for them. Tagamet can affect the liver, modifying the metabolism and elimination of a number of medications. Higher blood levels of such drugs may lead to increased toxicity, so check with your doctor and pharmacist if you take cimetidine with another medicine.

INSTRUCTIONS

Tagamet is usually taken with meals and/or at bedtime. Antacids may reduce absorption of Tagamet; do not take one for at least two hours after taking Tagamet.

BRAND NAME

Coumadin

GENERIC NAME

warfarin

DESCRIPTION

Warfarin slows the liver's production of factors essential for the formation of blood clots. It is prescribed when there is a risk that a dangerous clot could form in a deep vein or a blood vessel leading to the lung, heart, or brain. The most serious complication of anticoagulant treatment is excessive bleeding. The dosage must be individually adjusted, requiring daily blood tests at first, then tests every four to six weeks. Other side effects may include nausea, loss of appetite, rash, fever, yellow eyes and skin, prolonged painful erection, and hair loss.

INSTRUCTIONS

Warfarin tablets can be swallowed with food or on an empty stomach. Try to avoid large variations in the quantity of vitamin-K–containing vegetables—such as broccoli, cabbage, or spinach—that you eat each day. Consuming much more or less than usual could change the action of the drug.

INTERACTION

Although warfarin may cause nausea, loss of appetite, stomach cramping, or diarrhea, taking Tagamet to treat these symptoms might trigger serious problems. Tagamet affects metabolism and increases Coumadin's blood-thinning potential. This prolongs prothrombin time (a measure of clotting) and could lead to serious hemorrhaging. *The interaction is potentially lethal.* Experts warn against this combination of drugs. If an ulcer medicine is needed with warfarin, Axid, Pepcid, or Zantac may be a safer alternative than Tagamet. Prothrombin time should be monitored when taking warfarin with an ulcer drug.

Symptoms of Warfarin Overdose

There may be no early warning signs of danger. Blood tests are essential. Symptoms include any unusual bleeding, including rectal or urinary tract bleeding, excessive menstrual bleeding, nosebleeds, bleeding around gums, bruising, red or tar-black stools, vomiting blood, and red or dark-brown urine. Notify your doctor immediately if you suspect a problem.

Never take or stop medication without your doctor's advice.

INTERACTION

LIFE THREATENING

Ulcer Drug
(H₂ ANTAGONIST)

Asthma Drug
(THEOPHYLLINE)

BRAND NAME

Tagamet

GENERIC NAME

cimetidine

DESCRIPTION

Tagamet has revolutionized the treatment of ulcers and serious heartburn (esophagitis) by blocking special receptors (the histamine H_2 receptors), thereby reducing the acid environment of the stomach. Cimetidine is usually well tolerated, and has few side effects, although headaches, dizziness, and mild diarrhea are potential reactions. Some men complain of antitestosterone effects. At higher doses, this may lead to enlarged breasts or sexual problems. Older people and those who are very ill may experience depression, mental confusion, or disorientation. The dose may need to be adjusted for them. Tagamet can affect the liver, modifying the metabolism and elimination of a number of medications. Higher blood levels of such drugs may lead to increased toxicity, so check with your doctor and pharmacist if you take cimetidine with another medicine.

INSTRUCTIONS

Tagamet is usually taken with meals and/or at bedtime. Antacids may reduce absorption of Tagamet; do not take one for at least two hours after taking Tagamet.

BRAND NAME

Aerolate	Aquaphyllin	Asmalix
Bronkodyl	Elixomin	Elixophyllin
Quibron-T	Respbid	Slo-bid
Slo-Phyllin	Theobid	Theochron
Theoclear	Theo-Dur	Theolair
Theo-24	Theovent	Theo-X
T-Phyl	Uniphyl	

DESCRIPTION

Theophylline helps to open airways, so it is generally used to treat and prevent asthma attacks. It may also be prescribed for people with emphysema or other chronic breathing problems. Babies and elderly men may need lower doses. The dose is monitored with regular blood tests to ensure that levels are less than 20 mcg/ml.

INSTRUCTIONS

Theophylline interacts with food in complex ways, so discuss this issue thoroughly with your doctor and pharmacist. Theophylline may upset the stomach. In some cases this problem can be alleviated by taking the drug with food. See the table of Food and Drug Compatibility pages 59-73 for more information.

INTERACTION

One common side effect of theophylline is stomach upset, which may in some cases mimic the symptoms of an ulcer or chronic heartburn. If a patient taking theophylline is prescribed Tagamet for symptoms of stomach upset, blood levels of theophylline could reach toxic levels. *This interaction could be life threatening.*

Tagamet boosts blood levels of theophylline by a third to a half. Patients whose theophylline levels are already a bit high (over 15 mcg/ml) are at highest risk for trouble. Anyone who needs both of these medications should have blood levels of theophylline monitored closely. Notify your physician immediately of any symptoms of theophylline toxicity.

Symptoms of Theophylline Toxicity

Nausea, diarrhea, stomach pain, headache, insomnia, restlessness, and irritability. Severe toxicity (convulsions, heart rhythm changes, or death) may occur with no warning symptoms. Notify your doctor immediately if you suspect a problem.

INTERACTION

LIFE THREATENING

Ulcer Drug

(H₂ ANTAGONIST)

Cancer Treatment

BRAND NAME	GENERIC NAME
Tagamet	cimetidine

DESCRIPTION

Tagamet has revolutionized the treatment of ulcers and serious heartburn (esophagitis) by blocking special receptors, thereby reducing the acidity of the stomach. Cimetidine usually has few side effects, although headaches, dizziness, and mild diarrhea are potential reactions. Some men complain of antitestosterone effects. At higher doses, this may lead to enlarged breasts or sexual problems. Older people and those who are very ill may experience depression, mental confusion, or disorientation. The dose may need to be adjusted. Tagamet can affect the liver, modifying the metabolism and elimination of a number of medications. Higher blood levels of such drugs may lead to increased toxicity, so check with your doctor and pharmacist if you take cimetidine with another medicine.

INSTRUCTIONS

Tagamet is usually taken with meals and/or at bedtime. Antacids may reduce absorption of Tagamet; do not take one for at least two hours after taking Tagamet.

BRAND NAME	GENERIC NAME
BiCNU	carmustine

DESCRIPTION

BiCNU is a chemotherapeutic agent used to treat a number of difficult tumors. It has been employed by itself or in combination with other compounds to control a number of brain tumors as well as blood-based cancers such as multiple myeloma, Hodgkin's disease, and non-Hodgkin's lymphomas.

Because of its significant toxicity, patients receiving BiCNU must be monitored very carefully. They require frequent blood, liver, kidney, eye, and lung tests. Nausea and vomiting are common side effects.

INSTRUCTIONS

Like many chemotherapeutic drugs, BiCNU is given intravenously. Antinausea medicine can help reduce nausea and vomiting.

INTERACTION

BiCNU is a heavy-duty drug. Toxicity is a tradeoff in the fight against cancer. The one thing cancer patients don't need is extra problems. Because of the digestive upset BiCNU can cause, it is understandable that physicians might consider an acid controller such as Tagamet. But there are reports that such a combination could cause increased BiCNU bone marrow toxicity. *This side effect could be life threatening.*

It is not clear how Tagamet increases bone marrow suppression. It may be that this ulcer drug blocks normal metabolism of BiCNU or it may have a direct effect on bone marrow itself. No matter what the mechanism, Tagamet should probably not be used with BiCNU unless there are compelling reasons to take such a risk.

Symptoms of BiCNU Toxicity

Bone marrow toxicity creates blood diseases. Anemia, bleeding, and increased susceptibility to infections are signs of serious danger.

Never take or stop medication without your doctor's advice.

INTERACTION

LIFE THREATENING

Ulcer Drug

(H₂ ANTAGONIST)

Anticonvulsants

BRAND NAME	GENERIC NAME
Tagamet	cimetidine

DESCRIPTION

Tagamet has revolutionized the treatment of ulcers and serious heartburn (esophagitis) by blocking special receptors, thereby reducing the acidity of the stomach. Cimetidine usually has few side effects, although headaches, dizziness, and mild diarrhea are potential reactions. Some men complain of antitestosterone effects. At higher doses, this may lead to enlarged breasts or sexual problems. Older people and those who are very ill may experience depression, mental confusion, or disorientation. The dose may need to be adjusted. Tagamet can affect the liver, modifying the metabolism and elimination of a number of medications. Higher blood levels of such drugs may lead to increased toxicity, so check with your doctor and pharmacist if you take cimetidine with another medicine.

INSTRUCTIONS

Tagamet is usually taken with meals and/or at bedtime. Antacids may reduce absorption of Tagamet; do not take one for at least two hours after taking Tagamet.

BRAND NAME	GENERIC NAME
Dilantin	phenytoin
Mesantoin	mephenytoin
Peganone	ethotoin
Tegretol	carbamazepine

DESCRIPTION

Tegretol, Dilantin, and other epilepsy medicines help control a number of different seizure disorders through mechanisms that are as yet somewhat mysterious. Dilantin and Tegretol have also been used to treat a painful nerve condition in the face called trigeminal neuralgia. Tegretol has also been used (without official FDA sanction) to treat restless leg syndrome (cramping and pain that occur at night) and certain psychiatric disorders. These drugs have the potential to produce many side effects. Drowsiness, dizziness, unsteady gait, digestive tract upset, and blood disorders are possible complications. Careful monitoring is essential.

INSTRUCTIONS

These drugs are best taken with food to reduce the likelihood of stomach upset.

INTERACTION

Tagamet appears to modify the metabolism of Dilantin and Tegretol. The same reaction seems likely also to affect Mesantoin and Peganone, although it has not yet been documented in the medical literature. The problem is that Tagamet affects liver enzymes so that they may be less capable of processing these anticonvulsants. As a result, blood levels can rise. This could lead to toxicity.

While Tagamet and Tegretol seem less likely to interact if Tegretol has been taken for longer than four weeks, physicians should be cautious when considering such a combination. Dilantin blood levels have climbed significantly when Tagamet was added to the regimen. Symptoms of overdose have been noted.

Symptoms of Dilantin or Tegretol Toxicity

Uncontrollable eye movements, unsteadiness on the feet, slurred speech, dizziness, muscle twitching, and confusion may be signs of toxicity. Notify your physician promptly of any symptoms.

Never take or stop medication without your doctor's advice.

INTERACTION

DANGEROUS

Ulcer Drugs

(H₂ ANTAGONISTS)

Antifungal Agent

BRAND NAME	GENERIC NAME
Axid	nizatidine
Pepcid	famotidine
Tagamet	cimetidine
Zantac	ranitidine

DESCRIPTION

Axid, Pepcid, Tagamet, and Zantac cure ulcers and relieve serious heartburn (reflux esophagitis) by blocking special receptors (the histamine H₂ receptors), thereby reducing the acidity of the stomach. These medicines are often prescribed in larger doses for the first six to eight weeks to facilitate healing of ulcers. Then an evening maintenance dose may be employed to prevent recurrences.

These drugs have relatively few side effects, although some men complain of Tagamet's antitestosterone actions. At higher doses this may lead to enlarged breasts or sexual problems. Older people and those who are very ill may experience depression, mental confusion, or disorientation.

INSTRUCTIONS

These drugs can be taken with food or on an empty stomach.

BRAND NAME	GENERIC NAME
Nizoral	ketoconazole

DESCRIPTION

Fungi can cause serious health problems, especially for those with weakened immune systems. Hard-to-treat infections of the mouth, throat, lungs, blood, brain, reproductive tract, skin, and nails have been fought with new and more powerful antifungal drugs such as Nizoral. Although relatively rare, liver damage is a very serious adverse event associated with this medication. Liver enzymes should be monitored regularly and if symptoms develop (jaundice, fatigue, nausea, loss of appetite, pale stools, vomiting, dark urine), your physician should be contacted immediately.

INSTRUCTIONS

Nizoral is best taken with food to reduce stomach upset.

INTERACTION

Nizoral is often reserved for serious fungal infections because of its potential for liver toxicity. Some of these infections can be devastating or possibly even life threatening if not treated successfully.

Nizoral requires an acid environment to be absorbed effectively from the stomach. Drugs that make the stomach less acidic (Axid, Pepcid, Tagamet, and Zantac) appear to dramatically reduce absorption of Nizoral. This could lead to diminished effectiveness. Antacids and another acid-suppressing drug, Prilosec, could also hamper normal Nizoral absorption. One reference recommends that doctors who must treat people who require Nizoral and a medication for ulcers consider the drug Carafate (sucralfate), which does not affect acidity.

INTERACTION

DANGEROUS

Ulcer Drug

(H₂ ANTAGONIST)

Heart Medications

BRAND NAME	GENERIC NAME
Tagamet	cimetidine

DESCRIPTION

Tagamet has revolutionized the treatment of ulcers and serious heartburn (esophagitis) by blocking special receptors, thereby reducing the acidity of the stomach. Cimetidine usually has few side effects, although headaches, dizziness, and mild diarrhea are potential reactions. Some men complain of antitestosterone effects. At higher doses, this may lead to enlarged breasts or sexual problems. Older people and those who are very ill may experience depression, mental confusion, or disorientation. The dose may need to be adjusted. Tagamet can affect the liver, modifying the metabolism and elimination of a number of medications. Higher blood levels of such drugs may lead to increased toxicity, so check with your doctor and pharmacist if you take cimetidine with another medicine.

INSTRUCTIONS

Tagamet is usually taken with meals and/or at bedtime. Antacids may reduce absorption of Tagamet; do not take one for at least two hours after taking Tagamet.

BRAND NAME	GENERIC NAME
Cardioquin	quinidine
Cordarone	amiodarone
Ethmozine	moricizine
Procan SR	procainamide
Pronestyl	procainamide
Quinaglute	quinidine
Quinidex	quinidine
Quinora	quinidine
Tambocor	flecainide

DESCRIPTION

These medications are prescribed to control serious arrhythmias (irregular heart rhythms). Unfortunately, they can also promote arrhythmias. They may prolong the QT interval (electrocardiograhic readings). Because of this, cardiologists often reserve them for life-threatening arrhythmias.

INSTRUCTIONS

Quinidine is best taken with food to reduce stomach upset. Procainamide is absorbed better on an empty stomach but it causes GI problems and may be taken at mealtime. Check with your physician and pharmacist on proper dosing for all these drugs; the dose must be individualized and timed carefully. Ethmozine should be started only in a hospital.

INTERACTION

Tagamet appears to have the potential to boost blood levels of these anti-arrhythmic medicines. When the ulcer drug is taken together with any of these heart medications, the potential for increased toxicity may rise. Because the dose is so critical to successful treatment with these powerful heart medications, anything that modifies the usual pattern could present a serious problem. *Arrhythmias might result, which could be life threatening.*

Experts recommend avoiding this combination unless it is essential. If Tagamet must be added to one of these heart medicines, blood levels must be monitored carefully, electrocardiographic tests considered, and dosage adjustments made if necessary.

Symptoms of Heart Medicine Toxicity

Except for subtle changes on an electrocardiogram, there may be no warning signs of serious danger. Heart palpitations, dizziness, fainting, chest discomfort, or shortness of breath require emergency treatment.

Never take or stop medication without your doctor's advice.

INTERACTION

DANGEROUS

Ulcer Drug

(H₂ ANTAGONIST)

Alcohol

BRAND NAME **Tagamet**

GENERIC NAME cimetidine

DESCRIPTION

Tagamet has revolutionized the treatment of ulcers and serious heartburn (esophagitis) by blocking special receptors (the histamine H_2 receptors), thereby reducing the acidity of the stomach. Tagamet has few side effects, but some men complain of antitestosterone actions. At higher doses this may lead to enlarged breasts or sexual problems. Older people and those who are very ill may experience depression, mental confusion, or disorientation. Tagamet can affect the liver, modifying the metabolism and elimination of a number of medications. Higher blood levels of such drugs may lead to increased toxicity.

INSTRUCTIONS

Tagamet can be taken with food or on an empty stomach. Antacids may reduce absorption; wait two hours after taking Tagamet if one is needed.

NAME
beer
liquor
wine
medicines that contain alcohol

DESCRIPTION

Alcohol comes in many guises. The obvious ones are liquor, beer, and wine. But you can also find substantial amounts of alcohol in certain medicines. Over-the-counter cough and cold products can contain up to 40 or 50 proof (20 to 25 percent by volume), which is a higher alcohol content than you would find in beer or wine. "Nighttime" remedies such as NyQuil, Nytcold Medicine, and Pertussin PM Liquid are as much as 50 proof. This may not be a problem if all you take is a spoonful before bedtime, but some drugs may interact poorly with even modest amounts of alcohol.

INSTRUCTIONS

The absorption and effects of alcohol are magnified if you drink on an empty stomach. Fatty food can delay alcohol absorption. If you drink, do so in moderation, and never drive.

INTERACTION

This interesting interaction is extremely controversial. Some researchers have demonstrated that people taking Tagamet have higher blood alcohol levels after several drinks than subjects not taking Tagamet. This reaction seems to affect only men because they have an enzyme in the stomach called alcohol dehydrogenase that breaks down some of the alcohol from a drink even before it is absorbed into the bloodstream. The data suggest that Tagamet deactivates this enzyme and enhances alcohol absorption. If this were true, people might have higher blood alcohol levels than they expect. But other research has contradicted this conclusion. An expert panel for the FDA decided that, although more work would be helpful, there is no reason to issue a warning at this time. Where does this leave patients? At this time there are no firm answers. If you take Tagamet and drink, be cautious . . . your blood alcohol levels might be higher than you think.

Symptoms of Alcohol Overdose

This interaction, if it occurs at all, probably has a modest effect on alcohol levels. Disorientation, unsteadiness, or loss of motor coordination would be symptoms to watch for.

INTERACTION
TROUBLESOME

Ulcer Drug
(H₂ ANTAGONIST)

Anti-Anxiety Drugs
(BENZODIAZEPINES)

BRAND NAME	GENERIC NAME
Tagamet	cimetidine

DESCRIPTION
Tagamet has revolutionized the treatment of ulcers and serious heartburn (esophagitis) by blocking special receptors (the histamine H_2 receptors), thereby reducing the acidity of the stomach. Tagamet has few side effects, but some men complain of antitestosterone actions. At higher doses this may lead to enlarged breasts or sexual problems. Older people and those who are very ill may experience depression, mental confusion, or disorientation. Tagamet can affect the liver, modifying the metabolism and elimination of a number of medications. Higher blood levels of such drugs may lead to increased toxicity.

INSTRUCTIONS
Tagamet can be taken with food or on an empty stomach. Antacids may reduce absorption; wait two hours after taking Tagamet if one is needed.

BRAND NAME	GENERIC NAME
Ativan	lorazepam
Dalmane	flurazepam
Doral	quazepam
Halcion	triazolam
Klonopin	clonazepam
Librium	chlordiazepoxide
Paxipam	halazepam
ProSom	estazolam
Restoril	temazepam
Serax	oxazepam
Tranxene	clorazepate
Valium	diazepam
Versed	midazolam
Xanax	alprazolam

DESCRIPTION
Benzodiazepines are used primarily to treat anxiety disorders and insomnia. Some have also been employed to relieve panic attacks, seizures, and muscle cramps. Anesthesiologists often use such medications before certain surgical procedures. Prolonged use may lead to dependence. Sudden withdrawal can produce unpleasant side effects and should always be supervised by a physician.

INSTRUCTIONS
These drugs may be taken with food, especially if they upset the digestive tract.

INTERACTION

Tagamet can increase blood levels of benzodiazepines and prolong their stay in the body. Sedation and impairment could result, especially for older people. This interaction remains controversial since the data are contradictory. Be vigilant for any drowsiness or incoordination. Unsteadiness is a possible complication.

Symptoms of Benzodiazepine Overdose
This interaction could lead to symptoms of overdose such as disorientation, unsteadiness, confusion, slurred speech, drowsiness, dizziness, amnesia, and loss of motor coordination. Some other benzodiazepines may also be affected by cimetidine. Contact your physician if such symptoms occur.

Never take or stop medication without your doctor's advice.

INTERACTION

TROUBLESOME

Ulcer Drug

(H₂ ANTAGONIST)

Antidepressants

(TRICYCLIC)

BRAND NAME	GENERIC NAME
Tagamet	cimetidine

DESCRIPTION

Tagamet has revolutionized the treatment of ulcers and serious heartburn (esophagitis) by blocking special receptors (the histamine H_2 receptors), thereby reducing the acidity of the stomach. Tagamet has few side effects, but some men complain of antitestosterone actions. At higher doses this may lead to enlarged breasts or sexual problems. Older people and those who are very ill may experience depression, mental confusion, or disorientation. Tagamet can affect the liver, modifying the metabolism and elimination of a number of medications. Higher blood levels of such drugs may lead to increased toxicity.

INSTRUCTIONS

Tagamet can be taken with food or on an empty stomach. Antacids may reduce absorption; wait two hours after taking Tagamet if one is needed.

BRAND NAME	GENERIC NAME
Adapin, Sinequan	doxepin
Anafranil	clomipramine
Asendin	amoxapine
Aventyl, Pamelor	nortriptyline
Elavil, Endep	amitriptyline
Norpramin, Pertofrane	desipramine
Tofranil	imipramine
etc.	

DESCRIPTION

Tricyclic antidepressants became popular during the 1970s and 1980s although they often caused unpleasant side effects (constipation, weight gain, sexual dysfunction, sluggishness, increased sun sensitivity, etc.) Some of these drugs have been used for other purposes (though not with FDA approval) such as chronic pain, panic disorders, eating disorders (bulimia), and hives. Anafranil has been approved for the treatment of obsessive-compulsive disorder.

INSTRUCTIONS

Usually these medications are better taken with food. A high-fiber diet may interfere with absorption, however. See page 20 for details.

INTERACTION

There is convincing evidence that Tagamet can increase blood levels of tricyclic antidepressants. This probably happens because the ulcer drug interferes with normal metabolism. Patients have reported increased side effects after such a combination. Symptoms included dizziness, drowsiness, and even psychosis.

Other ulcer medications (such as Zantac) have not been shown to have this effect. If Tagamet must be prescribed in combination with a tricyclic antidepressant, it is important to have blood levels of the antidepressant checked periodically.

Symptoms of Antidepressant Toxicity

People vary in their response to higher doses of tricyclics. Side effects may include confusion, dilated pupils, flushing, dry mouth, hallucinations, heart palpitations, and agitation. Older people may be especially vulnerable. Notify your physician of any symptoms.

Never take or stop medication without your doctor's advice.

INTERACTION

TROUBLESOME

Ulcer Drug
(H₂ ANTAGONIST)

Heart/Blood Pressure Drugs
(BETA-BLOCKERS)

BRAND NAME	GENERIC NAME
Tagamet	cimetidine

DESCRIPTION

Tagamet revolutionized the treatment of ulcers and serious heartburn by blocking special receptors, thereby reducing the acidity of the stomach. Cimetidine usually has few side effects, although headaches, dizziness, and mild diarrhea are potential reactions. Some men complain of antitestosterone effects. At higher doses, this may lead to enlarged breasts or sexual problems. Older people and those who are very ill may experience depression, mental confusion, or disorientation. The dose may need to be adjusted for them. Tagamet may modify the metabolism of a number of medications, so check with your doctor and pharmacist if you take cimetidine with another medicine.

INSTRUCTIONS

Tagamet is usually taken with meals and/or at bedtime. Antacids may reduce absorption of Tagamet; do not take one for at least two hours after taking Tagamet.

BRAND NAME	GENERIC NAME
Inderal	propranolol
Lopressor	metoprolol
Normodyne, Trandate	labetalol

DESCRIPTION

Beta-blockers such as these are often used to lower blood pressure, stabilize irregular heartbeats, relieve angina, or prevent migraines. Despite the great usefulness and versatility of these medicines, in general they are not appropriate for people with chronic breathing problems, because they can trigger airway tightening. Other side effects include changes in heart rate, cold hands and feet, and depression.

INSTRUCTIONS

Inderal and Lopressor are best taken with meals, but consistency is the most important factor. They should be taken at roughly the same time every day. Do not stop these medicines suddenly except on doctor's orders. Serious side effects could result.

INTERACTION

Tagamet appears to affect the liver's ability to metabolize certain beta-blockers such as Inderal and Lopressor. These drugs may not be eliminated as efficiently as expected, leading to increased blood levels. One study noted a doubling or even tripling impact on propranolol. The effect on metoprolol is more complicated. Some research has shown increased blood levels while other data show there is no problem. With such contradictory information, all we can suggest is prudent caution.

When blood levels of beta-blockers are substantially increased, there could be unwanted side effects. There have been reports of very slow heart rate and low blood pressure. If there is a compelling reason to take both Tagamet and Inderal or Lopressor simultaneously, blood pressure and pulse should be closely monitored. A physician may wish to reevaluate the standard dose of beta-blocker as well.

Symptoms of Beta-Blocker Toxicity

If beta-blocker blood levels get too high, people may experience side effects such as low blood pressure, dizziness, very slow heart rate, breathing difficulties, or heart failure. Notify your physician promptly of any symptoms.

Never take or stop medication without your doctor's advice.

INTERACTION

TROUBLESOME

Ulcer Drug

(H₂ ANTAGONIST)

Heart/Blood Pressure Drugs

(CALCIUM CHANNEL BLOCKERS)

BRAND NAME	GENERIC NAME
Tagamet	cimetidine

DESCRIPTION

Tagamet has revolutionized the treatment of ulcers and serious heartburn (esophagitis) by blocking special receptors (the histamine H_2 receptors), thereby reducing the acidity of the stomach. Cimetidine is usually well tolerated and has few side effects, although headaches, dizziness, and mild diarrhea are potential reactions. Some men complain of anti-testosterone effects. At higher doses, this may lead to enlarged breasts or sexual problems. Older people and those who are very ill may experience depression, mental confusion, or disorientation. The dose may need to be adjusted for them. Tagamet can affect the liver, modifying the metabolism and elimination of a number of medications. Higher blood levels of such drugs may lead to increased toxicity, so check with your doctor and pharmacist if you take cimetidine with another medicine.

INSTRUCTIONS

Tagamet is usually taken with meals and/or at bedtime. Antacids may reduce absorption of Tagamet; do not take one for at least two hours after taking Tagamet.

BRAND NAME	GENERIC NAME
Adalat, Procardia	nifedipine

DESCRIPTION

Calcium channel blockers such as Procardia are popular drugs for lowering blood pressure and treating angina. Drugs in this class have been prescribed to prevent migraine or cluster headaches, ward off exercise-induced asthma, or treat congestive heart failure.

INSTRUCTIONS

These drugs come in a variety of doses; follow the doctor's directions. Taking Adalat or Procardia with grapefruit juice could boost blood levels of the drug unexpectedly. See the table of Food and Drug Compatibility on pages 59-73. If the drug must be discontinued, follow your doctor's instructions for gradual tapering.

INTERACTION

Cimetidine affects the liver's ability to metabolize many drugs. Nifedipine is vulnerable to this interaction. This combination of medications can lead to blood levels of nifedipine that are substantially higher than normal. This could lead to an exaggerated response to the blood pressure medicine. *This interaction could be troublesome.*

Studies on other calcium channel blockers are contradictory. It is possible that Tagamet increases levels of other calcium channel blockers such as verapamil or diltiazem slightly, but it does not appear that the effectiveness of these medications is likely to be affected.

Symptoms of Nifedipine Toxicity

Headaches, facial flushing, low blood pressure, nausea, dizziness, confusion, fluid retention, nervousness, weakness, sleep problems, changes in heart rate or irregular heartbeat, and palpitations. Notify the physician of any symptoms.

Never take or stop medication without your doctor's advice.

INTERACTION

TROUBLESOME

About the Authors

Joe Graedon

Pharmacologist Joe Graedon is a best-selling author, nationally syndicated newspaper columnist, host of an award-winning internationally syndicated radio talk show, and lecturer at the University of North Carolina School of Pharmacy. He is president of Graedon Enterprises, Inc., a corporation providing pharmaceutical and health care information services.

Joe Graedon received his B.S. from Pennsylvania State Univer sity in 1967 and went on to do research on mental illness, sleep, and basic brain physiology at the New Jersey Neuropsychiatric Institute in Princeton. In 1971 he received his M.S. in pharmacology from the University of Michigan. Following his medical anthropologist wife Teresa to Mexico, he taught clinical pharmacology to second-year medical students at the Benito Juárez Unversity of Oaxaca. While in Mexico, he started work on *The People's Pharmacy* (St. Martin's Press, 1976; revised 1985), a popular book on medicines that would eventually go on to become a *New York Times* number one best-seller.

Joe's other books, coauthored with Dr. Terry Graedon, include *The People's Pharmacy-2* (Avon, 1980), *The New People's Pharmacy #3: Drug Breakthroughs of the '80s* (Bantam, 1985), *Totally New and Revised The People's Pharmacy* (St. Martin's Press, 1985), *50+: The Graedons' People's Pharmacy for Older Adults* (Bantam, 1988), and *Graedons' Best Medicine: From Herbal Remedies to High-Tech R$_x$ Breakthroughs* (Bantam, 1991). *No Deadly Drug* (Pocket Books, 1992), coauthored with Dr. Tom Ferguson, is Graedon's first novel. Joe and Terry's most recent work, also coauthored with Dr. Ferguson, is *The Aspirin Handbook: A User's Guide to the Breakthrough Drug of the '90s* (Bantam, 1993). The total number of the Graedons' books in print well exceeds two million.

Joe has lectured at Duke University School of Nursing, the University of California School of Pharmacy (UCSF), and the University of North Carolina School of Pharmacy. He served as a consultant to the **Federal Trade Commission** from 1978 to 1983, and was on the Advisory Board for the **Drug Studies Unit** at UCSF from 1983 to 1989. He is a member of the **Board of Visitors** of the School of Pharmacy at the University of North Carolina, Chapel Hill. He is a member of the **American Association for the Advancement of Science**, the **Society for Neuroscience**, the **New York Academy of Science**, and the **Mystery Writers of America**. For more than a decade Joe and Terry contributed a regular column on self-medication for the journal *Medical Self Care*. Joe is an editorial adviser to *Men's Health Newsletter.* Joe and Terry's newspaper column, **The People's Pharmacy**, is syndicated nationally by King Features. *The People's Pharmacy* radio show won a Silver Award from the Corporation for Public Broadcasting in 1992. It is syndicated to more than 500 radio stations in the United States and 134 countries on public radio, the In Touch Radio Reading Service, and the U.S. Armed Forces Radio and Television Network.

Joe's features on health and pharmaceuticals have been syndicated nationally to public television stations via Intraregional Program Service member exchange. He is considered the country's leading drug expert for consumers. He has been a guest expert on *Donahue, 20/20, Geraldo, The Oprah Winfrey Show, Sally Jessy Raphael, Live with Regis and Kathie Lee, Today, Good Morning America, CBS Morning News, Sonia Live, The Home Show, Everyday with Joan Lunden, The Larry King Show*, and *The Tonight Show with Johnny Carson*. He lives in Durham, North Carolina, with his wife and coauthor, Teresa, and their two children. Joe speaks frequently on issues of pharmaceuticals, nutrition, and self-care.

Teresa Graedon

Medical anthropologist Teresa Graedon is a best-selling author, syndicated newspaper columnist, and host of an award-winning internationally syndicated radio talk show. Teresa Graedon received her A.B. from Bryn Mawr College in 1969, graduating magna cum laude with a major in anthropology. She attended graduate school at the University of Michigan, receiving her A.M. in 1971. She received a fellowship from the Institute for Environmental Quality (1972–1975), which enabled her to pursue doctoral research on health and nutritional status in a migrant community in Oaxaca, Mexico. Her doctorate was awarded in 1976.

Teresa taught at Duke University School of Nursing with an adjunct appointment in the Department of Anthropology from 1975 to 1979. Since that time she has taught courses periodically in medical anthropology and international health at Duke University. From 1982 to 1983 she pursued postdoctoral training in medical anthropology at the University of California, San Francisco.

Dr. Graedon has coauthored with Joe Graedon the following books: *The People's Pharmacy-2* (Avon, 1980), *The New People's Pharmacy #3: Drug Breakthroughs of the '80s* (Bantam, 1985), *Totally New and Revised The People's Pharmacy* (St. Martin's Press, 1985), *50+: The Graedons' People's Pharmacy for Older Adults* (Bantam, 1988), *Graedons' Best Medicine: From Herbal Remedies to High-Tech R_x Breakthroughs* (Bantam, 1991), and *The Aspirin Handbook: A User's Guide to the Breakthrough Drug of the '90s* (Bantam Books, 1993). The total number of her books in print exceeds two million.

Teresa is a member of the **Society for Applied Anthropology**, the **American Anthropological Association**, the **Society for Medical Anthropology**, and the **American Public Health Association**. The newspaper column she writes with Joe, **The People's Pharmacy**, is syndicated nationally by King Features. In 1992 *The People's Pharmacy* radio show won a Silver Award from the Corporation for Public Broadcasting. It is syndicated nationally by MIR Productions, Inc., and is heard on more than 500 radio stations in the United States and 134 countries on public radio, the In Touch Radio Reading Service, and the U.S. Armed Forces Radio and Television Network.

Index

For greater ease in locating the interactions of interest to you, please note that entries in the Guides to Dangerous Drug Interactions are indicated in red. Entries in tables are indicated in italics. Brand names are designated with boldface type throughout.

A

Abitrexate 27
Accupril 26, 50, *89*
Accupril, drug interactions
    with aspirin/arthritis drugs 260, 329
    with diabetes drugs 293, 333
    with diuretics 297, 312, 327, 334
    with gout medicine 330
    with lithium 331
    with potassium 328
    with transplant drugs 332
    with tuberculosis drugs 335
Accurbron *133*
Accutane *59, 86*
ACE (angiotensin-converting enzyme) inhibitors *89*, 107-9, *110*
    drug interactions guide 260, 293, 297, 312, 326-35
    see also specific drugs
Acebutolol *111*
Acetaminophen 107
    alcohol and *114*, 143, *146*
    birth control pills and *115*, 127
    drug/food compatibility 56-57, *59*
    drugs interacting with *114-15*
    gas medication and *105, 114*
    see also specific products
Acetaminophen, drug interactions
    with anticonvulsants 234
Acetaminophen with hydrocodone, drug interactions
    with anticonvulsants 234
Acetaminophen
    with propoxyphene *70*

Acetaminophen with propoxyphene, drug interactions
    with anticonvulsants 234
Acetazolamide *59, 112*
Acetohexamide, drug interactions
    with antibiotics 172, 285
    with heart/blood pressure drugs 293, 333
    with phenylbutazone 283
Acetylsalicylic acid. *See* Aspirin
Achromycin *87*
Achromycin V *25*, 52, *59*, 81, 103, *105, 129*
Achromycin V, drug interactions
    with anticoagulants 186
    with heart drugs 320
Acne medicine *86*, 103, 136
Actifed 23, *59*, 106
Actifed Plus *99*
Actifed Sinus Daytime/Nighttime *99*
Actifed Syrup *99*
Activated charcoal 105 *105, 110, 114*
Acutrim 23
Acutrim Late Day Strength Appetite Suppressant *99*
Acutrim 16 Hour Steady Control Appetite Suppressant *99*
Acutrim II Maximum Strength Appetite Suppressant *99*
Adalat *25*, 41, *59*
Adalat, drug interactions
    with antidepressants 246, 363
    with asthma drugs 270, 357
    with barbiturates 365
    with grapefruit juice 368
    with heart/blood pressure drugs 322, 346, 355, 358, 359
    with ulcer drugs 369, 381
Adapin 4, *59*
Adapin, drug interactions
    with anticonvulsants 203
    with antidepressants 241
    with diabetes drugs 287
    with ulcer drugs 379
Additive interactions 3

F

J

K